Clinical Applications of Metronomic Chemotherapy

Clinical Applications of Metronomic Chemotherapy

Editors

Guido Bocci
Giulio Francia

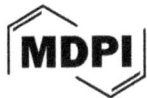

Basel • Beijing • Wuhan • Barcelona • Belgrade • Novi Sad • Cluj • Manchester

Editors
Guido Bocci
Department of Clinical and
Experimental Medicine
University of Pisa
Pisa, Italy

Giulio Francia
Border Biomedical
Research Center
University of Texas at El Paso
El Paso, TX, USA

Editorial Office
MDPI
St. Alban-Anlage 66
4052 Basel, Switzerland

This is a reprint of articles from the Special Issue published online in the open access journal *Journal of Clinical Medicine* (ISSN 2077-0383) (available at: https://www.mdpi.com/journal/jcm/special_issues/Metronomic_Chemotherapy).

For citation purposes, cite each article independently as indicated on the article page online and as indicated below:

Lastname, A.A.; Lastname, B.B. Article Title. *Journal Name* **Year**, *Volume Number*, Page Range.

ISBN 978-3-0365-9280-0 (Hbk)
ISBN 978-3-0365-9281-7 (PDF)
doi.org/10.3390/books978-3-0365-9281-7

© 2023 by the authors. Articles in this book are Open Access and distributed under the Creative Commons Attribution (CC BY) license. The book as a whole is distributed by MDPI under the terms and conditions of the Creative Commons Attribution-NonCommercial-NoDerivs (CC BY-NC-ND) license.

Contents

About the Editors vii

Stefania Orecchioni, Paolo Falvo, Giovanna Talarico, Giulia Mitola, Giulia Bravetti, Patrizia Mancuso, et al.
Vinorelbine and Intermittent Cyclophosphamide Sensitize an Aggressive Myc-Driven B-Cell Lymphoma to Anti-PD-1 by an Immunological Memory Effective against Tumor Re-Challenge
Reprinted from: *J. Clin. Med.* 2023, 12, 2535, doi:10.3390/jcm12072535 1

Camille Winnicki, Pierre Leblond, Franck Bourdeaut, Anne Pagnier, Gilles Paluenzela, Pascal Chastagner, et al.
Retrospective National "Real Life" Experience of the SFCE with the Metronomic MEMMAT and MEMMAT-like Protocol
Reprinted from: *J. Clin. Med.* 2023, 12, 1415, doi:10.3390/jcm12041415 15

Anna Buda-Nowak, Łukasz Kwinta, Paweł Potocki, Anna Michałowska-Kaczmarczyk, Agnieszka Słowik, Kamil Konopka, et al.
Metronomic Chemo-Endocrine Therapy (FulVEC) as a Salvage Treatment for Patients with Advanced, Treatment-Refractory ER+/HER2-Breast Cancer—A Retrospective Analysis of Consecutive Patients Data
Reprinted from: *J. Clin. Med.* 2023, 12, 1350, doi:10.3390/jcm12041350 29

Guido Bocci, Sabrina Pelliccia, Paola Orlandi, Matteo Caridi, Marta Banchi, Gerardo Musuraca, et al.
Remarkable Remission Rate and Long-Term Efficacy of Upfront Metronomic Chemotherapy in Elderly and Frail Patients, with Diffuse Large B-Cell Lymphoma
Reprinted from: *J. Clin. Med.* 2022, 11, 7162, doi:10.3390/jcm11237162 41

Marta Banchi, Elisabetta Fini, Stefania Crucitta and Guido Bocci
Metronomic Chemotherapy in Pediatric Oncology: From Preclinical Evidence to Clinical Studies
Reprinted from: *J. Clin. Med.* 2022, 11, 6254, doi:10.3390/jcm11216254 55

Marina Elena Cazzaniga, Serena Capici, Nicoletta Cordani, Viola Cogliati, Francesca Fulvia Pepe, Francesca Riva and Maria Grazia Cerrito
Metronomic Chemotherapy for Metastatic Breast Cancer Treatment: Clinical and Preclinical Data between Lights and Shadows
Reprinted from: *J. Clin. Med.* 2022, 11, 4710, doi:10.3390/jcm11164710 89

Piotr J. Wysocki, Maciej T. Lubas and Malgorzata L. Wysocka
Metronomic Chemotherapy in Prostate Cancer
Reprinted from: *J. Clin. Med.* 2022, 11, 2853, doi:10.3390/jcm11102853 107

Benjamin Carcamo and Giulio Francia
Cyclic Metronomic Chemotherapy for Pediatric Tumors: Six Case Reports and a Review of the Literature
Reprinted from: *J. Clin. Med.* 2022, 11, 2849, doi:10.3390/jcm11102849 121

Shruti Parshad, Amanjot K. Sidhu, Nabeeha Khan, Andrew Naoum and Urban Emmenegger
Metronomic Chemotherapy for Advanced Prostate Cancer: A Literature Review
Reprinted from: *J. Clin. Med.* 2022, 11, 2783, doi:10.3390/jcm11102783 141

Nai-Wen Su and Yu-Jen Chen
Metronomic Therapy in Oral Squamous Cell Carcinoma
Reprinted from: *J. Clin. Med.* 2021, 10, 2818, doi:10.3390/jcm10132818 155

About the Editors

Guido Bocci

Guido Bocci, MD PhD, is currently an Associate Professor of Pharmacology at the University of Pisa, with an Italian qualification of Full Professor. He is a European Certified Pharmacologist (EuCP). He manages his own laboratory at the Dept. of Clinical and Experimental Medicine. He maintains relevant international collaborations with various groups in Europe and North America. His international experience is closely related to a 3-year post-doctoral fellowship at the University of Toronto in Kerbel's Laboratory, with whom he continued to work in subsequent decades on numerous projects on metronomic chemotherapy. He has been a PI of various projects granted by AIRC, ITT and foundations. He is on the editorial board of various journals, and he has been a grant reviewer for the UK Association for Cancer Research, South Plains Foundation (USA), French National Cancer Institute (France), Genesis Oncology Trust (New Zealand), Innsbruck Medical University (Austria), United States–Israel Binational Science Foundation, and the German Israeli Foundation. Prof. Bocci is author of 4 national and 3 international patents; he has published 181 articles in international journals, 22 chapters, and 1 international book as an editor on metronomic chemotherapy. H index: 50 - Total Citations: 8690 - i10-index: 133.

He has been deeply involved in the birth and development of metronomic chemotherapy concepts in both pre-clinical and clinical trials. In recent years, Prof. Bocci and his group has set up a collaboration with Dr. Christina Cox to develop metronomic chemotherapy in hematological neoplasms, including B and T non-Hodgkin's lymphomas.

Giulio Francia

Giulio attended Bristol University in the United Kingdom where he earned a bachelor's degree in Biochemistry. He obtained his Ph.D. from the Imperial Cancer Research Fund, working in Ian Hart's Biology of Metastasis lab at St. Thomas' Hospital in London, UK. He then started postdoctoral training with Bob Kerbel at the University of Toronto, Canada. He joined UTEP as a faculty member in 2012.

Giulio studies new treatment strategies that can delay the growth of cancers that have spread to other organs. In 2002, he worked with Shan Man on the application of low-dose (metronomic) chemotherapy administered via drinking water as a new cancer treatment strategy. A year later, with Dr. Guido Bocci, he discovered that metronomic chemotherapy can induce a response that slows the formation of blood vessels that feed tumors. He has spent 28 years studying and developing models of late-stage cancer. In 2012 he joined UTEP, where he is now Associate Professor, and he works with his students Diana Prospero, Hector Padilla, Alejandro Sanchez and Saeedeh Darvishi on the anti-tumor effects of combinations of metronomic chemotherapy with targeted therapies.

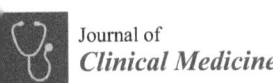

Article

Vinorelbine and Intermittent Cyclophosphamide Sensitize an Aggressive Myc-Driven B-Cell Lymphoma to Anti-PD-1 by an Immunological Memory Effective against Tumor Re-Challenge

Stefania Orecchioni [1,2,†], Paolo Falvo [1,2,†], Giovanna Talarico [1,2], Giulia Mitola [1,2], Giulia Bravetti [1,2], Patrizia Mancuso [1,2], Paola Nicoli [3] and Francesco Bertolini [1,2,*]

1 Laboratory of Hematology-Oncology, European Institute of Oncology IRCCS, Via Ripamonti 435, 20141 Milan, Italy
2 Onco-Tech Lab, European Institute of Oncology IRCCS and Politecnico di Milano, 20141 Milan, Italy
3 Department of Experimental Oncology, European Institute of Oncology IRCCS, Via Adamello 16, 20137 Milan, Italy
* Correspondence: francesco.bertolini@ieo.it
† These authors contributed equally to this work.

Abstract: We have previously shown in triple-negative breast cancer (TNBC) models that a triple therapy (TT) including intermittent cyclophosphamide (C), vinorelbine (V), and anti-PD-1 activates antigen-presenting cells (APC) and generates stem like-T cells able to control local and metastatic tumor progression. In the present manuscript, we report the generation of a highly aggressive, anti-PD-1 resistant model of a high-grade, Myc-driven B-cell non-Hodgkin's lymphoma (NHL) that can be controlled in vivo by TT but not by other chemotherapeutic agents, including cytarabine (AraC), platinum (P), and doxorubicin (D). The immunological memory elicited in tumor-bearing mice by TT (but not by other treatments) can effectively control NHL re-challenge even at very high inoculum doses. TT re-shaped the landscape of circulating innate NK cells and adaptive immune cells, including B and T cells, and significantly reduced exhausted $CD4^+$ and $CD8^+$ $TIM3^+PD-1^+$ T cells in the spleens of treated mice.

Keywords: lymphoma; cyclophosphamide; vinorelbine; metronomic chemotherapy; checkpoint inhibitors

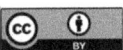

1. Introduction

Immune checkpoint inhibitors (ICI) such as anti-CTLA-4, anti-PD-1, and anti-PD-L1 monoclonal antibodies have been successfully introduced in the therapy of a variety of cancer types [1]. However, at the present time, only a fraction of cancer patients benefit from ICIs, and in the large majority of cases, the clinical benefit is limited in time [2].

Cancer genomic and microenvironmental complexity suggests that in almost all patients only a combinatorial therapeutic approach can be successful [3]. For this reason, intense preclinical and clinical research is currently ongoing to define and validate in patients the best synergic strategy for ICI incorporation in cancer therapy.

We have described that a "two-hit" triple therapy (TT) [4,5], involving antigen-presenting cell (APC) activation by a vinca alkaloid such as vinorelbine (V) and the generation of new TCF1+ stem cell-like T cell (scT) clones by an intermittent dosage of the alkylating agent cyclophosphamide (C140), can significantly improve the efficacy of anti-PD-1 in two triple-negative breast cancer (TNBC) models otherwise poorly sensitive to ICIs. The TT effect was dependent upon C dosage and schedule, and due to T cells, as it was abrogated by the in vivo depletion of $CD3^+CD4^+$ and/or $CD3^+CD8^+$ cells [4–6].

To confirm that this approach can also be effective in different types of cancer and to investigate whether TT may generate an immunological anti-cancer memory, in the present study we describe a model of a very aggressive neoplasia resistant to anti-PD-1, i.e., a disseminated, orthotopic, Myc-driven B-cell lymphoma, and compared TT with other therapies currently used in the clinic for this disease. TT, but not other therapies, sensitized lymphoma cells to anti-PD-1, controlled lymphoma progression, and generated an immunological memory that in the large majority of mice avoided lymphoma generation even when lymphoma cells were re-injected in numbers significantly higher than in the previous inoculum.

2. Materials and Methods

2.1. Cell Lines

The LY27805 cell line was kindly provided by Bruno Amati's group [7] at the European Institute of Oncology–Italian Foundation for Cancer Research (FIRC) Institute of Molecular Oncology (IEO–IFOM, Milan, Italy) campus, expanded and stored according to their instructions. Specifically, LY27805 cells were plated at 2×10^5 cells/mL in B cell medium: 50:50 mixture of DMEM and IMDM (Euroclone, Pero (MI), Italy), 10% FBS (Euroclone, Pero (MI), Italy), 2 mM L-glutamine (Euroclone, Pero (MI), Italy), 1% penicillin/streptomycin (Euroclone, Pero (MI), Italy), 50 µM β-mercaptoethanol (Euroclone, Pero (MI), Italy), and non-essential amino acid (NEEA) (Euroclone, Pero (MI), Italy). Phoenix-Ampho cells were cultured with DMEM (Euclone, Pero (MI), Italy), 10%FBS (Euclone, Pero (MI), Italy), 2 mM L-glutamine (Euclone, Pero (MI), Italy), 1% penicillin/streptomycin (Euclone, Pero (MI), Italy).

Cells were tested and authenticated by the StemElite ID System (Promega, Madison, WI, USA). Cells were tested every six months for Mycoplasma by means of the ATCC Universal Mycoplasma Detection Kit 30-1012, cultured for no more than two weeks, and used for no longer than 15 passages.

2.2. Cell Line Infection

The LY27805 cell line was thoroughly transduced with retroviral vectors expressing stably luciferase under the control of a promoter: pRetro MI-Luciferase-IRES-mCherry (Addagene plasmid #75020). Phoenix-Ampho cells were co-transfected with 10 µg of retroviral vector, 6 µg of pKAT2 vector (helping retroviral particle-producing vector) using the Calcium Phosphate transfection system. After 16 h, media was removed and replaced with 5 mL of fresh medium to increase viral load.

Viral supernatant was then collected at 24 and 48 h and added directly to the LY27805 cell lines plated. In detail, viral supernatant was collected with a 0.22 µm sterile syringe filter and added directly to 2×10^5 LY27805 cells supplemented with 8 µg/mL of polybrene (Sigma-Aldrich Merck, St. Louis, MO, USA). Spin Infection was performed for 1 h at 37 °C twice at 1800 rpm in a day for two separate days. Infection efficiency was then assessed using a fluorescence microscope (EVOS cells imaging system, Promega, Madison, WI, USA). Infected cells were then sorted using FACS Jazz (BD Bioscience, Franklin Lakes, NJ, USA).

2.3. In Vivo Experiments

Experiments involving animals were approved by the Italian Ministry of Health and have been performed in accordance with the applicable Italian laws (D.L. vo 26/14 and following amendments), the Institutional Animal Care and Use Committee, the institutional guidelines at the European Institute of Oncology, and the ARRIVE guidelines. In vivo studies were carried out in 8-week-old immune-competent C57BL/6J female mice (Envigo) in the animal facility at the IEO-IFOM campus.

To generate a syngeneic model of Non-Hodgkin lymphoma, 5×10^4 to 2.5×10^5 LY27805-RFP$^+$Luc$^+$ cells were injected intravenously (IV) in the tail vein of C57BL/6J mice. Tumor growth was monitored weekly using the In Vivo Imaging System (IVIS; PerkinElmer, Whaltam, MA, USA). Briefly, mice were intraperitoneally (IP) injected with 150 mg/kg of XenoLight D-Luciferin–K+ Salt Bioluminescent Substrate (PerkinElmer Whaltam, MA, USA). After 10 min, animals were anaesthetized with isofluorane apparatus and images acquired using Living Image Software (PerkinElmer Whaltam, MA, USA).

Radiant efficiency was calculated on the basis of the epifluorescence signal, as indicated in the user manual. Treatment started about 7–10 days from tumor injection, when a bioluminescence signal was detectable in each individual mouse. Mice were observed daily throughout the treatment period for signs of morbidity/mortality.

2.4. In Vivo Therapy

C57BL/6J tumor-bearing mice (n = 5 per study arm) were treated with different drugs used as single agents or in combination. Drug dosages used in this study are the standard chemotherapeutic drugs for Non-Hodgkin lymphoma and doses were based on the literature data associated with no or acceptable toxicity, as well as no significant changes in mouse weight. Blood was collected at different time points from the tail vein, and circulating immune cells were determined by multiparametric, 10-colour flow cytometry. Cyclophosphamide was used at 140 mg/kg (C140) as already shown in Refs. [4,8,9]. Vinorelbine (V) was used at 9 mg/Kg as we have previously shown in Refs. [4,9]; Doxorubicin (D) was used at 2.9 mg/kg [4,10], Cisplatin (P) was used at 0.25 mg/kg [4,10], and Cytarabine (ara-C) was used at 15 mg/kg [11]. Chemotherapeutic drugs were dissolved in PBS and IP administrated once a week, every 6 days for 3 weeks. Mouse monoclonal anti-PD-1 targeting antibody was purchased from Bioxcell (Lebanon, NH, USA) (clone RMP1-14) and was administered IP 0.2 mg/mouse every 2 days for a total of 5 doses [4]. The therapeutic scheme is presented in Supplementary Figure S1.

2.5. Flow Cytometry

At least 100,000 cells per sample were acquired using a 3-laser, 10-color flow cytometer (Navios-Ex; Beckman Coulter, Brea, CA, USA) for T-cell receptor analysis or using a 13-color FACS Celesta (BD Bioscience) for immune cell population analyses. The antibodies list and gating strategies are summarized in the Supplementary Table S1. Lymphocytes and myeloid cells were characterized using state-of-the-art markers. Specifically, cells were gated for size, singlets, and then by positive and negative markers: $CD3^+CD4^+$ and $CD3^+CD8^+$ T cells, $CD3-CD335^+$ NKs, $CD19^+$ B cells, $Gr1^-CD11b^+CD11c^+$ monocytes, $SSC^{high}CD11b^+Gr1^+$ granulocytes, $CD11c^+CD11b^-Gr1^-$ antigen-presenting cells (APC), $SSC^{low}CD11b^+Gr1^+$ myeloid-derived suppressor cells (MDSC), and T cells were further analyzed to investigate the exhaustion status ($Tim3^+PD-1^+$).

2.6. T Cell Receptor Clonality

T-cell receptor (TCR) clonality was analyzed in the spleen using the FITC Hamster Anti-Mouse Beta TCR Kit (BD Biosciences, clone H57-597), following the manufacturer's protocol. Briefly, the spleen was mechanically dissociated and 2×10^5 cells were stained with an antibody cocktail mix containing: 7AAD (Beckman Coulter, Brea, CA, USA), CD45 PE-Cy7 (BD Biosciences, clone 30-F11), CD3 APC (BD Biosciences, clone 145-2C11), CD4 PE (BD Biosciences, clone GK1.5), CD8 APC-Cy7 (BD Biosciences, clone 53-6.7), and a specific region of VDJ beta chain rearrangement. Viable cells ($7-AAD^-$) were gated for CD45/CD3/CD4 and CD45/CD3/CD8 positivity, and among them, we evaluated for each β chain rearrangement the percentage of positivity. Fold increase was determined by dividing the percentage of positive cells revealed in each experimental condition versus the untreated control. Finally, not engrafted mice were normalized to the engrafted ones.

2.7. Statistical Analysis

Data were expressed as means ± sem (in case of normal distribution). Normal distribution was assessed using the Shapiro Wilk's normality test. To compare two sample groups, either the Student's t-test or the Mann-Whitney U-test was used based on normal or not normal distribution. To test differences in survival, the Mantel-Cox test was performed. Statistical analysis was carried out with Prism 9.3.1. (GraphPad).

3. Results

3.1. TT Sensitizes an Aggressive Myc-Driven B-Cell Lymphoma to Anti-PD-1 and Prevents Lymphoma Growth In Vivo

In our previous work [4,5], we demonstrated that TT, including C140, V, and anti-PD-1, eradicates tumor growth in two murine models of TNBC. We investigated whether the same TT combinatorial therapy can also be effective against a highly aggressive murine lymphoma model. To achieve this aim, we took advantage of a previous Myc-driven B-cell non-Hodgkin's lymphoma cell line characterized by Bruno Amati's laboratory [7].

These cells were retrovirally infected with pRetro MI-Luciferase-IRES-mCherry (Addagene plasmid #75020) plasmids carrying both an RFP gene (for in vitro selection) and a Luc gene (for in vivo tracking), herein called Ly27085-Luc. To characterize the latency and the penetrance of this lymphoma, mice were IV inoculated with three scalar concentrations of Ly27085-Luc cells (5×10^4, 1×10^5, and 2×10^5) (Figure 1A). As shown, all mice died of lymphoma shortly after tumor inoculation (on average 20 days). Paradoxically, the higher number of cells did not correlate with higher aggressiveness, and with shorter latency. Moreover, taking advantage from the RFP selective marker, we assessed that very low percentages of lymphoma cells within the spleen were sufficient to kill the animal (Figure 1B). Taken together, these results indicate that Ly27805-Luc is an aggressive MYC-driven lymphoma model with very short latency (20 days on average) and high penetrance (100%).

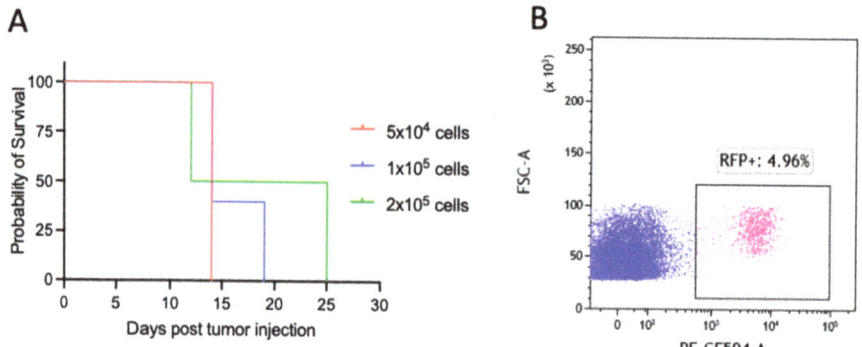

Figure 1. Ly27085-Luc is a lymphoma model with high penetrance and low latency. (**A**) Kaplan-Meier survival analysis of mice injected intravenously with 5×10^4 (red line), 1×10^5 (blue line), and 2×10^5 (green line) Ly27805-Luc cells. The Mantel-Cox test was performed to assess statistical differences in survival between the three groups (n = 5 per experimental condition). (**B**) Representative flow cytometry plots showing percentage of RFP+ cells within the spleen of a control mouse. Cells were gated according to physical parameters.

To assess the efficacy of our TT approach [4,5], we injected C57BL/6J mice with 1×10^5 Ly27805-Luc cells and treated them with several chemotherapeutic agents used in the clinic for B-cell lymphoma therapy, the anti-PD-1 ICI, and chemotherapeutic agents combined to ICI. We measured tumor growth by bioluminescence signals as shown in Figure 2A,B. In vivo studies indicated that intermittent (i.e., every 6 days, in a metronomic fashion) C140 was more effective than any other combinatorial regimens including ICI plus AraC, D, or P at their regular preclinical dosages. Both C140 alone and TT initially abrogated tumor growth, in line with our previous studies on TNBC [4,9]. Therefore, after interrupting the treatments, we prolonged the experimental observational time to more than 80 days and we found that the TT association with V and anti-PD-1 significantly increased the preclinical efficacy of C140 ($p < 0.01$). In addition, TT dramatically improved the overall survival rate compared with other combinatorial therapies (Figure 2C). All the C140-treated mice succumbed around 30–40 days after tumor injection, whereas the TT-treated mice were alive and without any signs of lymphoma ($p < 0.0001$) up to day 80, at the end of the observational study. At the end of the experiment, the animals were sacrificed, and the RFP signal was evaluated in the spleen, as shown in Figure 2D. In accordance with the luciferase signal, RFP-positive cells dramatically dropped after TT.

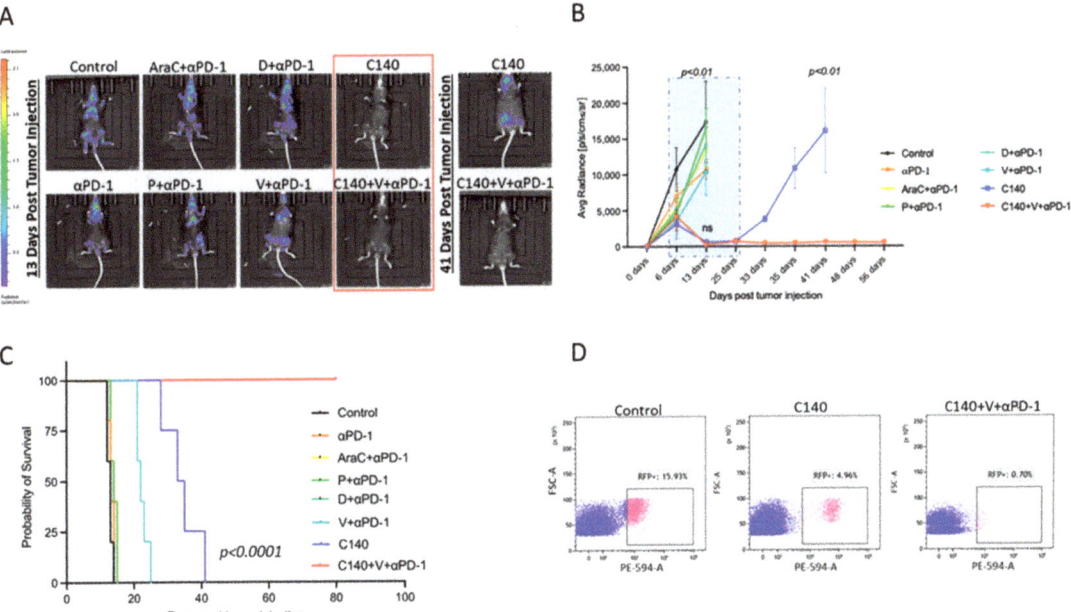

Figure 2. Ly27085-Luc lymphoma growth control by TT vs. other therapies. (**A**) In vivo live imaging of Ly27805-Luc tumors of mice treated with different experimental conditions. On the left is shown the luminescence/radiance bar. Red indicates a higher luminescence signal while blue is the lowest one. Mice were injected with 1×10^5 Ly27805-Luc cells and monitored by IVIS. Images were taken 13 days after tumor injection. Mice in the red square did not show any difference, thus the mice were monitored for a longer period. On the right is shown the image 41 days after tumor injection. (**B**) Ly27085-Luc tumor growth curve of mice treated with chemotherapeutic agents, ICI, or chemotherapeutic agents combined with ICI. The dashed blue square represents the treatment period (from day 7 until day 28 post lymphoma injection). The Shapiro–Wilk test was performed to define normal distribution, and a 2-tail T Student's test was applied. Statistical analysis was done for each condition compared with C140+V+anti-PD-1 (n = 5 per experimental condition). (**C**) Kaplan-Meier survival analysis of Ly27085-Luc-injected mice treated with chemotherapeutic agents, ICI, or chemotherapeutic agents combined with ICI. The Mantel-Cox test was performed to assess statistical differences in survival between the three groups (n = 5 per experimental condition). (**D**) Representative flow cytometry plots showing the percentage of RFP$^+$ cells within the spleen of a control (left panel), C140- (middle) and C140+V+anti-PD-1-treated mouse. Cells were gated according to physical parameters.

3.2. TT Reshapes the Intratumoral Immune Cell Landscape and Targets Terminally Exhausted T Cells

We and others have previously demonstrated that anti-PD-1 favors the selection of progenitor-exhausted T cells, with crucial effects over tumor growth [4–6]. Progenitor-exhausted T cells are defined to be Tcf1$^+$ [12], whereas terminally exhausted T cells, which have poor anticancer function, are defined as PD-1$^+$Tim3$^+$ [13].

To determine whether anti-PD-1 might also have a similar function within our lymphoma model, we analyzed by flow cytometry the immune cell populations in the spleen of control, C140, and TT-treated mice. Animals (n = 5 per study arm) were inoculated IV with 1×10^5 Ly27085-Luc cells and treated with C140 alone, TT (C140+V+anti-PD-1), or without any treatment. Control and C140-treated mice were sacrificed when moribund, TT-treated mice after 80 days, and the T cell composition within the spleen was analyzed (Figure 3).

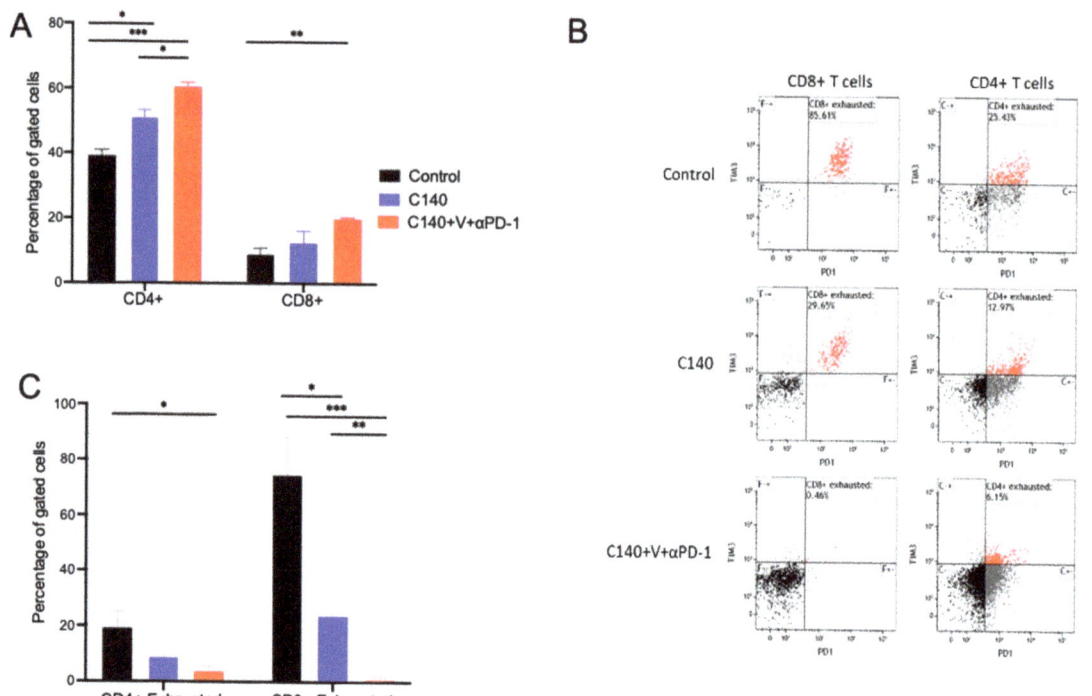

Figure 3. TT reshapes tumor infiltrating lymphocytes and reduces exhausted $CD3^+CD4^+$ and $CD3^+CD8^+$ T cells. (**A**) Percentage of $CD3^+CD4^+$ and $CD3^+CD8^+$ cells in the spleen of control (black), C140- (blue), and C140+V+anti-PD-1-treated mice (red). The Shapiro–Wilk test was performed to assess normal distribution, and thus 2-tails Student's t test' was applied. (* $p < 0.05$, ** $p < 0.01$, *** $p < 0.001$) (n = 5 per experimental condition). (**B**) Representative flow cytometry plots showing the percentage of exhausted $CD3^+CD8^+$ cells (defined as $CD3^+CD8^+PD-1^+TIM3^+$, on the left) and of exhausted $CD3^+CD4^+$ cells (defined as $CD3^+CD4^+PD-1^+TIM3^+$, on the right) within the spleen of a control (upper panel), C140- (middle), and C140+V+anti-PD-1-treated mouse (bottom panel). Cells were gated according to physical parameters. (**C**) Quantification of exhausted $CD3^+CD8^+$ cells (defined as $CD3^+CD8^+PD-1^+TIM3^+$) and of exhausted $CD3^+CD4^+$ cells (defined as $CD3^+CD4^+PD-1^+TIM3^+$) within the spleen of control, C140-treated, and C140+V+anti-PD-1-treated mice. The Shapiro–Wilk test was performed to define normal distribution, and thus 2-tails Student's t test' was applied (* $p < 0.05$, ** $p < 0.01$, *** $p < 0.001$) (n = 5 per experimental condition).

As shown in Figure 3A, we observed that C140 alone and TT increase the percentage of $CD3^+CD4^+$ and $CD3^+CD8^+$ cells in the spleen. This increase is larger when one compares controls versus TT-treated mice (40% of $CD3^+CD4^+$ in the control versus 60% in the TT, $p < 0.001$ and 10% of $CD3^+CD8^+$ in the control versus 20% in the TT, $p < 0.01$). A statistically significant increase ($p < 0.05$) was observed also for $CD3^+CD4^+$ T cells between C140 and TT-treated mice.

We then analyzed terminally exhausted T cells, defined as $CD3^+CD4^+/CD8^+$ PD-1^+TIM3^+ T cells. Surprisingly, we observed that terminally exhausted T cells were abundant in the control and decreased in the treated samples. This decrease was more profound in TT-treated mice. Specifically, we confirmed that TT was associated with a significant decrease in exhausted $CD3^+CD8^+$ T cells compared to controls ($p < 0.001$) and C140-treated mice ($p < 0.01$). A similar trend was also observed for exhausted $CD3^+CD4^+$ T cells (Figure 3B,C).

In line with results observed in TNBC models [4–6], these results in the lymphoma model suggest that TT reshapes the T cell landscape and selects for anti-tumor effective T cells.

3.3. TT Orchestrates the Activation of T Cell Antitumor Memory in Mice

As we previously demonstrated that T cells are the most likely mediators of the anti-tumor TT effect, we asked whether an immune cell memory was generated in TT-treated mice. To answer this question, we performed a tumor re-challenge experiment, as illustrated in Figure 4A. Briefly, mice were injected with 1×10^5 Ly27805-Luc cells and the presence of lymphoma cells was assessed by IVIS analyses 10 days after tumor injection (Figure 4B, top panel). Mice were then randomized into two experimental groups, treated with C140 or TT. When C140 and TT were administered to lymphoma-bearing mice, tumors were completely eradicated after the first infusion (Figure 4B, middle panel). When we re-challenged TT- and C140-cured mice with a 2.5-fold higher number of lymphoma cells on day 9 after the end of the treatment (day 40 after tumor injection), all control (i.e., untreated) mice (5/5) developed signs of lymphoma about 10 days post tumor re-challenge. Three out of five C140-treated mice presented signals in the limbs with a growth kinetic similar to controls. Remarkably, only one out of five TT-treated mice presented lymphoma signs (Figure 4B, bottom panel, Figure 4 C,D). At the end of the study, all control mice, 3/5 C140-treated, and only 1/5 triple-treated mice died of lymphoma ($p < 0.01$) (Figure 4E).

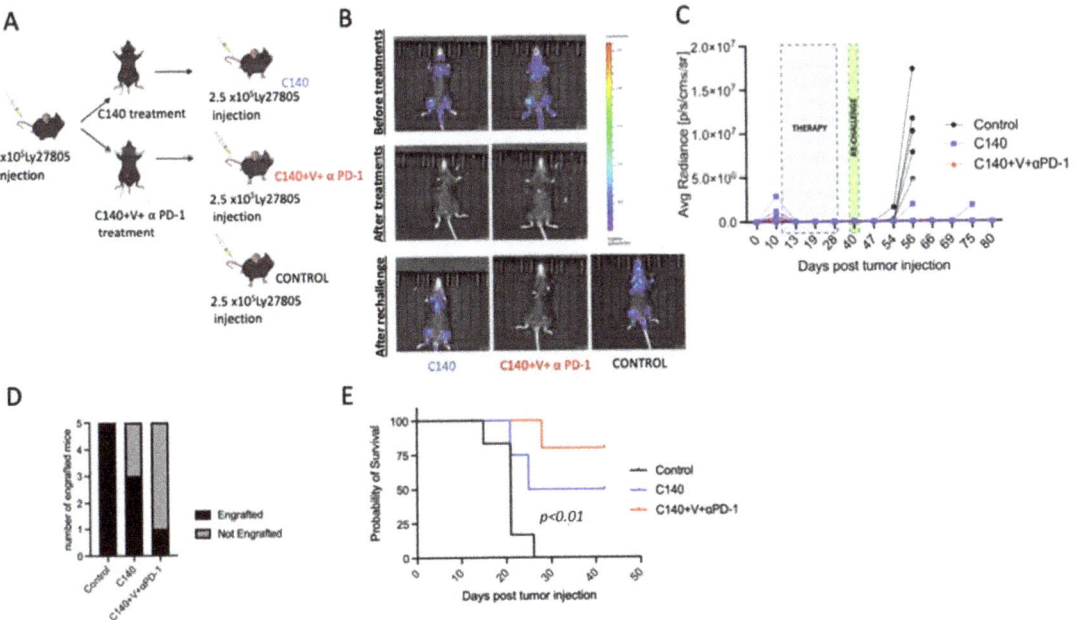

Figure 4. TT generates an anti-tumor immune memory. (**A**) Schematic representation of the tumor re-challenge experiment. Briefly, 10 C57BL/6J mice were injected IV with 1×10^5 Ly27085-Luc cells; on day 10 post lymphoma injection, once systemic engraftment was confirmed, mice were randomized

to receive different treatments (n = 5 per experimental condition) up to day 31; on day 40 post tumor injection, TT- and C140-treated mice were re-challenged with 2.5 × 10⁵ Ly27085-Luc cells (i.e., a 2.5-fold higher inoculum of lymphoma cells); in parallel, 5 C57BL/6J mice were injected with 2.5 × 10⁵ Ly27085-Luc cells as control.). Graphic representation present was carried out with the Biorender software (https://app.biorender.com, accessed on 18 January 2023). (**B**) In vivo live imaging of Ly27805-Luc tumors in TT- and C140-treated and control mice. On the right is shown the luminescence/radiance bar. Red indicates a higher luminescence signal while blue is the lowest one. Images were taken before (upper panel), at the end of the treatment (middle panel), and after 2.5 × 10⁵ Ly27805-Luc lymphoma re-challenge (bottom panel). (**C**) Ly27085-Luc tumor growth of single re-challenged mice (black line control, blue line C140-cured and red line TT cured mice (n = 5 per experimental condition). The dashed blue square represents the treatment period (from day 10 until day 31 post lymphoma injection). The dashed green square represents Ly27805-Luc re-challenge on day 40 post-tumor injection. (**D**) Bar graph showing the number of lymphoma-engrafted mice (in black) over the number of not engrafted mice (in gray). (**E**) Kaplan-Meier analysis of re-challenged Ly27085-Luc mice. The Mantel-Cox test was performed to assess statistical differences in survival between the three groups (n = 5 per experimental condition).

These results suggest that TT efficiently generated some memory immune responses persisting after lymphoma eradication.

3.4. The Immune Cell Landscape in the Peripheral Blood Is Altered after Lymphoma Re-Challenge

As we have evidence that TT activates an immunological memory, we asked which types of immune cell subsets were altered during therapy and after the re-challenge with tumor cells. To this purpose, we analyzed by flow cytometry, at different time points, the percentages of circulating immune populations in the peripheral blood of untreated, TT- and C140-treated mice (Figure 5).

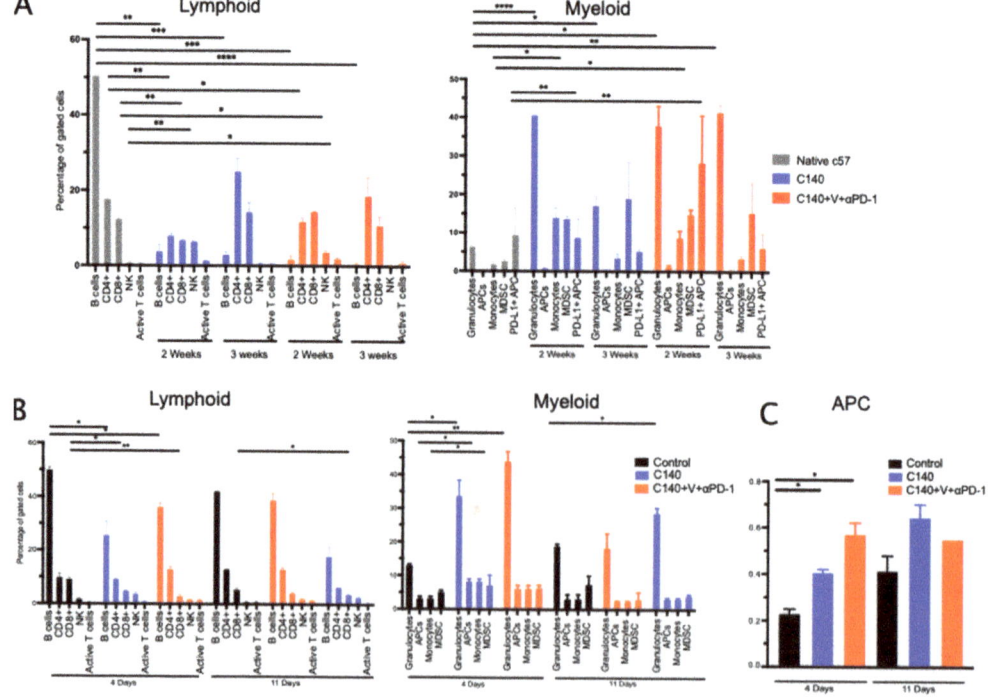

Figure 5. TT reshapes the immune cell landscape in the peripheral blood (PB). (**A**) Flow cytometry analysis in Ly27085-Luc bearing mice treated with C140 and TT at two different time points (two and

three weeks after tumor injection). In the graph, major lymphoid (on the left panel) and myeloid cell subpopulations (on the right panel) are shown. Lymphoid comprises B cells (CD19$^+$), CD3$^+$CD4$^+$ and CD3$^+$CD8$^+$ T cells, NK cells (CD335$^+$), and activated CD8$^+$T cells (CD3$^+$CD8$^+$CD69$^+$CD25$^+$). Myeloid cells include granulocytes (CD11b$^+$Gr1$^+$), APCs (CD11b$^-$Gr1$^-$D11c$^+$), monocytes (CD11b$^+$Gr1$^-$CD11c$^+$), myeloid-derived suppressor cells (MDSC) (CD11b$^+$Gr1$^+$), and PD-L1$^+$APC (PD-L1$^+$CD11b$^-$Gr1$^-$D11c$^+$). The Shapiro-Wilk Test was applied to define normal distribution. A 2-tails Student's t test' was applied. Statistic is referred to each condition compared to un-treated and not injected C57/BL6 mice (in grey in the graph). (* $p < 0.05$, ** $p < 0.01$, *** $p < 0.001$, **** $p < 0.0001$). (**B**) Flow cytometry analysis in Ly27085-Luc re-challenged mice at two different time points (4 and 11 days after tumor re-challenge). In the graph major lymphoid (on the left panel) and myeloid cell subpopulations (on the right panel) are shown. Lymphoid comprises B cells (CD19$^+$), CD3$^+$CD4$^+$ and CD3$^+$CD8$^+$ T cells, NK cells (CD335$^+$), and activated CD8$^+$T cells (CD3$^+$CD8$^+$CD69$^+$CD25$^+$). Myeloid cells include granulocytes (CD11b$^+$Gr1$^+$), APCs (CD11b$^-$Gr1$^-$D11c$^+$), monocytes (CD11b$^+$Gr1$^-$CD11c$^+$), myeloid-derived suppressor cells (MDSC) (CD11b$^+$Gr1$^+$), and PD-L1$^+$APC (PD-L1$^+$CD11b$^-$Gr1$^-$D11c$^+$). The Shapiro-Wilk Test was applied to define normal distribution. A 2-tails Student's t test' was applied. Statistic is referred to each condition compared to untreated Ly27805-Luc injected C57/BL6 mice (in black in the graph). (* $p < 0.05$, ** $p < 0.01$). (**C**) Flow cytometry analysis in Ly27085-Luc re-challenged mice at two different time points (4 and 11 days after tumor re-challenge) for APC cells (defined as CD11b$^-$Gr1$^-$D11c$^+$). The Shapiro-Wilk Test was applied to define normal distribution. A 2-tails Student's t test' was applied. Statistic is referred to each condition compared to untreated Ly27805-Luc injected C57/BL6 mice (in black in the graph). (* $p < 0.05$).

We first focused on the changes at two different time points (2 and 3 weeks) within the myeloid and lymphoid cell compartments after C140 or TT treatments (Figure 5A). As a control, we investigated five un-injected, untreated mice. We then focused on the same populations 4 and 11 days after the lymphoma re-challenge (Figure 5B,C).

B cells decreased after the treatments and increased after lymphoma re-challenge ($p < 0.0001$). This is consistent with our previous observations in TNBC and lymphoma models [4,9]. NK cells had a different kinetic, they initially increased during the TT (2 weeks) but were reduced in number after tumor re-challenge. We also analyzed the percentage of active T cells, defined as CD25$^+$CD69$^+$CD8$^+$cells. Albeit not statistically significant, we observed an increase of active T cells after lymphoma re-challenge. These data deserve further molecular and phenotypic investigations, as they suggest an activation of T cells upon re-encounter with the antigens present on tumor cells.

Regarding the myeloid compartment, we did not observe any significant alterations in the peripheral blood for antigen-presenting cells (APC), monocytes, and myeloid-derived suppressor cells (MDSC). PD-L1$^+$ APC significantly increased during the V-containing regimen ($p < 0.01$), while APC increased as previously described (Figure 5C) [4].

We observed that granulocyte numbers had a significant increase after treatment and after lymphoma re-challenge. We have observed a similar kinetic in another model of murine lymphoma [9], and these data deserve further investigation.

3.5. TT Decreases Terminally Exhausted T Cells upon Tumor Re-Challenge and Induces Specific T-Cell Clonal Selection

As already shown in Figures 1B and 2D, lymphoma cells localize in the spleen. As we have not observed significant differences among adaptive immune cells in the peripheral blood of treated animals after tumor re-challenge, we focused our attention on splenic immune cell populations.

We analyzed by flow cytometry the percentage of exhausted CD3$^+$CD4$^+$ and CD3$^+$CD8$^+$ T cells along with PD-1$^+$TIM3$^+$ subpopulations in the spleen of lymphoma-engrafted and not engrafted mice. Exhausted T cells dramatically increased in the CD3$^+$CD4$^+$ and CD3$^+$CD8$^+$ subpopulations in lymphoma-bearing animals. At variance, in mice where lymphoma did not grow, we observed very few exhausted T cells (PD-1$^+$TIM3$^+$CD4$^+$ were <2% and PD-1$^+$TIM3$^+$CD8$^+$ were <1% of all gated cells). These data suggest a reduction of the suppressive immune response, in favor of an anti-tumoral activity. This evidence suggests that in the spleen, after lymphoma re-challenge, there is a selection for anti-tumor T cells (Figure 6A,B).

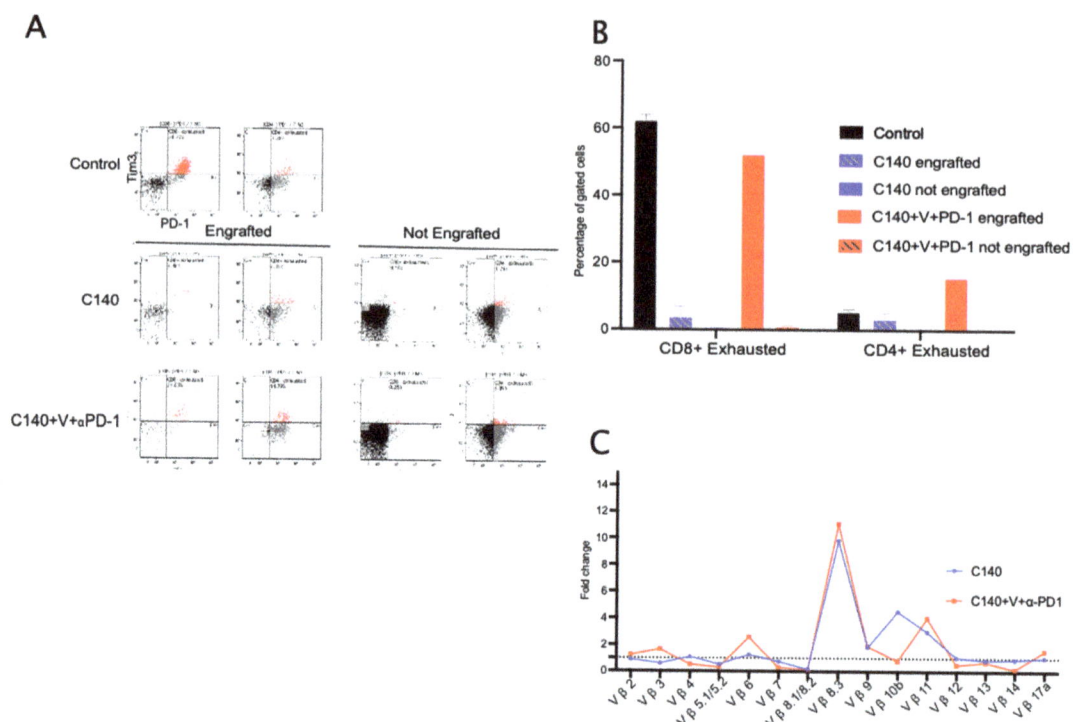

Figure 6. TT in tumor re-challenged mice selects for proliferative and oligoclonal T cells. (**A**) Representative flow cytometry plots showing the percentage of exhausted CD3$^+$CD8$^+$ cells (defined as CD3$^+$CD8$^+$PD-1$^+$TIM3$^+$, on the left) and of exhausted CD3$^+$CD4$^+$ cells (defined as CD3$^+$CD4$^+$PD-1$^+$TIM3$^+$, on the right) from the spleen of a control (upper panel), C140-engrafted (middle on the left), C140-not-engrafted (middle on the right), C140+V+anti-PD-1-engrafted (bottom on the left) C140+V+anti-PD-1-not engrafted (bottom on the right) mouse. Cells were gated according to physical parameters. (**B**) Quantification of exhausted CD3$^+$CD8$^+$ cells (defined as CD3$^+$CD8$^+$PD-1$^+$TIM3$^+$) and of exhausted CD3$^+$CD4$^+$ cells (defined as CD3$^+$CD4$^+$PD-1$^+$TIM3$^+$) from the spleen of a control (black), C140-engrafted (dashed blue), C140-not-engrafted (blue), and C140+V+anti-PD-1-engrafted (dashed red) and C140+V+anti-PD-1-not engrafted (red graph) mice. Two C140-treated mice did not engraft the lymphoma, one TT-treated mouse had lymphoma. (**C**) CD3$^+$CD8$^+$ TCR clonality in the spleen of lymphoma re-challenged mice. On the x-axis, 15 common Vβ chain recombinations are present, whereas on the y-axis the fold change increase is compared with engrafted mice (represented as dashed lines in the graph).

We then performed a T cell receptor (TCR) clonal analysis on CD3$^+$CD8$^+$ T cells collected from the spleen. We investigated, by flow cytometry, 15 common rearrangements of the TCR. In the case of a specific rearrangement, one evident peak is generated. As shown in Figure 6C, after tumor re-challenge we detected two specific peaks in mice resistant to lymphoma—corresponding to variants vβ8.3 and vβ11—when normalized over engrafted mice. These data indicate a switch towards oligoclonality in T cells.

Taken together, these data suggest that, in the tumor-infiltrated spleen, T cells might have a crucial role in the anti-tumor immunological memory elicitation, by inducing a shift towards more proliferative and anti-tumor T cells, and to an oligoclonal selection of T cells.

4. Discussion

ICI's clinical impact on cancer therapy has been so far very relevant: in the past 10 years, eight immune checkpoint blockers against CTLA-4, PD-1, or PD-L1 have been approved for clinical use in more than 85 oncology indications [1,2]. However, at the present time, only a fraction of cancer patients benefit from ICI as a single therapy, and there is increasing evidence that, to improve ICI's clinical efficacy, a combinatorial therapy is needed. The TT approach we have recently described in two TNBC models [4–6] includes drugs already in use in the oncology clinic for different indications and involves (a) APC activation by the vinca alkaloid vinorelbine and (b) the generation of new ScT clones by intermittent cyclophosphamide (i.e., every 6 days, in a metronomic fashion) [8] to overcome TNBC resistance to the anti-PD-1 ICI.

The kinetics of immune cell subsets during TT vs. other therapies have been described in Ref. [4]. Significant differences in the innate (myeloid and lymphoid) and adaptive subsets observed during these therapies might explain—at least in part—resistance to therapies other than TT and will be investigated in future studies.

V effects over APC activation have been previously described by us [9] and by the Takashima lab [14]. In the latter study, in a panel of 54 anti-cancer drugs, vinca alkaloids were ranked as the most prominent inducer of APC maturation; they increased CD40, CD80, CD86, and MHC II expression, triggered IL-1β, IL-6, and IL-12 p40 production, and augmented the capacity to activate T cells. The major hypothesis, still to be confirmed in mechanistic studies, is that partial and temporal disruption of intracellular microtubule networks by vinca alkaloids may be sensed by APCs as intrinsic danger signals.

The role of different dosages of the alkylating agent cyclophosphamide in improving ICI activity [15] and in generating an inflammatory neoplastic microenvironment that may foster $CD3^+CD4^+$ T-cell activity and an IFN/TNFalpha gene signature have also been recently described [16].

The present study shows that TT is also preclinically active in another type of otherwise ICI-resistant neoplastic disease, a high-grade, Myc-driven B-cell lymphoma. It should be noted that, in randomized clinical trials, TNBC patients seem to benefit from the association of ICIs with several chemotherapeutics including cyclophosphamide [17], whereas so far high-grade B-cell non-Hodgkin's lymphoma patients have not been reported to receive a significant clinical benefit from ICIs, alone or in combinatorial therapies, apart from the case of mediastinal large-B cell lymphoma where the anti-PD-1 antibody is clinically active [18]. Thus, our data might be used to design future clinical trials in the non-Hodgkin's lymphoma field. Notably, metronomic chemotherapy based on V and C has significant activity in patients with aggressive B-cell lymphomas, as long-lasting remissions were observed [19]. The tumoricidal activity of this combination may add to its immune-mediated effect, and this double effect may lay the groundwork for clinical translation.

In this context, Yu and colleagues [20] have recently suggested in single-cell studies that coinhibitory signals from the immune checkpoint molecules TIGIT and TIM-3 may drive T cell exhaustion in this disease. As clinically effective antibodies against TIGIT and TIM-3 are currently tested in trials, these ICI might deserve investigation in this neoplastic disease along with TT.

Another finding from the data reported here might be of interest for future clinical applications: we have found in the TNBC preclinical studies that TT efficacy was abrogated when $CD3^+CD4^+$ and/or $CD3^+CD8^+$ T cells were crippled in vivo by neutralizing monoclonal antibodies. Along a similar line, Zhang and colleagues [21] have recently identified subpopulations of $CD3^+CD4^+CXCL13^+$ and $CD3^+CD8^+CXCL13^+$ T cells that predict effective responses to ICI. In the present lymphoma model, we enlarge these observations with the finding that TT (and, to a significantly lesser extent, C140 alone) generate a preclinically active immunological memory against lymphoma re-challenge at doses 2.5 higher than the first lymphoma inoculum. We are now planning studies in TNBC and lymphoma models to pinpoint what immune cell subpopulation(s) is/are involved and crucial for this immunological memory. When phenotypically defined and purified, these cells might be transplanted for possible cellular therapies of TNBC, lymphoma, or other types of neoplastic diseases.

A possible caveat of the present study is related to differences in the immune systems of rodents and humans. We are now planning TT clinical trials that will be instrumental to confirm TT mechanisms of action in humans.

Supplementary Materials: The following supporting information can be downloaded at: https://www.mdpi.com/article/10.3390/jcm12072535/s1. Table S1: Antibodies and gating strategies used in the study. Cell type is indicated in the first column, the phenotype in the second, fluorophores in the third, the clone and the distributors of the antibody in the fourth and fifth respectively. Figure S1: Therapeutic scheme used in this study.

Author Contributions: Methodology, S.O., P.F., G.T., P.M. and F.B.; Validation, P.F., S.O. and P.N.; Formal analysis, S.O., P.F., G.T. and P.M.; Investigation, S.O. and P.F.; Resources, S.O, P.F. and F.B.; Data curation, S.O., P.F., G.T., G.M., G.B. and P.M.; Writing—original draft, S.O., P.F. and F.B.; Supervision, S.O., P.F. and F.B.; Project administration, F.B.; Funding acquisition, F.B. All authors have read and agreed to the published version of the manuscript.

Funding: This research was funded by AIRC (IG 20109) and the Italian Ministry of Health.

Institutional Review Board Statement: The animal study protocol was approved by the Institutional Review Board (or Ethics Committee) by Italian Ministry of health (protocol code 639-2019 approved on 9 April 2019).

Informed Consent Statement: Not applicable.

Data Availability Statement: Data are available upon reasonable request.

Acknowledgments: Supported in part by AIRC and the Italian Ministry of Health. Authors would like to Bruno Amati and Iros Barozzi for their helpful suggestions, IEO imaging facility, in particular Simona Ronzoni for sorting experiments, IEO cell culture, in particular Cristina Spinelli, Manuela Moia, and Donatella Genovese for cells technical supports.

Conflicts of Interest: The authors declare no conflict of interest.

References

1. Robert, C. A decade of immune-checkpoint inhibitors in cancer therapy. *Nat. Commun.* **2020**, *11*, 3801. [CrossRef] [PubMed]
2. Beaver, J.A.; Pazdur, R. The wild west of checkpoint inhibitor development. *N. Engl. J. Med.* **2022**, *386*, 1297–1301. [CrossRef] [PubMed]
3. Bertolini, F.; Sukhatme, V.P.; Bouche, G. Drug repurposing in oncology—Patient and health systems opportunities. *Nat. Rev. Clin. Oncol.* **2015**, *12*, 732–742. [CrossRef]
4. Falvo, P.; Orecchioni, S.; Hillje, R.; Raveane, A.; Mancuso, P.; Camisaschi, C.; Luzi, L.; Pelicci, P.; Bertolini, F. Cyclophosphamide and vinorelbine activate stem-like CD8+ T cells and improve anti-PD-1 efficacy in triple-negative breast cancer. *Cancer Res.* **2021**, *81*, 685–697. [CrossRef]
5. Falvo, P.; Orecchioni, S.; Raveane, A.; Mitola, G.; Bertolini, F. A "two-hit"(chemo) therapy to improve checkpoint inhibition in cancer. *Oncoscience* **2021**, *8*, 55. [CrossRef]
6. Carpen, L.; Falvo, P.; Orecchioni, S.; Mitola, G.; Hillje, R.; Mazzara, S.; Mancuso, P.; Pileri, S.; Raveane, A.; Bertolini, F. A single-cell transcriptomic landscape of innate and adaptive intratumoral immunity in triple negative breast cancer during chemo-and immunotherapies. *Cell Death Discov.* **2022**, *8*, 106. [CrossRef] [PubMed]
7. D'Andrea, A.; Gritti, I.; Nicoli, P.; Giorgio, M.; Doni, M.; Conti, A.; Bianchi, V.; Casoli, L.; Sabò, A.; Mironov, A. The mitochondrial translation machinery as a therapeutic target in Myc-driven lymphomas. *Oncotarget* **2016**, *7*, 72415. [CrossRef]
8. Wu, J.; Waxman, D.J. Metronomic cyclophosphamide eradicates large implanted GL261 gliomas by activating antitumor Cd8$^+$ T-cell responses and immune memory. *Oncoimmunology* **2015**, *4*, e1005521. [CrossRef]
9. Orecchioni, S.; Talarico, G.; Labanca, V.; Calleri, A.; Mancuso, P.; Bertolini, F. Vinorelbine, cyclophosphamide and 5-FU effects on the circulating and intratumoural landscape of immune cells improve anti-PD-L1 efficacy in preclinical models of breast cancer and lymphoma. *Br. J. Cancer* **2018**, *118*, 1329–1336. [CrossRef] [PubMed]

20. Pfirschke, C.; Engblom, C.; Rickelt, S.; Cortez-Retamozo, V.; Garris, C.; Pucci, F.; Yamazaki, T.; Poirier-Colame, V.; Newton, A.; Redouane, Y. Immunogenic chemotherapy sensitizes tumors to checkpoint blockade therapy. *Immunity* **2016**, *44*, 343–354. [CrossRef]
21. Budak-Alpdogan, T.; Alpdogan, O.; Banerjee, D.; Wang, E.; Moore, M.A.; Bertino, J.R. Methotrexate and cytarabine inhibit progression of human lymphoma in NOD/SCID mice carrying a mutant dihydrofolate reductase and cytidine deaminase fusion gene. *Mol. Ther.* **2004**, *10*, 574–584. [CrossRef] [PubMed]
22. Visan, I. TCF-1+ progenitors. *Nat. Immunol.* **2022**, *23*, 988. [CrossRef] [PubMed]
23. Wang, D.; Fang, J.; Wen, S.; Li, Q.; Wang, J.; Yang, L.; Dai, W.; Lu, H.; Guo, J.; Shan, Z. A comprehensive profile of TCF1$^+$ progenitor and TCF1− terminally exhausted PD-1$^+$ CD8$^+$ T cells in head and neck squamous cell carcinoma: Implications for prognosis and immunotherapy. *Int. J. Oral Sci.* **2022**, *14*, 8. [CrossRef] [PubMed]
24. Tanaka, H.; Matsushima, H.; Mizumoto, N.; Takashima, A. Classification of chemotherapeutic agents based on their differential in vitro effects on dendritic cells. *Cancer Res.* **2009**, *69*, 6978–6986. [CrossRef] [PubMed]
25. Zsiros, E.; Lynam, S.; Attwood, K.M.; Wang, C.; Chilakapati, S.; Gomez, E.C.; Liu, S.; Akers, S.; Lele, S.; Frederick, P.J. Efficacy and safety of pembrolizumab in combination with bevacizumab and oral metronomic cyclophosphamide in the treatment of recurrent ovarian cancer: A phase 2 nonrandomized clinical trial. *JAMA Oncol.* **2021**, *7*, 78–85. [CrossRef]
26. Tilsed, C.M.; Principe, N.; Kidman, J.; Chin, W.L.; Morales, M.L.O.; Zemek, R.M.; Chee, J.; Islam, R.; Fear, V.S.; Forbes, C. CD4$^+$ T cells drive an inflammatory, TNF-α/IFN-rich tumor microenvironment responsive to chemotherapy. *Cell Rep.* **2022**, *41*, 111874. [CrossRef]
27. Røssevold, A.H.; Andresen, N.K.; Bjerre, C.A.; Gilje, B.; Jakobsen, E.H.; Raj, S.X.; Falk, R.S.; Russnes, H.G.; Jahr, T.; Mathiesen, R.R.; et al. Atezolizumab plus anthracycline-based chemotherapy in metastatic triple-negative breast cancer: The randomized, double-blind phase 2b ALICE trial. *Nat. Med.* **2022**, *28*, 2573–2583. [CrossRef]
28. Davoodi-Moghaddam, Z.; Jafari-Raddani, F.; Noori, M.; Bashash, D. A systematic review and meta-analysis of immune checkpoint therapy in relapsed or refractory non-Hodgkin lymphoma; a friend or foe? *Transl. Oncol.* **2023**, *30*, 101636. [CrossRef]
29. Bocci, G.; Pelliccia, S.; Orlandi, P.; Caridi, M.; Banchi, M.; Musuraca, G.; Di Napoli, A.; Bianchi, M.P.; Patti, C.; Anticoli-Borza, P.; et al. Remarkable Remission Rate and Long-Term Efficacy of Upfront Metronomic Chemotherapy in Elderly and Frail Patients, with Diffuse Large B-Cell Lymphoma. *J. Clin. Med.* **2022**, *11*, 7162. [CrossRef]
30. Ye, X.; Wang, L.; Nie, M.; Wang, Y.; Dong, S.; Ren, W.; Li, G.; Li, Z.M.; Wu, K.; Pan-Hammarström, Q. A single-cell atlas of diffuse large B cell lymphoma. *Cell Rep.* **2022**, *39*, 110713. [CrossRef]
31. Zhang, Y.; Chen, H.; Mo, H.; Hu, X.; Gao, R.; Zhao, Y.; Liu, B.; Niu, L.; Sun, X.; Yu, X.; et al. Single-cell analyses reveal key immune cell subsets associated with response to PD-L1 blockade in triple-negative breast cancer. *Cancer Cell* **2021**, *39*, 1578–1593. [CrossRef] [PubMed]

Disclaimer/Publisher's Note: The statements, opinions and data contained in all publications are solely those of the individual author(s) and contributor(s) and not of MDPI and/or the editor(s). MDPI and/or the editor(s) disclaim responsibility for any injury to people or property resulting from any ideas, methods, instructions or products referred to in the content.

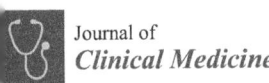

Retrospective National "Real Life" Experience of the SFCE with the Metronomic MEMMAT and MEMMAT-like Protocol

Camille Winnicki [1], Pierre Leblond [2], Franck Bourdeaut [3], Anne Pagnier [4], Gilles Paluenzela [5], Pascal Chastagner [6], Gwenaelle Duhil-De Benaze [7], Victoria Min [1], Hélène Sudour-Bonnange [8], Catherine Piette [9], Natacha Entz-Werle [10], Sylvie Chabaud [11] and Nicolas André [1,12,13,*]

1. Department of Pediatric Immunology, Hematology and Oncology, Children Hospital of La Timone, Assistance Publique Hôpitaux de Marseille, 13005 Marseille, France
2. Department of Pediatric Oncology, Institut d'Hématologie et d'Oncologie Pédiatrique, Centre Léon Bérard, 69008 Lyon, France
3. SIREDO Pediatric Oncology Center, Curie Institute, 75005 Paris, France
4. Department of Pediatric Immunohematology and Oncology, University Hospital, 38043 Grenoble, France
5. Department of Pediatric Hematology-Oncology, Centre Hospitalo-Universitaire de Montpellier, 34000 Montpellier, France
6. Pediatric Oncology, University Hospital of Nancy, 54000 Nancy, France
7. Department of Pediatric Oncology, Centre Hospitalier Universitaire, University Côte d'Azur, 06108 Nice, France
8. Oscar-Lambret Center, Department of Pediatric Oncology & AYA Unit, 59020 Lille, France
9. Department of Pediatric Oncology, Centre Hospitalo-Universitaire de Liège, 4000 Liège, Belgium
10. Pediatric Onco-Hematology Department-Pediatrics III, University Hospital of Strasbourg, 67091 Strasbourg, France
11. Department of Statistics, Centre Léon Bérard, 69373 Lyon, France
12. Centre de Recherche en Cancérologie de Marseille, Aix-Marseille Université, Inserm, CNRS, 13273 Marseille, France
13. Metronomics Global Health Initiative, 13385 Marseille, France
* Correspondence: nicolas.andre@ap-hm.fr

Abstract: Background: Relapses in pediatric high-risk brain tumors remain unmet medical needs. Over the last 15 years, metronomic chemotherapy has gradually emerged as an alternative therapeutic approach. Patients and Methods: This is a national retrospective study of patients with relapsing pediatric brain tumors treated according to the MEMMAT or MEMMAT-like regimen from 2010 to 2022. Treatment consisted of daily oral thalidomide, fenofibrate, and celecoxib, and alternating 21-day cycles of metronomic etoposide and cyclophosphamide associated with bevacizumab and intraventricular chemotherapy. Results: Forty-one patients were included. The most frequent malignancies were medulloblastoma (22) and ATRT (8). Overall, the best responses were CR in eight patients (20%), PR in three patients (7%), and SD in three patients (7%), for a clinical benefit rate of 34%. The median overall survival was 26 months (IC95% = 12.4–42.7), and median EFS was 9.7 months (IC95% = 6.0–18.6). The most frequent grade $\frac{3}{4}$ toxicities were hematological. Dose had to be adjusted in 27% of the cases. There was no statistical difference in outcome between full or modified MEMMAT. The best setting seems to be when MEMMAT is used as a maintenance and at first relapse. Conclusions: The metronomic MEMMAT combination can lead to sustained control of relapsed high-risk pediatric brain tumors.

Keywords: pediatric oncology; brain tumors; metronomic chemotherapy; pharmacology; medulloblastoma; ATRT; angiogenesis; immunotherapy

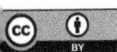

1. Introduction

Central nervous system (CNS) cancers are the most frequent group of solid tumors in children and represent almost 3000 patients per year in Europe [1–4]. Initial treatments usually include primary surgery, radiation therapy, and chemotherapy [1,2,5,6]. Targeted molecules are gaining growing interest in some specific situations such as BRAF pathway-altered glioma [7,8] or NTRK-altered brain tumors [9,10]. Nevertheless, overall survival remains poor in some tumors, and this is even more critical for relapsed or resistant malignancies such as high-grade gliomas or medulloblastoma. Consequently, new therapeutic strategies are needed. One such potential therapeutic approach is metronomic chemotherapy (MC). MC relies on the frequent administration of a low dose of chemotherapy without long breaks [11,12]. It is frequently combined with drug repurposing to generate metronomics. Its mechanism of action is complex and based on multi-target effects. Indeed, MC was initially reported to be anti-angiogenic, but its pro-immune anti-tumoral effect are being increasingly described [13–15]. Additionally, direct effects on anti-cancer and anti-cancer stems cells seem to contribute to the activity of MC [16].

In children, several reports have indicated the potential of various metronomic combinations to control relapsing/refractory tumors [11,17–20], and its interest during maintenance is well-known in leukemia and growing in solid tumors such as rhabdomyosarcoma [21]. Of note, the use of MC also seems to be a promising and well-suited strategy for low- and middle-income countries [19,22,23].

Among many metronomic regimens, the four-drug regimen initially reported by Kieran et al. in a phase 2 trial showed a good safety profile as well as sustained tumor control, especially in ependymoma [17]. This combination was then completed with the addition of fenofibrate, which did not seem to significantly improve its efficacy, as reported in a larger phase 2 trial [24]. The combination was then further enriched by the addition of intra-ventricular (IVe) chemotherapy (etoposide and aracytine) and bevacizumab to generate the so-called MEMMAT combination for metronomic multitarget anti-angiogenic therapy [25,26]. Intra-ventricular chemotherapy was introduced to target meningeal disease that does not seem to be angiogenic-dependent. Bevacizumab was added to further strengthen the anti-angiogenic effect of the combination, as previously reported in the initial metronomic preclinical publications [27]. The initial pilot study reported promising results especially in medulloblastoma [26]. An international state-of-the-art phase II study is ongoing (NCT01356290).

In France, several centers have started treating pediatric patients with refractory/relapsing brain tumors according to the MEMMAT regimen outside of the trial. Interestingly, physicians also sometimes used lighter versions of this protocol, for instance, by not using intra-ventricular chemotherapy, bevacizumab, or thalidomide. We report here the retrospective experience of the French Society for Children with Cancer (SFCE).

2. Materials and Methods

2.1. Patients and Data Collection

In this retrospective study, data from patients younger than 19 years treated in pediatric oncology units of the SCFE from 2010 to 2022 who received the MEMMAT combination were collected. All 41 patients had relapsed or refractory CNS brain tumors. A full medical history was obtained from the electronic medical chart including neurological examination; performance status evaluation; and routine laboratory tests including blood chemistry, urine analysis, CSF analysis, and MRI scans. MRI scans were repeated at least every 2–3 months during treatment and during follow-up until progression.

2.2. The MEMMAT Regimen

Treatment consisted of a continuous oral regimen including the following:
- Daily oral thalidomide (3 mg/kg/d);
- Daily oral fenofibrate (90 mg/m^2/d);
- Twice daily oral celecoxib (100 to 400 mg 2x/d);
- Alternating 21-day cycles of low-dose oral etoposide (50 mg/m^2/d) and cyclophosphamide (2.5 mg/kg/d) [24].
- Intra-venous Bevacizumab (10 mg/kg) every two weeks;

- IVe therapy consisting of alternating etoposide (0.25 mg to 0.5 mg/d) for five consecutive days [28], alternating with liposomal cytarabine (25–50 mg) in combination with oral steroids to prevent chemical meningitis every 3 weeks [29]. When liposomal cytarabine was no longer available, it was switched for standard aqueous aracytine.

The MEMMAT-like regimen was defined as MEMMAT without IVe therapy, without bevacizumab, and/or without thalidomide. The planned treatment duration was 1 year. In cases of toxicity, dose reductions were recommended to try to avoid treatment breaks at the discretion of the local treating physician. Additional radiotherapy concomitant to or at the end of MEMMAT was allowed in case of a response.

2.3. Evaluation

2.3.1. Response to Treatment

T1- or T2-weighted images of the target lesions on MRI were used to evaluate the length of the 2 longest tumor dimensions. Complete response (CR) was defined as the complete disappearance of a measurable disease, a partial response (PR) was defined as $\geq 50\%$ decrease in the product of the two maximum perpendicular diameters compared with the baseline evaluation, and stable disease was defined as $\leq 50\%$ decrease and $\leq 25\%$ increase in the product of diameters. Progressive disease (PD) was defined as a $\geq 25\%$ increase in the product of diameters or the appearance of new lesions (RAPNO) [30].

2.3.2. Evaluation of Toxicity

Side effects were retrospectively collected and evaluated according to the Common Terminology Criteria for Adverse Events (CTCAE) v. 4.0.

2.4. Statistical Methods

Progression-free survival (PFS) was defined as time elapsed from recurrence that triggered the initiation of the "MEMMAT" regimen to the date of relapse, progression, or death from any cause or, for patients without any events, to the date of last follow-up. Overall survival (OS) was defined as the time elapsed from the date of relapse that triggered the initiation of the "MEMMAT" regimen to the date of death from any cause or, for survivors, to the date of last follow-up.

PFS and OS were estimated using the Kaplan–Meier method and described in terms of median along with the associated 2-sided 95% CIs. Survival distributions were compared according to the type of malignancy; the number of previous lines of treatments; and the type of regime, full or MEMMAT-like, using a Log-Rank test, supported by a Cox regression. The hazard ratios between subgroups, along with the associated 2-sided 95% CIs for the estimates, were determined. Statistical analysis was conducted using SAS statistical software version 9.4.

3. Results

Forty-one patients were identified and included in this series. The characteristics of the patients are detailed in Table 1. All 41 patients had relapsed or refractory CNS brain tumors, mostly medulloblastoma (22 pts—54%) or ATRT (8 pts—27%). Thirty-three patients (80%) received MEMMAT for a relapsed/progressing tumor, and eight patients (20%) received treatment as part of maintenance. The MEMMAT treatment was given as a second-line treatment in 32% of the patients and as third- to fifth-line treatments in 68% of the patients. Almost all patients had anterior chemotherapy (95%—39 pts) and/or radiotherapy (95%—39 pts) and/or surgery (98%—40 patients). The full MEMMAT was given in 39% of the patients. Fourteen and ten patients did not receive IVe therapy and bevacizumab, respectively. Of note, seven patients also received radiotherapy during or after completing their MEMMAT treatment.

Table 1. Patients characteristics.

Patient Characteristics	Frequency N = 41	
Age (years)		
Median age (min; max)	14 (1; 19)	
Gender		
Female	20	(48.8%)
Male	21	(51.2%)
Type of malignancy		
Medulloblastoma	22	(53.7%)
Atypical Teratoid Rhabdoid Tumor	8	(19.5%)
Ependymoma	5	(12.2%)
Others	6	(14.6%)
Number of previous lines of treatment		
1	13	(31.7%)
2	17	(41.5%)
3	5	(12.2%)
4	6	(14.6%)
Type of treatment previously received		
Chemotherapy	39	(95.1%)
Surgery	40	(97.6%)
Radiotherapy	39	(95.1%)
Immunotherapy	0	(0%)
Targeted therapies	3	(7.3%)
MEMMAT received		
Full-type	16	(39.0%)
Modified-type	25	(61.0%)
Drugs not administrated in modified MEMMAT		
Bevacizumab	10	(24.4%)
Intrathecal injections	14	(34.1%)
Thalidomide	13	(31.7%)

The median duration of treatment was 32 weeks (range 4–156), and the mean time to response was 75 days (+/− 97). Treatment was overall well tolerated. Grade 3 or 4 toxicities were reported in 68% of the patients. The most frequent grade 3–4 toxicities were hematological. Details of the grade 3–4 are presented in Table 2. Dose had to be adjusted in 27% of the cases.

With a mean follow-up of 28 months, the best responses were CR in eight patients (20%), PR in three patients (7%), and SD in three patients (7%), for a clinical benefit rate of 34%. Progressive disease was observed in 56% of the cases and was either local (20%) or metastatic (46%). Twenty-one patients died of disease during the follow-up period. The median overall survival was 26 months (IC95% = 12.4–42.7), and median EFS was 9.7 months (IC95% = 6.0–18.6) (Figure 1).

Table 2. Observed grade III and IV toxicities.

Toxicity (Grade 3–4)	Number of Patients N = 41
Hematological toxicity	
-Neutropenia	20 (49%)
-Thrombopenia	4 (10%)
-Anemia	2 (5%)
Neurological disorder	
-Neuropathy	7 (17%)
-Status epilepticus	2 (4%)
-Hemiparesis	1 (2%)
-Cerebellitis	1 (2%)
Hemorrhagic disorder	
-Macroscopic hematuria	1 (2%)
-Rectal bleeding	1 (2%)
Intraventricular reservoir disorder	3 (7%)
Infections	2 (5%)
Others	
-Mucositis	2 (5%)
-Rhinitis	2 (5%)
-Thyroiditis	1 (2%)

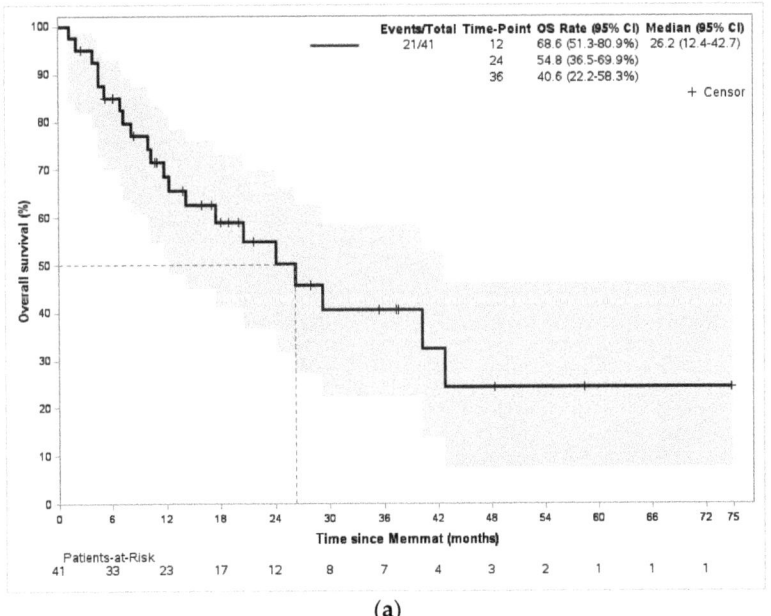

(a)

Figure 1. Cont.

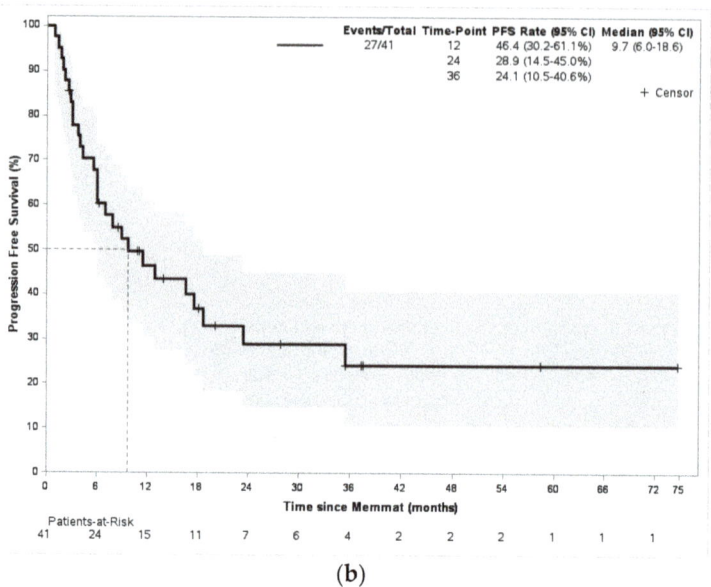

Figure 1. Overall survival and event-free survival of the whole population. (**a**) Overall survival; (**b**) event-free survival.

When considering the underlying malignancy, EFS for ATRT and medulloblastoma were, respectively, 6 months and 9.7 months. Interestingly, for the five ependymoma patients, the median EFS was not reached and only one event was reported (Figure 2). Among the seven patients who received radiotherapy during or at the end of the MEMMAT regimen, we observed two complete remissions, one partial remission, one stable disease, and three progressive diseases.

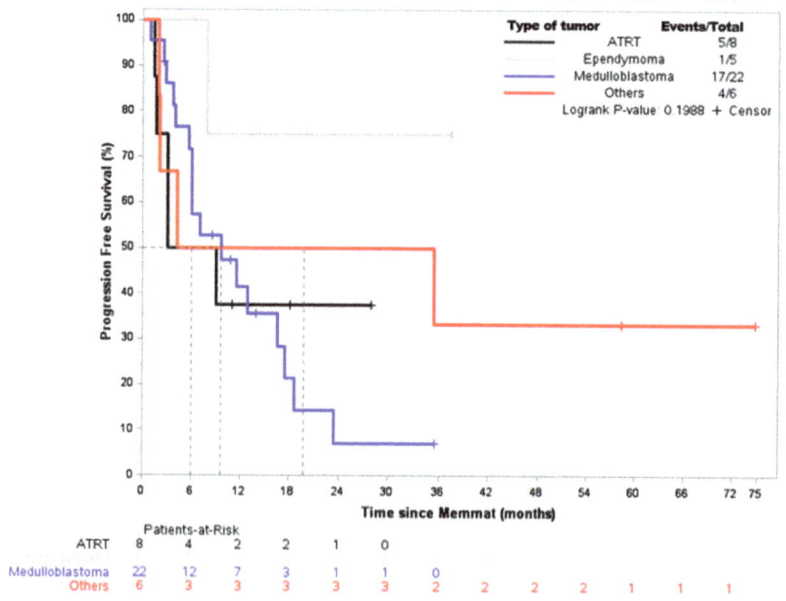

Figure 2. Event-free survival according to tumor type.

Since a significant proportion of the patients did not receive the full MEMMAT regimen, we investigated whether this had a significant impact on survival. As shown in Figure 3, there was no impact on event-free survival when comparing full versus adapted MEMMAT (7 months (4.1-NE)) vs. 13 months ((3.0–35) $p = 0.9$)). Interestingly, when looking at further details of the impact of IVe therapy or bevacuzimab on EFS, we did not find any difference either (bevacizumab (7.4 months (1.4-NE) vs. 11.5 months (6.0–18.6) $p = 0.68$) or IVe therapy (16.6 (3–35) vs. 8 months (3.9-NE) $p = 0.73$)). Lastly, a similar specific analysis run on the medulloblastoma population did not show any difference for PFS either (17 months (1–26) vs. 20 (4.5—not reached) $p = 0.44$)).

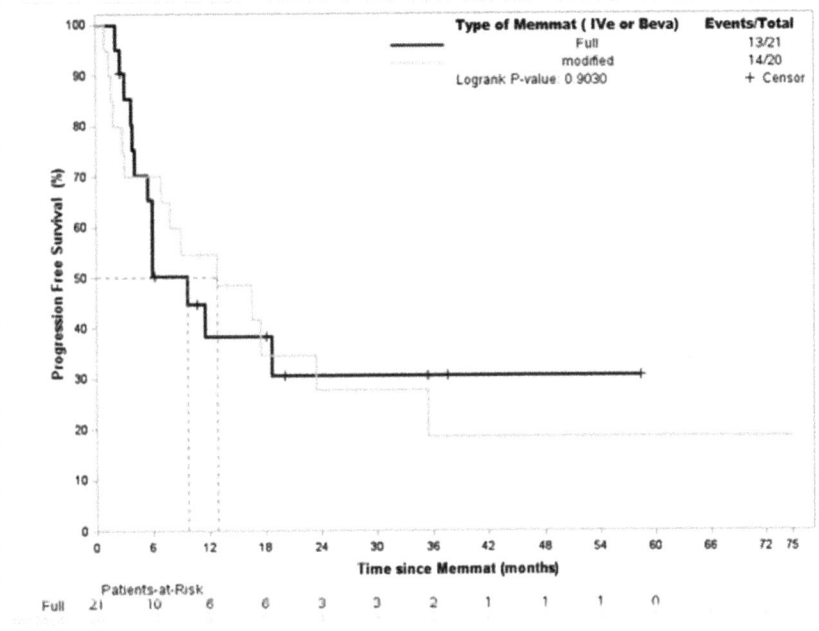

Figure 3. EFS according to treatment with full MEMMAT or modified MEMMAT.

To try to identify patients more likely to benefit from the MEMMAT regimen, we investigated the impact of the number of previous lines of treatment and the setting of initiation of MEMMAT (maintenance vs. progressive disease). As shown in Figure 4, the number of previous lines of treatment was associated with a statistically significant impact on EFS. Indeed, when patients received MEMMAT as a second line of treatment, EFS was not reached vs. 6.4 months (5.7–12.9; $p = 0.0076$) for patients receiving MEMMAT as a third or higher line of treatment. Similarly, when MEMMAT was initiated as part of maintenance, EFS was significantly better in the maintenance arm (median EFS was not reached versus 7.8 months (4–17) when compared with patients with progressive disease at initiation of MEMMAT). These results suggest that MEMMAT should be used as a means of maintenance during the first relapse. Among the patients who received MEMMAT as part of maintenance, three had medulloblastoma, two had ependymoma, and three patients had other types of tumors. Out of the eight patients, four had metastatic relapse. All patients but one previously received a combination of surgery, radiotherapy, and chemotherapy. One patient out of eight was in complete remission at the initiation of MEMMAT. At last follow-up, one patient presented a progressive disease; three and two patients were in complete remission and partial remission, respectively; and two patients had a stable disease.

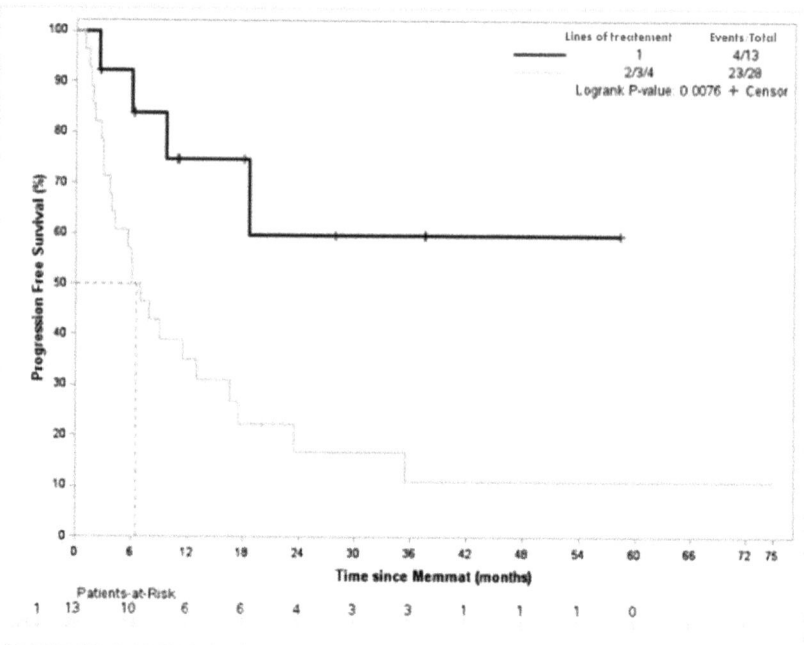

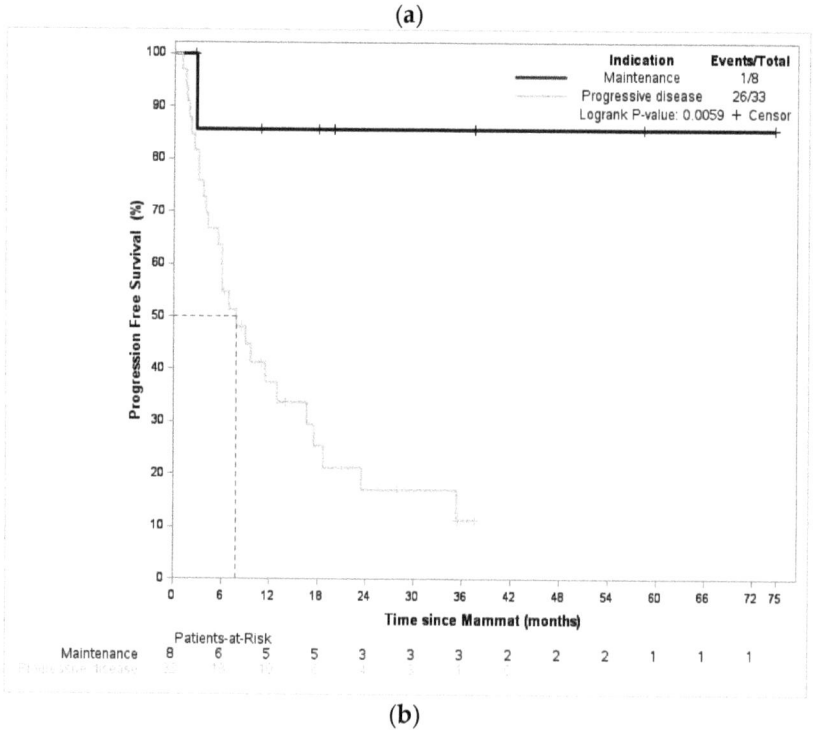

Figure 4. Event-free survival according to the number of previous lines of treatment and setting (progressive disease vs. maintenance). (**a**) EFS according to number of previous lines of treatment (1 vs. >1). (**b**) EFS according to the setting at the initiation of MEMMAT (maintenance vs. relapse).

Lastly, as limited data are available about the use of MEMMAT of ependymoma, we then focused on the patients with ependymoma. The details are provided in Table 3. All patients had progressive disease after at least one line of treatment and previously received at least radiotherapy, except one patient who received MEMMAT as part of maintenance. Only one patient with metastatic disease progressed while on MEMMAT given as a fourth line of treatment.

Table 3. Characteristics of patients with ependymomas.

	Diagnosis	Tumor Status Prior to MEMMAT	nb Previous Lines of Treatment	Type of Treatment Previously Received	Time to Progression Prior to MEMMAT (days)	Time to Progression with MEMMAT (days)
Patient #1, 7 y-o	Anaplastic grade 3	local disease	1	Surgery, chemotherapy, radiation therapy	0	0
Patient #2, 21 y-o	Grade 2	local disease	3	Surgery, chemotherapy, radiation therapy	122	0
Patient #3, 1 y-o	Anaplastic grade 3	Metastatic disease, CSF positive	4	Surgery, chemotherapy, radiation therapy	240	34
Patient #4, 9 y-o	Anaplastic grade 3	Metastatic disease	1	Surgery, radiation therapy	452	0
Patient #5, 4 y-o	No data	Metastatic disease	1	Surgery, chemotherapy, radiation therapy	55	0

4. Discussion

We report here the experience of the SFCE with the "real life" use of the MEMMAT or MEMMAT-like regimen outside of a clinical trial in 41 pediatric patients with refractory or relapsing brain tumors. The combination appears to be safe and to display efficacy in patients with ependymoma, ATRT, and medulloblastoma. Indeed, 25% of the patients were alive without a progressive disease after 3 years.

Among the 17 patients with medulloblastoma, we observed 10% overall survival at 24 months after initiating the MEMMAT treatment. This does not seem to be as good as the initial report of the MEMMAT regimen [26]. The Vienna team has also further reported that, out of 29 patients with medulloblastoma treatment with MEMMAT, 9 patients were alive, with a median of 44 months after recurrence [31]. Five out of nine surviving patients are currently in CR between 96 and 164 months after starting MEMMAT therapy. Of note, in this series, five patients died of another cause (accident, leukemia, and septicemia). OS was $44 \pm 10\%$ at 5 years and $39 \pm 10\%$ at 10 years, and PFS was $33 \pm 10\%$ at 5 years and $28 \pm 9\%$ at 10 years. It is not clear why the results we report here are not as good. First, at last follow-up, five patients were still under treatment in hopes that, with a longer follow-up, overall outcome might improve. Additionally, the main difference from the Vienna experience is that a significant proportion of the patients we report here did not receive the full MEMMAT regimen. Anyhow, when looking more closely at the impact of not receiving the full MEMMAT regimen, we could not find any difference in survival both in the global population or in the medulloblastoma sub-population. These findings shall nevertheless be considered cautiously because the reasons for not giving full MEMMAT (i.e., no meningeal disease and frail patients) might have induced a strong bias and could have not led to us trying to use the MEMMAT-like regime until our findings were confirmed. This study is also retrospective and was not well equipped to demonstrate the differences between the full and adapted MEMMAT. Anyhow, as the statistical analysis did not reveal significant differences in the patients receiving the full MEMMAT or MEMMAT-like regimen (i.e., without IVe therapy, thalidomide, or bevacizumab), the fact that some patients can reach sustained CR without the full regimen raises the question of an optimal design of the combination. Indeed, the results we report here seem to be anyhow better than the previous versions of the MEMMAT backbone protocol relying on a four-drug combination or five-drug combination [17,24]. The mechanism of action of MEMMAT is rooted in the metronomic concept; it was therefore designed as an antiangiogenic treatment [26,32], and IVe therapy was added to avoid resistance in the metastatic meningeal disease, which is not sensitive to MC. Furthermore, MC has been demonstrated to restore the anti-cancer properties of the immune system and to directly target cancer cells and cancer stem cells [20]. Ultimately, the MEMMAT regimen may be regarded as a treatment that targets cancer as a system, suggesting that the treatment might work differently according to the disease patients, and setting (i.e., bulky disease vs. minimum residual disease) so that all agents may not be mandatory for all patients. Noteworthy from this perspective is that survival is better when MEMMAT is given as maintenance of maintenance after additional treatment at relapse (i.e., surgery, re-irradiation, and chemotherapy), although several treatments make it impossible to formally demonstrate the respective impacts of the different parts of the treatment on the outcome.

We also report an interesting outcome in patients with relapsed ATRT or ependymoma. The two groups of tumors represent tumors with unmet needs, and innovative therapies such as targeted therapies and immunotherapies have had quite a limited impact so far. While the number of patients remains small and shall be confirmed, MC has previously been reported to be of interest in these two types of tumors [33–36]. For ependymoma, the articulation of a metronomic MEMMAT method of maintenance may be of high value after second surgery and/or re-irradiation.

A significant proportion of the patients presented with grade 3 or grade 4 toxicities. The most frequent types were hematological toxicities that required dose adjustments. This is in part related to previous heavy treatment with craniospinal radiotherapy and/or high-dose chemotherapy followed by peripheral stem cell transplantation, but this treatment, although metronomic, has an intrinsic toxicity, as previously reported by Peyrl et al. [26] or Porkholm et al. in a modified version of the MEMMAT protocol for patients with relapsing DIPG/HGG [37]. Pediatric patients living in low- and middle-income countries (LMIC) are potentially interested in MC given its low cost and low toxicity [22]. Anyhow, the addition of bevacizumab or thalidomide, and the requirements of IT therapy make it not fully adapted for this setting. Whether a lighter MEMMAT-like protocol would be of interest for LMIC remains an open question.

We also need to acknowledge the limitations of this series. It is retrospective, despite a detailed and precise protocol; as mentioned above, the treatment is heterogenous, and several types of disease have been included. Additionally, physicians may have chosen to add IVe therapy when meningeal disease was evidenced, creating bias. Lastly, we did not have precise molecular subgroups for most patients. Group 4 medulloblastoma, for instance, has been reported to have a less aggressive behavior [38]. The repartition of the molecular subtypes of brain tumors included might therefore influence the EFS in this series. Anyhow, in the series from Slavc et al. [31] among the 23 patients whose tumors underwent molecular subgrouping classification using a DNA methylation array and brain classifier mnp-V12.5, group 4 medulloblastomas seem to group 4 have better outcome than group 3 medulloblastoma (median survival: 43 months (14–71) vs. not reached). As group 3 medulloblastomas are commonly accepted as displaying worse prognoses, the findings reported by Slavc et al. [31] seem to further highlight the potential of MEMMAT for both relapsing Group 3 and 4 medulloblastomas, which represent medical unmet needs. Moreover, the lack of molecular profiling for most of our patients should not diminish the interesting outcomes reported despite not furthering research in precision medicine. Nevertheless, this series represents real-life data from patients who have not been highly selected as it would be the case for an early phase clinical trial, and it provides valuable additional information regarding the potential of this combination.

5. Conclusions

Our series confirms the capacity of the MEMMAT regimen to control relapsing/refractory pediatric brain malignancies beyond medulloblastomas. It seems that it would lead to better outcome if used as a second-line treatment and as part of maintenance. Performing additional state-of-the-art studies is mandatory to confirm or question our results.

Author Contributions: Conceptualization, N.A. and P.L.; methodology, N.A., P.L. and S.C.; validation, N.A., P.L. and S.C.; formal analysis, N.A., C.W., P.L. and S.C.; investigation, all authors.; resources, N.A. and P.L.; data curation, C.W., N.A. and S.C.; writing—original draft preparation, C.W. and N.A.; writing—review and editing, all authors; supervision, N.A.; project administration, N.A. All authors have read and agreed to the published version of the manuscript."

Funding: This research received no external funding.

Institutional Review Board Statement: The study was conducted in accordance with the Declaration of Helsinki. Ethical review and approval were waived for this study as the data were generated as part of routine care. Access to the patients' biological and registry data issued from the hospital information system was approved by the data protection committee (DPD) of Centre Leon Bérard (R201-004-217) on 8 February 2022.

Informed Consent Statement: Informed consent from all parents and children, if competent to give consent depending on their age.

Data Availability Statement: The data will be available upon reasonable request to the authors.

Acknowledgments: We thank RESOP, LN La Vie, Fondation Flavien, Cancéropole PACA, Fondation Mont Ventoux, and Au nom d'Andréa for their support.

Conflicts of Interest: The authors declare no conflict of interest.

References

1. Ostrom, Q.T.; de Blank, P.M.; Kruchko, C.; Petersen, C.M.; Liao, P.; Finlay, J.L.; Stearns, D.S.; Wolff, J.E.; Wolinsky, Y.; Letterio, J.J.; et al. Alex's Lemonade Stand Foundation Infant and Childhood Primary Brain and Central Nervous System Tumors Diagnosed in the United States in 2007–2011. *Neuro-Oncol.* **2015**, *16*, x1–x36. [CrossRef] [PubMed]
2. Pollack, I.F.; Agnihotri, S.; Broniscer, A. Childhood Brain Tumors: Current Management, Biological Insights, and Future Directions. *J. Neurosurg. Pediatr.* **2019**, *23*, 261–273. [CrossRef] [PubMed]
3. Pollack, I.F. Brain Tumors in Children. *N. Engl. J. Med.* **1994**, *331*, 1500–1507. [CrossRef]
4. Pritchard-Jones, K.; Kaatsch, P.; Steliarova-Foucher, E.; Stiller, C.A.; Coebergh, J.W.W. Cancer in Children and Adolescents in Europe: Developments over 20 Years and Future Challenges. *Eur. J. Cancer* **2006**, *42*, 2183–2190. [CrossRef]
5. Packer, R.J.; Gajjar, A.; Vezina, G.; Rorke-Adams, L.; Burger, P.C.; Robertson, P.L.; Bayer, L.; LaFond, D.; Donahue, B.R.; Marymont, M.H.; et al. Phase III Study of Craniospinal Radiation Therapy Followed by Adjuvant Chemotherapy for Newly Diagnosed Average-Risk Medulloblastoma. *J. Clin. Oncol.* **2006**, *24*, 4202–4208. [CrossRef]
6. Bailey, S.; André, N.; Gandola, L.; Massimino, M.; Rutkowski, S.; Clifford, S.C. Clinical Trials in High-Risk Medulloblastoma: Evolution of the SIOP-Europe HR-MB Trial. *Cancers* **2022**, *14*, 374. [CrossRef]
7. Banerjee, A.; Jakacki, R.I.; Onar-Thomas, A.; Wu, S.; Nicolaides, T.; Young Poussaint, T.; Fangusaro, J.; Phillips, J.; Perry, A.; Turner, D.; et al. A Phase I Trial of the MEK Inhibitor Selumetinib (AZD6244) in Pediatric Patients with Recurrent or Refractory Low-Grade Glioma: A Pediatric Brain Tumor Consortium (PBTC) Study. *Neuro-Oncol.* **2017**, *19*, 1135–1144. [CrossRef]
8. Fangusaro, J.; Onar-Thomas, A.; Poussaint, T.Y.; Wu, S.; Ligon, A.H.; Lindeman, N.; Campagne, O.; Banerjee, A.; Gururangan, S.; Kilburn, L.B.; et al. A Phase II Trial of Selumetinib in Children with Recurrent Optic Pathway and Hypothalamic Low-Grade Glioma without NF1: A Pediatric Brain Tumor Consortium Study. *Neuro-Oncol.* **2021**, *23*, 1777–1788. [CrossRef] [PubMed]
9. Desai, A.V.; Robinson, G.W.; Gauvain, K.; Basu, E.M.; Macy, M.E.; Maese, L.; Whipple, N.S.; Sabnis, A.J.; Foster, J.H.; Shusterman, S.; et al. Entrectinib in Children and Young Adults with Solid or Primary CNS Tumors Harboring NTRK, ROS1 or ALK Aberrations (STARTRK-NG). *Neuro-Oncol.* **2022**, *24*, 1776–1789. [CrossRef]
10. Tauziède-Espariat, A.; Dangouloff-Ros, V.; Figarella-Branger, D.; Uro-Coste, E.; Nicaise, Y.; André, N.; Scavarda, D.; Testud, B.; Girard, N.; Rousseau, A.; et al. Clinicopathological and Molecular Characterization of Three Cases Classified by DNA-Methylation Profiling as "Glioneuronal Tumors, NOS, Subtype A". *Acta Neuropathol.* **2022**, *144*, 1179–1183. [CrossRef]
11. André, N.; Carré, M.; Pasquier, E. Metronomics: Towards Personalized Chemotherapy? *Nat. Rev. Clin. Oncol.* **2014**, *11*, 413–431. [CrossRef]
12. Kerbel, R.S.; Kamen, B.A. The Anti-Angiogenic Basis of Metronomic Chemotherapy. *Nat. Rev. Cancer* **2004**, *4*, 423–436. [CrossRef]
13. Yang, M.-Y.; Lee, H.-T.; Chen, C.-M.; Shen, C.-C.; Ma, H.-I. Celecoxib Suppresses the Phosphorylation of STAT3 Protein and Can Enhance the Radiosensitivity of Medulloblastoma-Derived Cancer Stem-Like Cells. *Int. J. Mol. Sci.* **2014**, *15*, 11013–11029. [CrossRef] [PubMed]
14. Nars, M.S.; Kaneno, R. Immunomodulatory Effects of Low Dose Chemotherapy and Perspectives of Its Combination with Immunotherapy. *Int. J. Cancer* **2013**, *132*, 2471–2478. [CrossRef] [PubMed]

15. Hao, Y.-B.; Yi, S.-Y.; Ruan, J.; Zhao, L.; Nan, K.-J. New Insights into Metronomic Chemotherapy-Induced Immunoregulation. *Cancer Lett.* **2014**, *354*, 220–226. [CrossRef]
16. André, N.; Tsai, K.; Carré, M.; Pasquier, E. Metronomic Chemotherapy: Direct Targeting of Cancer Cells after All? *Trends Cancer* **2017**, *3*, 319–325. [CrossRef]
17. Kieran, M.W.; Turner, C.D.; Rubin, J.B.; Chi, S.N.; Zimmerman, M.A.; Chordas, C.; Klement, G.; Laforme, A.; Gordon, A.; Thomas, A.; et al. A Feasibility Trial of Antiangiogenic (Metronomic) Chemotherapy in Pediatric Patients with Recurrent or Progressive Cancer. *J. Pediatr. Hematol. Oncol.* **2005**, *27*, 573–581. [CrossRef]
18. Zapletalova, D.; André, N.; Deak, L.; Kyr, M.; Bajciova, V.; Mudry, P.; Dubska, L.; Demlova, R.; Pavelka, Z.; Zitterbart, K.; et al. Metronomic Chemotherapy with the COMBAT Regimen in Advanced Pediatric Malignancies: A Multicenter Experience. *Oncology* **2012**, *82*, 249–260. [CrossRef] [PubMed]
19. Fousseyni, T.; Diawara, M.; Pasquier, E.; Andre, N. Children Treated With Metronomic Chemotherapy in a Low-Income Country: METRO-MALI-0. *J. Pediatr. Hematol. Oncol.* **2011**, *33*, 31–34. [CrossRef]
20. André, N.; Abed, S.; Orbach, D.; Alla, C.A.; Padovani, L.; Pasquier, E.; Gentet, J.C.; Verschuur, A. Pilot Study of a Pediatric Metronomic 4-Drug Regimen. *Oncotarget* **2011**, *2*, 960–965. [CrossRef] [PubMed]
21. André, N.; Orbach, D.; Pasquier, E. Metronomic Maintenance for High-Risk Pediatric Malignancies: One Size Will Not Fit All. *Trends Cancer* **2020**, *6*, 819–828. [CrossRef]
22. André, N.; Banavali, S.; Snihur, Y.; Pasquier, E. Has the Time Come for Metronomics in Low-Income and Middle-Income Countries? *Lancet Oncol.* **2013**, *14*, e239–e248. [CrossRef]
23. Revon-Rivière, G.; Banavali, S.; Heississen, L.; Gomez Garcia, W.; Abdolkarimi, B.; Vaithilingum, M.; Li, C.-K.; Leung, P.C.; Malik, P.; Pasquier, E.; et al. Metronomic Chemotherapy for Children in Low- and Middle-Income Countries: Survey of Current Practices and Opinions of Pediatric Oncologists. *J. Glob. Oncol.* **2019**, *5*, 1–8. [CrossRef] [PubMed]
24. Robison, N.J.; Campigotto, F.; Chi, S.N.; Manley, P.E.; Turner, C.D.; Zimmerman, M.A.; Chordas, C.A.; Werger, A.M.; Allen, J.C.; Goldman, S.; et al. A Phase II Trial of a Multi-Agent Oral Antiangiogenic (Metronomic) Regimen in Children with Recurrent or Progressive Cancer. *Pediatr. Blood Cancer* **2014**, *61*, 636–642. [CrossRef] [PubMed]
25. Pasquier, E.; Kieran, M.W.; Sterba, J.; Shaked, Y.; Baruchel, S.; Oberlin, O.; Kivivuori, M.S.; Peyrl, A.; Diawarra, M.; Casanova, M.; et al. Moving Forward with Metronomic Chemotherapy: Meeting Report of the 2nd International Workshop on Metronomic and Anti-Angiogenic Chemotherapy in Paediatric Oncology. *Transl. Oncol.* **2011**, *4*, 203–211. [CrossRef]
26. Peyrl, A.; Chocholous, M.; Kieran, M.W.; Azizi, A.A.; Prucker, C.; Czech, T.; Dieckmann, K.; Schmook, M.-T.; Haberler, C.; Leiss, U.; et al. Antiangiogenic Metronomic Therapy for Children with Recurrent Embryonal Brain Tumors. *Pediatr. Blood Cancer* **2012**, *59*, 511–517. [CrossRef] [PubMed]
27. Klement, G.; Baruchel, S.; Rak, J.; Man, S.; Clark, K.; Hicklin, D.J.; Bohlen, P.; Kerbel, R.S. Continuous Low-Dose Therapy with Vinblastine and VEGF Receptor-2 Antibody Induces Sustained Tumor Regression without Overt Toxicity. *J. Clin. Investig.* **2000**, *105*, R15–R24. [CrossRef]
28. Fleischhack, G.; Reif, S.; Hasan, C.; Jaehde, U.; Hettmer, S.; Bode, U. Feasibility of Intraventricular Administration of Etoposide in Patients with Metastatic Brain Tumours. *Br. J. Cancer* **2001**, *84*, 1453–1459. [CrossRef] [PubMed]
29. Peyrl, A.; Sauermann, R.; Chocholous, M.; Azizi, A.A.; Jäger, W.; Höferl, M.; Slavc, I. Pharmacokinetics and Toxicity of Intrathecal Liposomal Cytarabine in Children and Adolescents Following Age-Adapted Dosing. *Clin. Pharm.* **2014**, *53*, 165–173. [CrossRef]
30. Warren, K.E.; Vezina, G.; Poussaint, T.Y.; Warmuth-Metz, M.; Chamberlain, M.C.; Packer, R.J.; Brandes, A.A.; Reiss, M.; Goldman, S.; Fisher, M.J.; et al. Response Assessment in Medulloblastoma and Leptomeningeal Seeding Tumors: Recommendations from the Response Assessment in Pediatric Neuro-Oncology Committee. *Neuro-Oncol.* **2018**, *20*, 13–23. [CrossRef]
31. Slavc, I.; Mayr, L.; Stepien, N.; Gojo, J.; Aliotti Lippolis, M.; Azizi, A.A.; Chocholous, M.; Baumgartner, A.; Hedrich, C.S.; Holm, S.; et al. Improved Long-Term Survival of Patients with Recurrent Medulloblastoma Treated with a "MEMMAT-like" Metronomic Antiangiogenic Approach. *Cancers* **2022**, *14*, 5128. [CrossRef]
32. Pasquier, E.; Kavallaris, M.; André, N. Metronomic Chemotherapy: New Rationale for New Directions. *Nat. Rev. Clin. Oncol.* **2010**, *7*, 455–465. [CrossRef]
33. Li, L.; Patel, M.; Nguyen, H.S.; Doan, N.; Sharma, A.; Maiman, D. Primary Atypical Teratoid/Rhabdoid Tumor of the Spine in an Adult Patient. *Surg. Neurol. Int.* **2016**, *7*, 27. [CrossRef]
34. Gotti, G.; Biassoni, V.; Schiavello, E.; Spreafico, F.; Antonelli, M.; Calareso, G.; Pecori, E.; Gandola, L.; Massimino, M. A Case of Relapsing Spinal Atypical Teratoid/Rhabdoid Tumor (AT/RT) Responding to Vinorelbine, Cyclophosphamide, and Celecoxib. *Childs Nerv. Syst.* **2015**, *31*, 1621–1623. [CrossRef] [PubMed]
35. Steinbügl, M.; Nemes, K.; Gruhle, M.; Johann, P.; Gil-da-Costa, M.J.; Ebinger, M.; Sehested, A.; Hauser, P.; Reinhard, H.; Hettmer, S.; et al. ATRT-09. Outcome and Therapeutic Interventions in Relapsed and Refractory ATRT—The EU-RHAB Perspective. *Neuro-Oncol.* **2022**, *24*, i4. [CrossRef]
36. Berland, M.; Padovani, L.; Rome, A.; Pech-Gourg, G.; Figarella-Branger, D.; André, N. Sustained Complete Response to Metronomic Chemotherapy in a Child with Refractory Atypical Teratoid Rhabdoid Tumor: A Case Report. *Front. Pharmacol.* **2017**, *8*, 792. [CrossRef] [PubMed]

7. Porkholm, M.; Toiviainen-Salo, S.; Seuri, R.; Lönnqvist, T.; Vepsäläinen, K.; Saarinen-Pihkala, U.M.; Pentikäinen, V.; Kivivuori, S.-M. Metronomic Therapy Can Increase Quality of Life during Paediatric Palliative Cancer Care, but Careful Patient Selection Is Essential. *Acta Paediatr.* **2016**, *105*, 946–951. [CrossRef] [PubMed]
8. Ramaswamy, V.; Remke, M.; Bouffet, E.; Bailey, S.; Clifford, S.C.; Doz, F.; Kool, M.; Dufour, C.; Vassal, G.; Milde, T.; et al. Risk Stratification of Childhood Medulloblastoma in the Molecular Era: The Current Consensus. *Acta Neuropathol.* **2016**, *131*, 821–831. [CrossRef]

Disclaimer/Publisher's Note: The statements, opinions and data contained in all publications are solely those of the individual author(s) and contributor(s) and not of MDPI and/or the editor(s). MDPI and/or the editor(s) disclaim responsibility for any injury to people or property resulting from any ideas, methods, instructions or products referred to in the content.

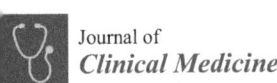

Article

Metronomic Chemo-Endocrine Therapy (FulVEC) as a Salvage Treatment for Patients with Advanced, Treatment-Refractory ER+/HER2-Breast Cancer—A Retrospective Analysis of Consecutive Patients Data

Anna Buda-Nowak [1], Łukasz Kwinta [1,2], Paweł Potocki [1,2], Anna Michałowska-Kaczmarczyk [1,2], Agnieszka Słowik [1], Kamil Konopka [1,2], Joanna Streb [1,2], Maciej Koniewski [3] and Piotr J. Wysocki [1,2,*]

1. Department of Oncology, Jagiellonian University Medical College, University Hospital, 30-501 Krakow, Poland
2. Department of Oncology, Jagiellonian University Medical College, 31-008 Krakow, Poland
3. Institute of Sociology, Jagiellonian University, 30-962 Krakow, Poland
* Correspondence: piotr.wysocki@uj.edu.pl

Abstract: Background: Breast cancer, with 2.3 million new cases and 0.7 million deaths every year, represents a great medical challenge worldwide. These numbers confirm that approx. 30% of BC patients will develop an incurable disease requiring life-long, palliative systemic treatment. Endocrine treatment and chemotherapy administered in a sequential fashion are the basic treatment options in advanced ER+/HER2- BC, which is the most common BC type. The palliative, long-term treatment of advanced BC should not only be highly active but also minimally toxic to allow long-term survival with the optimal quality of life. A combination of metronomic chemotherapy (MC) with endocrine treatment (ET) in patients who failed earlier lines of ET represents an interesting and promising option. Methods: The methodology includes retrospective data analyses of pretreated, metastatic ER+/HER2- BC (mBC) patients who were treated with the FulVEC regimen combining fulvestrant and MC (cyclophosphamide, vinorelbine, and capecitabine). Results: Thirty-nine previously treated (median 2 lines 1–9) mBC patients received FulVEC. The median PFS and OS were 8.4 and 21.5 months, respectively. Biochemical responses (CA-15.3 serum marker decline ≥50%) were observed in 48.7%, and any increase in CA-15.3 was observed in 23.1% of patients. The activity of FulVEC was independent of previous treatments with fulvestrant of cytotoxic components of the FulVEC regimen. The treatment was safe and well tolerated. Conclusions: Metronomic chemo-endocrine therapy with FulVEC regimen represents an interesting option and compares favorably with other approaches in patients' refractory to endocrine treatments. A phase II randomized trial is warranted.

Keywords: breast cancer; metronomic chemotherapy; chemo-endocrine therapy; FulVEC

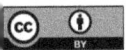

1. Introduction

Breast cancer (BC) is the most commonly diagnosed cancer type, accounting for one in eight cancer diagnoses worldwide. Over the last 30 years, the incidence of BC has continuously increased, while mortality demonstrated an opposite trend. There were about 2.3 million new breast cancer cases and 0.7 million breast cancer deaths worldwide in 2020. Breast cancer is the second most common cause of death from cancer in women in the United States and numbers fifth worldwide [1]. There is no doubt, that the majority of BC-related death is observed in patients with disseminated diseases. While only 5% of BC patients are initially diagnosed with metastatic disease, approx. 30% of BC survivors will ultimately metastasize [2]. Over the recent two decades, despite the introduction of many novel targeted therapies for mBC, the prognosis of advanced breast cancer patients is poor, and mBC remains an incurable, fatal condition.

Most BCs express estrogen receptors (ER), which act as a therapeutic target for endocrine therapies representing the central core of the initial systemic treatment in the majority of advanced BC ER+/HER2- patients [3]. The activity of endocrine therapy (ET), even when combined with novel targeted agents such as CDK4/6 inhibitors, PIK3CA, or mTOR inhibitors, is time-restricted, and ultimately, all metastatic BC patients treated with ET will progress. Globally, chemotherapy (CT) is the treatment of choice in ER+/HER2- patients resistant to ET [4]. Although novel approaches based on antibody-drug conjugates are emerging, their timely implementation in clinical practice may be limited by regulatory and financial issues. Most advanced, ET-resistant BCs are treated with single-drug chemotherapy regimens administered intravenously or orally on a long-term (until progression) basis. However, the heterogeneity of advanced BC represents a tremendous clinical challenge in that various metastatic lesions may develop distinct resistance mechanisms to ET and CT, thus making them susceptible to different therapeutic agents [5]. Therefore, combinatory approaches represent a promising treatment strategy for the better systemic control of the disseminated disease. While intravenous multi-drug regimens are usually highly toxic, the metronomic, orally administered polychemotherapy is much better tolerated, and due to its multidirectional activity (anti-proliferative, antiangiogenic, and immunomodulatory), it may provide superior clinical benefits in many tumor types, including breast cancer [6–8].

The combination of ET and CT is still controversial based on the non-conclusive evidence from numerous but old clinical studies. However, considering the highly positive data on the combination of ET with antiproliferative agents (CDK4/6i) and many biological similarities between CDK4/6i and metronomic chemotherapy, the combination of ET with CT deserves attention, especially in low- and middle-income countries for which many novel drugs are simply unaffordable [9].

This manuscript presents the results of a retrospective analysis that evaluated the safety and efficacy of a metronomic chemo-endocrine regimen (FulVEC) in advanced, pretreated ER+/HER2- patients.

2. Materials and Methods

2.1. Patients

We retrospectively collected data on consecutive, advanced BC patients treated with metronomic chemo-endocrine therapy (FulVEC) at Jagiellonian University-Medical College Hospital in Cracow between 2018 and 2022. Metronomic chemotherapy has been initially offered to pretreated, progressing (radiographic and biochemical progression) patients who were deemed unfit or refused further lines of standard intravenous chemotherapy regimens. Furthermore, the treatment was also offered to pretreated, progressing patients who were asymptomatic or mildly symptomatic and were reluctant toward the immediate initiation of intensive, intravenous chemotherapy. Eligible patients had histologically proven advanced (metastatic or locally recurrent) inoperable breast cancer and presented with a performance status of ECOG 0–2. The study has been approved by the local bioethical committee at Jagiellonian University.

2.2. Treatment

The metronomic chemo-endocrine therapy FulVEC consisted of fulvestrant 500 mg i.m. administered on days 1, 14, 28, and q1m thereof combined with metronomic, continuous polychemotherapy VEC (vinorelbine 40 mg three times a week, cyclophosphamide 50 mg p.o. qd, capecitabine 500 mg p.o. tid). Dose adjustments were performed based on the evaluation of treatment-emergent adverse events, and particular drug-related AE has led to a stepwise reduction in a given drug. Upon the occurrence of vinorelbine-induced AE, the dosage was reduced from 50 mg tiw to 30 mg q2d. Capecitabine-related AE led to a stepwise reduction from 500 mg tid to 500 mg bid and then to 500 mg qd. The single-step reduction in cyclophosphamide was based on decreased frequencies from 50 mg qd to 50 mg q2d. In the case of non-sufficient dose reduction, the treatment with a particular drug was withheld until the resolution of particular AEs.

Data on the following background characteristics of the patients were collected using standardized data collection instruments: age; ECOG performance status; clinical symptoms; serum tumor markers, including CA-15.3; tumor stage (locally advanced or metastatic); sites of distant metastases; pathological diagnosis including immunohistochemistry.

2.3. Analysis of Treatment Efficacy

Since the metronomic chemo-endocrine treatment was initially used as a last-resort therapy for heavily pretreated ER+ BC patients, an objective evaluation of tumor response by imaging modalities was not considered a critical aspect and a justified option in most treated individuals. Clinical decisions were based on the patient's performance status, disease-related symptoms intensity, and lab results involving blood morphology and the biochemical evaluation of organ functions. Treatment efficacy was analyzed retrospectively by the evaluation of overall survival (OS), progression-free survival (PFS), and treatment-induced changes in the CA-15.3 level. Biochemical response (bRR) was defined as $\geq 50\%$ serum marker reduction, biochemical stabilization (bSD) was defined as a $\leq 50\%$ reduction, and biochemical progression (bPD) was defined as any increase in CA-15.3 levels. The biochemical benefit (bBR) was defined as any decline in CA-15.3 concentrations.

2.4. Safety Analysis

Data on treatment-related myelotoxicity was obtained by the automatic analysis of laboratory results of the blood samples collected every four weeks during treatment with the FulVEC regimen. Data on other bone-marrow-unrelated AEs and on FulVEC dosage modifications or interruptions were derived directly from patients' medical history.

2.5. Statistical Considerations

Distributions of quantitative variables were summarized with mean, standard deviation, median and interquartile range, whereas distributions of qualitative variables were summarized with the number and percent of occurrence for each of their values.

Hazard ratios of death and progression were estimated for each predictor at interest in a univariate Cox proportional hazard model with Jackknife standard errors. Kaplan-Meier curves and Nelson-Aalen curves were estimated for the overall data and compared with log-rank test. The significance level for all statistical tests was set to 0.05. However, due to small sample size at hand, we also reported marginally significant effects with $p < 0.1$. Stata/MP 17 was used for computations..

3. Results

Between May 2018 and June 2022, 38 patients with advanced ER+/HER2- BC received palliative metronomic FulVEC chemo-endocrine treatments. The median age of patients at the FulVEC initiation was 46 years (30–80), and the median follow-up was 22 months. Most patients had bone (82%) and/or liver (66%) metastases, with only 8% of patients presenting bone-only disease. Almost half of the analyzed patients (47%) failed previous endocrine treatments with CDK4/6 inhibitors administered in the first line (27.7%) or $\geq$ second line of therapy (19.3%). Most patients failed previous endocrine treatments with fulvestrant (53%) and experienced progression during chemotherapy, including at least one cytotoxic agent used in the FulVEC regimen (48.7%). Detailed patients' characteristics are included in Table 1.

Table 1. Patients' characteristics.

Parameter	N (%)
Number of patients	38
Median age (range)	46 years (30–80)
Menopausal status	
Premenopausal	15 (39%)
Postmenopausal	24 (61%)
Previous neo/adjuvant chemotherapy	24 (63%)
Previous adjuvant endocrine therapy	23 (61%)
Locoregional relapse	11 (29%)
Disseminated disease	39 (100%)
Bone metastasis	31 (82%)
Bone-only disease	3 (7.7%)
Lung metastasis	13 (34%)
Liver metastasis	25 (66%)
CNS metastasis	3 (8%)
No. of previous systemic treatments	2 (median)
≤2	20 (53%)
3–4	8 (21%)
≥5	10 (26%)
Previously any FulVEC component	30 (77%)
Fulvestrant	20 (53%)
Vinorelbine	11 (29%)
Cyclophosphamide	12 (32%)
Capecitabine	13 (34%)
Previous treatment with CDK4/6i	18 (47%)
1st line	10 (59%)
≥1st line	7 (41%)

3.1. Efficacy

Biochemical response in the evaluable group (n:38) was observed in 19 (48.7%) patients, with the complete normalization of CA-15.3 confirmed in 8 patients (20.5%). In general, 30 patients (76.9%) experienced a decline in the serum marker (Figure 1). Patients who had previously received treatment based on any drugs included in the FulVEC regimen had non-significantly lower bRR and bSD compared to individuals not exposed to any FulVEC's component. The bRR and bSD rates were 70% and 20% in non-pretreated patients and 50% and 28.6% in pretreated patients, respectively (Figure 2A).

Previous treatments with fulvestrant were associated with a higher risk of biochemical progression—30% compared to 11.1% in fulvestrant-naïve patients (Figure 2B).

Biochemical stabilization (any decline in CA-15.3 levels) was observed in a similar percentage of patients irrespectively of previous exposure to any of the cytotoxic drugs used in the FulVEC regimen (73.7% in the pretreated and 89.5% in the non-pretreated population). However, the bRR was more often observed in non-pretreated patients (73.7%) than in patients who received any cytotoxic component of the FulVEC regimen (42.1%) (Figure 2C). There was no significant difference in the biochemical responses with respect to previous exposure to CDK4/6i. However, numerically, the risk of biochemical progression on FulVEC was at least twice as high in CDK4/6i non-pretreated patients than in pretreated patients (Figure 2D).

The median progression-free survival in the entire population was 8.4 months (95%CI 6.5–11.6) with 12- and 24-month PFS rates of 21% and 3%, respectively (Figure 3A). The median overall survival of FulVEC-treated patients was 21.5 (95%CI 16.7–27.6) with 12- and 24-month OS rates of 63% and 21%, respectively (Figure 3B).

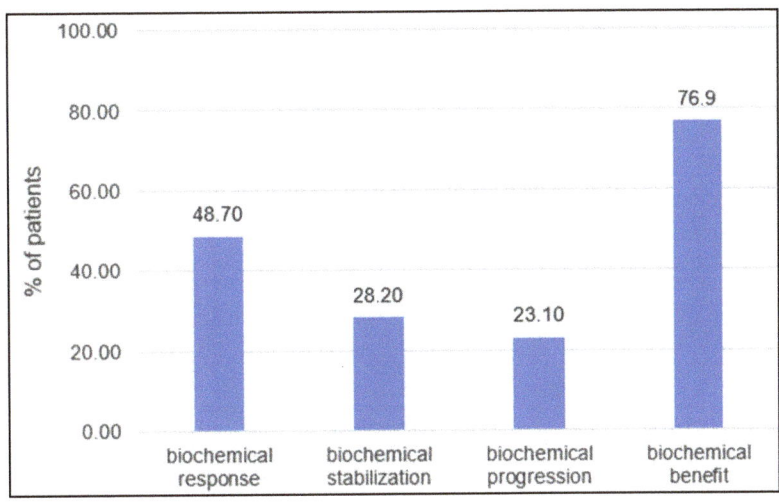

Figure 1. Biochemical efficacy of FulVEC (bRR—≥50% decline in CA-15.3; bSD—1–49% decline in CA-15.3; bPD—any increase in CA-15.3; bBR—any decline in CA-15.3).

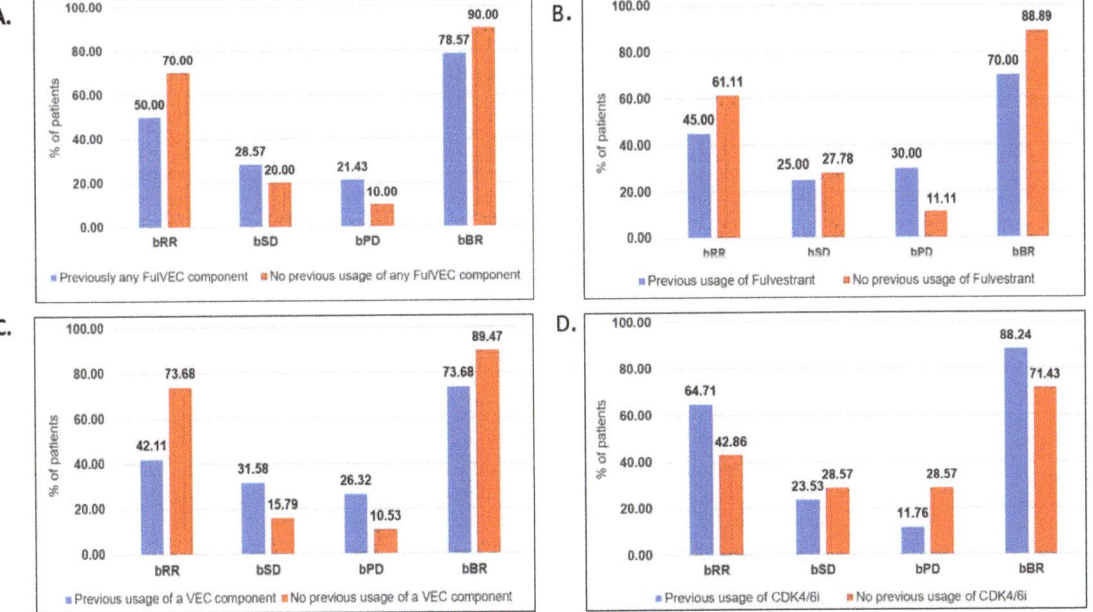

Figure 2. Biochemical efficacy of FulVEC according to previous therapy. (**A**). Previous use of any FulVEC component, (**B**). Previous use of fulvestrant, (**C**). Previous use of any VEC component, (**D**). Previous use of CDK4/6i. (bRR—≥50% decline in CA-15.3; bSD—1–49% decline in CA-15.3; bPD—any increase in CA-15.3; bBR—any decline in CA-15.3). No significant differences (chi-square test) in biochemical response rates in relationships relative to previous treatments were observed in (**A–D**).

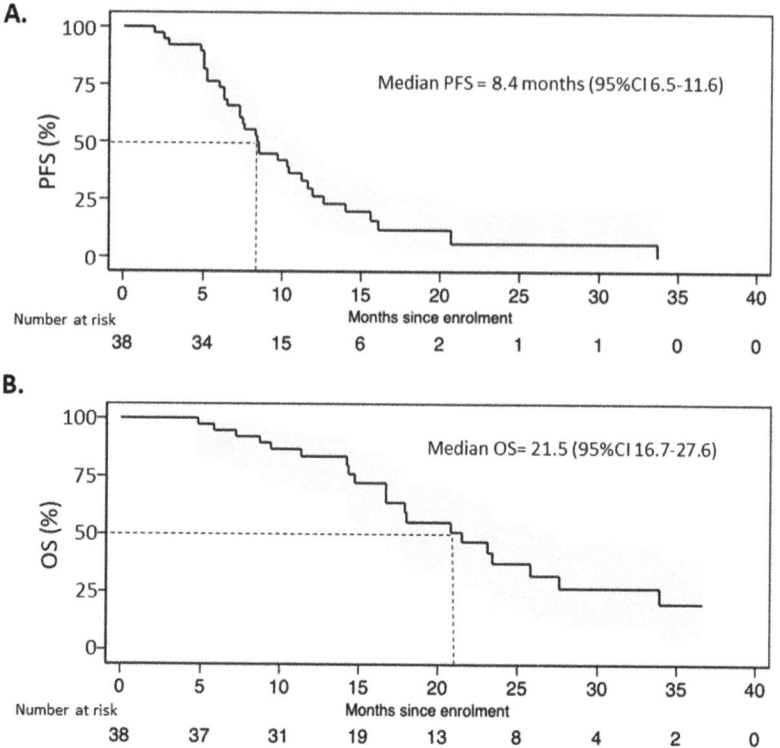

Figure 3. (**A**). Progression-free survival and (**B**) overall survival of patients treated with FulVEC.

There were no significant differences in PFS irrespective of previous exposure to CDK4/6i, fulvestrant, or FulVEC cytotoxic components (Figure 4A–C). However, patients pretreated with CDK4/6i had a higher median PFS of 9.7 months (95% CI, 5.2–11.6) compared to non-pretreated patients (7.3 months—95% CI, 6.0–14.0). Similarly to PFS, previous exposure to CDK4/6i, fulvestrant or FulVEC cytotoxic components had no impact on OS (Figure 4D–F).

3.2. Safety

The most frequent type of AE was myelotoxicity, with neutropenia observed in 41% of patients (G3-4 in 25.7%); however, no cases of neutropenic fever were observed (Table 2). Additionally, the most frequent non-hematologic AE was the capecitabine-related hand-foot syndrome (HFS), which occurred in 12.8% of patients (G3-4 in 2.5%). Treatment-related AEs leading to dose reduction in 46% of patients were most often associated with myelotoxicity (80%) or HFS (15%).

Table 2. Adverse events in patients treated with the FulVEC regimen.

Adverse Events	Any Grade	G3	G4
Any adverse event	51.3%	38.5%	10.3%
Neutropenia	41.0%	15.4%	10.3%
Anemia	12.8%	5.1%	0%
Thrombocytopenia	2.5%	0%	0%
Fatigue	7.7%	2.6%	0%
Hfs	12.8%	2.5%	0%
Hepatotoxicity	5.1%	2.5%	0%
Abdominal pain	2.5%	2.5%	0%

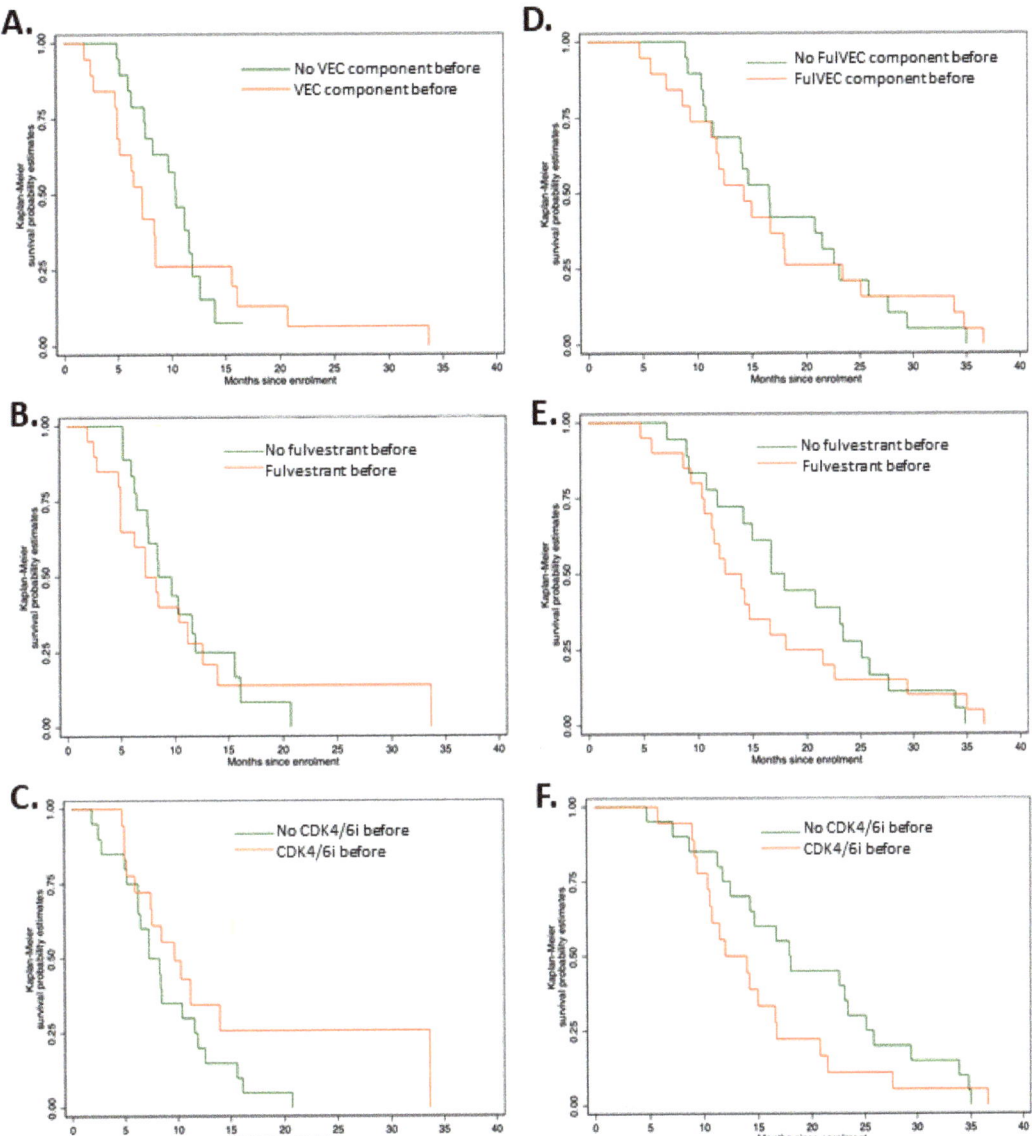

Figure 4. Progression-free survival and overall survival of patients treated with FulVEC. PFS of patients pretreated with (**A**) any cytotoxic component of FulVEC; $p = 0.502$; (**B**) fulvestrant; $p = 0.739$; (**C**) CDK4/6i; $p = 0.142$. Overall survival of patients treated with FulVEC and OS of patients pretreated with (**D**) any cytotoxic component of FulVEC; $p = 0.284$; (**E**) fulvestrant; $p = 0.898$; (**F**) CDK4/6i; $p = 0.929$. All log rank tests for the equality of survival functions (χ^2).

The AE-related temporary treatment interruption was required in 23% of patients and was again most often associated with myelotoxicity (70%) or HFS (25%). However, no patient required permanent treatment cessation due to FulVEC-associated toxicity, and all patients could continue the metronomic chemo-endocrine therapy, albeit with some dose reductions (Table 3).

Table 3. Interventions in patients experiencing AE during metronomic chemo-endocrine therapy.

Toxicity-Related Treatment Decisions	% (N)
Dose reduction	46% (18)
Myelotoxicity	80%
H&F syndrome	15%
Other	5%
Temporary treatment interruption	23% (9)
Myelotoxicity	70%
H&F syndrome	25%
Other	5%
Permanent treatment cessation due to AE	0% (0)

Treatment-related AEs were easily manageable by a precise, step-wise dose-adjustment approach of the FulVEC regimen (Figure 5). Such a precise mode of dose modification is a unique feature of multi-drug chemotherapy regimens, which allow for a minimal decrease in treatment intensity with the direct mitigation of particular treatment-emergent AE.

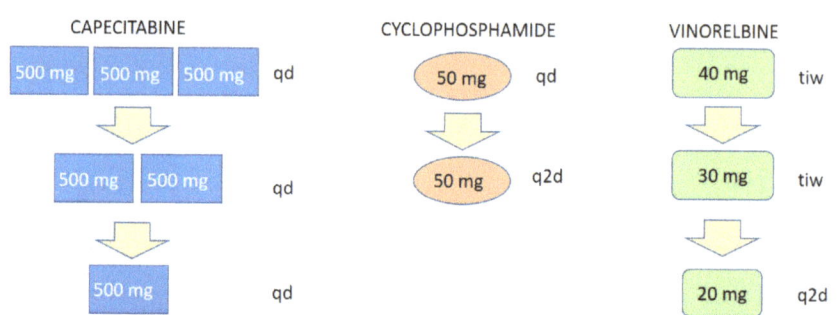

Figure 5. Scheme of a stepwise, particular AE-related dose reduction in FulVEC cytotoxic components. tid—three times a day; bid—two times a day; qd—every day; q2d—every second day; tiw—three times a week.

4. Discussion

Even though the concept of metronomic chemotherapy is relatively old, it has not been robustly evaluated in randomized clinical trials. Most available data on the utility of metronomic chemotherapy (MCT) in advanced breast cancer (ABC) come from single-arm, phase II clinical trials or retrospective analyses [10–16]. The results of a phase III study (METEORA), which were presented recently, demonstrate the superiority of metronomic chemotherapy VEX (VEC) over weekly paclitaxel in terms of PFS and time-to-treatment failure (TTF) endpoints [17]. The METEORA study has thus established the VEC regimen as a safe and active option of MCT for the treatment of advanced BC.

Compared to metronomic chemotherapy, there are even fewer data on the role of a combination of MCT with endocrine treatments. In a single-arm phase II study, 41 ABC patients following ≤1 line of endocrine treatment without previous chemotherapy received metronomic capecitabine combined with fulvestrant [18]. The administration of concurrent chemo-endocrine therapy (CET) induced 24.5% of objective responses and 58.5% of the clinical benefit rate. The median PFS and OS were 15.0 and 28.7 months, respectively, which compares favorably to the outcomes observed in pivotal clinical trials on CDK4/6i combined with fulvestrant. The treatment was well tolerated, with hand-foot syndrome being the most common G3 adverse event observed in 7.3% of patients. A retrospective study by Aurilio et al. evaluated the combination of fulvestrant with metronomic chemotherapy (cyclophosphamide + methotrexate) in 32 heavily pretreated ER+ ABC patients [19]. Concurrent CETs led to one partial response and disease stabilization in 17 patients (53%).

Again, the study revealed promising clinical activity of CET with an excellent safety profile. In a phase II study, Rashad et al. evaluated a combination of capecitabine-based chemotherapy with endocrine treatment (letrozole or tamoxifen) as the first-line treatment of ER+ ABC [20]. Concurrent CETs were associated with objective response and clinical benefit rates in 60% and 82.5% of patients, respectively. The median PFS and OS for the general population were 10.0 and 23.3 months, respectively. In patients treated with the capecitabine + letrozole combination, the median PFS and OS were higher, respectively, by 4.0 and 3.0 months than in the capecitabine + tamoxifen combination.

The results of our analysis compare favorably to the above-mentioned studies. FulVEC led to a high rate of clinical benefit (at least stabilization of serum marker with no signs of progression) in most patients who were previously resistant to ET and (in many cases) also to CT. Additionally, unlike other studies conducted in much less pretreated populations, the median PFS of 8.4 months and median OS of 21.5% underscores the activity of FulVEC regimen. Moreover, almost half of the patients treated with FulVEC regimen failed earlier endocrine therapy combined with CDK4/6i, which were not available when the older, above-mentioned studies on CET were conducted. Recent studies on the repeated administration of CDK4/6 inhibitors combined with other endocrine agents applied in patients who failed 1st line ET + CDK4/6i revealed at least some modest activity of such approaches. A phase II study (PACE) was conducted in patients who failed first-line treatment with CDK4/6i+IA. Patients were randomized into three arms: treatment with fulvestrant, fulvestrant + palbociclib, or fulvestrant + palbociclib + avelumab. The repeated administration of CDK4/6i has no impact on fulvestrant's efficacy with median PFS and OS of 4.6 months and 24.6 months (fulvestrant + palbociclib) and 4.8 months and 27.5 months (fulvestrant), respectively [21]. Another phase II, single-arm study, which evaluated the combination of fulvestrant + palbociclib in patients who failed IA + Palbociclib, demonstrated a short median PFS of 3.7 months [22].

Since phase III studies on the combination of fulvestrant + CDK4/6i in metastatic BC resistant to aromatase inhibitor alone demonstrated a median PFS within the range of 11.2–20.5 months and a median OS of 34.8–46.7 months [23–25], the CDK4/6i rechallenge does not represent a viable clinical option. In this context, the results of our analysis provide very promising data on the activity of the FulVEC regimen in metastatic BC patients irrespective of previous therapies (fulvestrant, chemotherapy or CDK4/6i). This phenomenon must be linked to the multidirectional activity of metronomic chemotherapy and the synergism of multi-drug chemotherapy combinations, as well as the simultaneous administration of cytotoxic and hormonal agents.

One of the most important aspects of the FulVEC-based treatment is its safety and the gradual development of treatment-emergent AEs. Despite the fact that some patients experienced G3-4 AEs (mainly neutropenia but without neutropenic fever), none were life-threatening, and all readily subsided after dose adjustments. This safety profile of FulVEC highly resembles the typical toxicity observed in patients treated with CDK4/6i combined with ET. It must be underscored that the construction of FulVEC allows for a uniquely precise and stepwise dose reduction in a particular drug responsible for a specific AE. The dose intensity of FulVEC can be thus be reduced by much smaller steps compared to CDK4/6i (Figure 5), where the relative dose intensity per dose reduction diminished by 20% (palbociclib) or 33% (ribociclib, abemaciclib). Therefore, only a few FulVEC-treated patients required treatment interruption, and none definitely stopped the MCT due to toxicity.

We admit that our analysis of FulVEC regimen has several limitations, and they are mainly related to its retrospective character and the diversity of the studied population. There are also insufficient data on objective tumor responses since regular imaging (outside prospective clinical trials) is rarely clinically meaningful in advanced, treatment-refractory, and often symptomatic patients who demonstrate clinical benefit from a palliative systemic treatment. Additionally, PIK3CA or ESR1 gene mutations, which may have had a significant impact on ET efficacy, have not been determined in the studied population. Nevertheless, the study provides a promising signal on the safety and efficacy of metronomic chemo-endocrine therapy in advanced, often heavily pretreated metastatic BC patients, of whom many exhausted all available treatment options and who represent a real-world population of patients with extremely poor outcomes. Such a population of BC patients desperately awaits novel, active and safe systemic therapies. The robust OS data observed in the FulVEC-treated population stay in conjunction with other endpoints of our analysis (biochemical responses and PFS). Based on the obtained results, a randomized, phase II study is warranted.

5. Conclusions

The promising OS data observed in the FulVEC-treated population stay in conjunction with other endpoints of our analysis (biochemical responses and PFS). Based on the obtained results, a randomized, phase II study is warranted.

Author Contributions: Conceptualization, A.B.-N. and P.J.W.; methodology, M.K. and P.J.W.; formal analysis, M.K.; investigation, A.B.-N.; resources, Ł.K., P.P., K.K., A.M.-K., A.S. and J.S.; data curation, A.B.-N.; writing—original draft preparation, P.J.W.; funding acquisition, P.J.W. All authors have read and agreed to the published version of the manuscript.

Funding: The research was funded by Jagiellonian University—Medical College grant no. N41/DBS/000706.

Institutional Review Board Statement: The study was conducted in accordance with the Declaration of Helsinki and approved by the Institutional Ethics Committee of Jagiellonian University (1072.6120.229.2022 issued on 12 October 2022).

Informed Consent Statement: Patient consent was waived due to the retrospective nature of the study according to the Local Bioethical Committee's opinion.

Data Availability Statement: Data is unavailable due to ethical restrictions.

Conflicts of Interest: The authors declare no conflict of interest.

References

1. Sung, H.; Ferlay, J.; Siegel, R.L.; Laversanne, M.; Soerjomataram, I.; Jemal, A.; Bray, F. Global Cancer Statistics 2020: GLOBOCAN Estimates of Incidence and Mortality Worldwide for 36 Cancers in 185 Countries. *CA Cancer J. Clin.* **2021**, *71*, 209–249. [CrossRef] [PubMed]
2. Redig, A.J.; Mcallister, S.S. Breast Cancer as a Systemic Disease: A View of Metastasis. *J. Intern. Med.* **2013**, *274*, 113. [CrossRef] [PubMed]
3. Rozeboom, B.; Dey, N.; De, P. ER+ Metastatic Breast Cancer: Past, Present, and a Prescription for an Apoptosis-Targeted Future. *Am. J. Cancer Res.* **2019**, *9*, 2821. [PubMed]
4. Gennari, A.; André, F.; Barrios, C.H.; Cortés, J.; de Azambuja, E.; DeMichele, A.; Dent, R.; Fenlon, D.; Gligorov, J.; Hurvitz, S.A.; et al. ESMO Clinical Practice Guideline for the Diagnosis, Staging and Treatment of Patients with Metastatic Breast Cancer. *Ann. Oncol.* **2021**, *32*, 1475–1495. [CrossRef] [PubMed]
5. Fumagalli, C.; Barberis, M. Breast Cancer Heterogeneity. *Diagnostics* **2021**, *11*, 1555. [CrossRef]
6. Cazzaniga, M.; Cordani, N.; Capici, S.; Cogliati, V.; Riva, F.; Cerrito, M. Metronomic Chemotherapy. *Cancers* **2021**, *13*, 2236. [CrossRef]
7. Cazzaniga, M.E.; Munzone, E.; Bocci, G.; Afonso, N.; Gomez, P.; Langkjer, S.; Petru, E.; Pivot, X.; Sánchez Rovira, P.; Wysocki, P.; et al. Pan-European Expert Meeting on the Use of Metronomic Chemotherapy in Advanced Breast Cancer Patients: The PENELOPE Project. *Adv. Ther.* **2019**, *36*, 381–406. [CrossRef]
8. Wysocki, P.J.; Lubas, M.T.; Wysocka, M.L. Metronomic Chemotherapy in Prostate Cancer. *J. Clin. Med.* **2022**, *11*, 2853. [CrossRef]
9. André, N.; Banavali, S.; Snihur, Y.; Pasquier, E. Has the Time Come for Metronomics in Low-Income and Middle-Income Countries? *Lancet Oncol.* **2013**, *14*, e239–e248. [CrossRef]
10. Cazzaniga, M.E.; Pinotti, G.; Montagna, E.; Amoroso, D.; Berardi, R.; Butera, A.; Cagossi, K.; Cavanna, L.; Ciccarese, M.; Cinieri, S.; et al. Metronomic Chemotherapy for Advanced Breast Cancer Patients in the Real World Practice: Final Results of the VICTOR-6 Study. *Breast* **2019**, *48*, 7–16. [CrossRef]
11. Cazzaniga, M.E.; Cortesi, L.; Ferzi, A.; Scaltriti, L.; Cicchiello, F.; Ciccarese, M.; della Torre, S.; Villa, F.; Giordano, M.; Verusio, C.; et al. Metronomic Chemotherapy with Oral Vinorelbine (MVNR) and Capecitabine (MCAPE) in Advanced HER2-Negative Breast Cancer Patients: Is It a Way to Optimize Disease Control? Final Results of the VICTOR-2 Study. *Breast Cancer Res. Treat.* **2016**, *160*, 501–509. [CrossRef] [PubMed]

2. Montagna, E.; Bagnardi, V.; Cancello, G.; Sangalli, C.; Pagan, E.; Iorfida, M.; Mazza, M.; Mazzarol, G.; Dellapasqua, S.; Munzone, E.; et al. Metronomic Chemotherapy for First-Line Treatment of Metastatic Triple-Negative Breast Cancer: A Phase II Trial. *Breast Care* **2018**, *13*, 177–181. [CrossRef] [PubMed]
3. Fedele, P.; Marino, A.; Orlando, L.; Schiavone, P.; Nacci, A.; Sponziello, F.; Rizzo, P.; Calvani, N.; Mazzoni, E.; Cinefra, M.; et al. Efficacy and Safety of Low-Dose Metronomic Chemotherapy with Capecitabine in Heavily Pretreated Patients with Metastatic Breast Cancer. *Eur. J. Cancer* **2012**, *48*, 24–29. [CrossRef] [PubMed]
4. Cazzaniga, M.E.; Torri, V.; Villa, F.; Giuntini, N.; Riva, F.; Zeppellini, A.; Cortinovis, D.; Bidoli, P. Efficacy and Safety of the All-Oral Schedule of Metronomic Vinorelbine and Capecitabine in Locally Advanced or Metastatic Breast Cancer Patients: The Phase I-II VICTOR-1 Study. *Int. J. Breast Cancer* **2014**, *2014*, 769790. [CrossRef] [PubMed]
5. Wang, Z.; Lu, J.; Leaw, S.; Hong, X.; Wang, J.; Shao, Z.; Hu, X. An All-Oral Combination of Metronomic Cyclophosphamide plus Capecitabine in Patients with Anthracycline- and Taxane-Pretreated Metastatic Breast Cancer: A Phase II Study. *Cancer Chemother. Pharm.* **2012**, *69*, 515–522. [CrossRef]
6. Taguchi, T.; Nakayama, T.; Masuda, N.; Yoshidome, K.; Akagi, K.; Nishida, Y.; Yoshikawa, Y.; Ogino, N.; Abe, C.; Sakamoto, J.; et al. Study of Low-Dose Capecitabine Monotherapy for Metastatic Breast Cancer. *Chemotherapy* **2010**, *56*, 166–170. [CrossRef]
7. Munzone, E.; Regan, M.M.; Cinieri, S.; Montagna, E.; Orlando, L.; Shi, R.; Campadelli, E.; Gianni, L.; De Giorgi, U.F.F.; Bengala, C.; et al. A Randomized Phase II Trial of Metronomic Oral Vinorelbine plus Cyclophosphamide and Capecitabine (VEX) vs Weekly Paclitaxel (P) as First- or Secon... | OncologyPRO. In *Proceedings of the ESMO Annual Meeting*; Elsevier: Amsterdam, The Netherlands, 2022.
8. Schwartzberg, L.S.; Wang, G.; Somer, B.G.; Blakely, L.J.; Wheeler, B.M.; Walker, M.S.; Stepanski, E.J.; Houts, A.C. Phase II Trial of Fulvestrant with Metronomic Capecitabine for Postmenopausal Women with Hormone Receptor-Positive, HER2-Negative Metastatic Breast Cancer. *Clin. Breast Cancer* **2014**, *14*, 13–19. [CrossRef]
9. Aurilio, G.; Munzone, E.; Botteri, E.; Sciandivasci, A.; Adamoli, L.; Minchella, I.; Esposito, A.; Cullurà, D.; Curigliano, G.; Colleoni, M.; et al. Oral Metronomic Cyclophosphamide and Methotrexate Plus Fulvestrant in Advanced Breast Cancer Patients: A Mono-Institutional Case-Cohort Report. *Breast J.* **2012**, *18*, 470–474. [CrossRef]
10. Rashad, N.; Abdelhamid, T.; Shouman, S.A.; Nassar, H.; Omran, M.A.; El Desouky, E.D.; Khaled, H. Capecitabine-Based Chemoendocrine Combination as First-Line Treatment for Metastatic Hormone-Positive Metastatic Breast Cancer: Phase 2 Study. *Clin. Breast Cancer* **2020**, *20*, 228–237. [CrossRef]
11. Mayer, E.L.; Ren, Y.; Wagle, N.; Ma, C.; DeMichele, A.; Cristofanilli, M.; Meisel, J. Palbociclib after CDK4/6i and Endocrine Therapy (PACE): A Randomized Phase II Study of Fulvestrant, Palbociclib, and Avelumab for Endocrine Pre-Treated ER+/HER2- Metastatic Breast Cancer. In Proceedings of the San Antonio Breast Cancer Symposium, San Antonio, TX, USA, 6–10 December 2022.
12. Tao, J.J.; Blackford, A.L.; Nunes, R.; Truica, C.I.; Mahosky, J.; Jones, M.K.; Leasure, N.C.; Cescon, T. Phase II Trial of Palbociclib with Fulvestrant in Individuals with Hormone Receptor-Positive, HER2-Negative Metastatic Breast Cancer with Disease Progression after Palbociclib with an Aromatase Inhibitor. In Proceedings of the San Antonio Breast Cancer Symposium, San Antonio, TX, USA, 6–10 December 2022.
13. Sledge, G.W., Jr.; Toi, M.; Neven, P.; Sohn, J.H.; Inoue, K.; Pivot, X.; Okera, M.; Masuda, N.; Kaufman, P.A.; Koh, H.; et al. Final overall survival analysis of Monarch 2: A phase 3 trial of Abemaciclib plus Fulvestrant in patients with hormone receptor-positive, HER2-negative advanced breast cancer. In Proceedings of the San Antonio Breast Cancer Symposium, San Antonio, TX, USA, 6–10 December 2022.
14. Lu, Y.S.; Im, S.A.; Colleoni, M.; Franke, F.; Bardia, A.; Cardoso, F.; Harbeck, N.; Hurvitz, S.; Chow, L.; Sohn, J.; et al. Updated Overall Survival of Ribociclib plus Endocrine Therapy versus Endocrine Therapy Alone in Pre- and Perimenopausal Patients with HR+/HER2- Advanced Breast Cancer in MONALEESA-7: A Phase III Randomized Clinical Trial. *Clin. Cancer Res.* **2022**, *28*, 851–859. [CrossRef]
15. Neven, P.; Fasching, P.A.; Chia, S.; Jerusalem, G.; Laurentiis, M.; Im, S.; Petrakova, K.; Bianchi, G.V.; Martin, M.; Nusch, A.; et al. LBA4 Updated Overall Survival (OS) Results from the First-Line (1L) Population in the Phase III MONALEESA-3 Trial of Postmenopausal Patients (PTS) with HR+/HER2− Advanced Breast Cancer (ABC) Treated with Ribociclib (RIB) + Fulvestrant (FUL). *Ann. Oncol.* **2022**, *33*, S194. [CrossRef]

Disclaimer/Publisher's Note: The statements, opinions and data contained in all publications are solely those of the individual author(s) and contributor(s) and not of MDPI and/or the editor(s). MDPI and/or the editor(s) disclaim responsibility for any injury to people or property resulting from any ideas, methods, instructions or products referred to in the content.

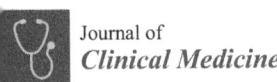

Article

Remarkable Remission Rate and Long-Term Efficacy of Upfront Metronomic Chemotherapy in Elderly and Frail Patients, with Diffuse Large B-Cell Lymphoma

Guido Bocci [1,*], Sabrina Pelliccia [2], Paola Orlandi [1], Matteo Caridi [3], Marta Banchi [1], Gerardo Musuraca [4], Arianna Di Napoli [5], Maria Paola Bianchi [2], Caterina Patti [6], Paola Anticoli-Borza [7], Roberta Battistini [8], Ivana Casaroli [9], Tiziana Lanzolla [10], Agostino Tafuri [2] and Maria Christina Cox [2,11,*]

1. Department of Clinical and Experimental Medicine, School of Medicine, University of Pisa, 56126 Pisa, Italy
2. UOC Ematologia, Azienda Ospedaliera Universitaria Sant'Andrea, 00189 Rome, Italy
3. Division of Hematology and Clinical Immunology, Department of Medicine, University of Perugia, 06125 Perugia, Italy
4. Hematology Unit, Istituto Scientifico Romagnolo per lo Studio e la Cura dei Tumori (IRST) Srl—IRCCS, 47014 Meldola, Italy
5. UOC Anatomia Patologica, Azienda Ospedaliera Universitaria Sant'Andrea & Department of Clinical and Molecular Medicine Sapienza University, 00185 Rome, Italy
6. UOC Oncoematologia, Azienda Villa Sofia-Cervello, 90146 Palermo, Italy
7. UOC Ematologia, Azienda Ospedaliera San Giovanni-Addolorata, 00184 Rome, Italy
8. UOC Ematologia, Azienda Ospedaliera San Camillo, 00152 Rome, Italy
9. Haematology Department, San Gerardo Hospital Monza, 20900 Monza, Italy
10. UOC Medicina Nucleare, Azienda Ospedaliera Universitaria Sant'Andrea, 00189 Rome, Italy
11. Hematology Unit, Fondazione Policlinico Tor Vergata, 00133 Rome, Italy
* Correspondence: guido.bocci@unipi.it (G.B.); mariacristina.cox@ptvonline.it (M.C.C.)

Abstract: The upfront treatment of very elderly and frail patients with diffuse large B-cell lymphoma (DLBCL) is still a matter of debate. Herein, we report results of the metronomic all-oral DEVEC [prednisolone/deltacortene®, vinorelbine (VNR), etoposide (ETO), cyclophosphamide] combined with i.v. rituximab (R). This schedule was administered as a first line therapy in 22 elderly/frail DLBCL subjects (median age = 84.5 years). In 17/22 (77%) patients, the Elderly-IPI-score was high. After a median follow-up of 24 months, 15 patients had died: seven (50%) for causes unrelated to DLBCL or its treatment, six (40%) for progression, and two (13%) for multiorgan failure. Six treatment-pertinent serious-adverse-events occurred. At the end of induction, 14/22 (64%) achieved complete remission; overall survival and event-free survival at 24 months were both 54% (95% CI = 32–72%), while the disease-free survival was 74% (95% CI = 48–88%). Furthermore, antiproliferative and proapoptotic assays were performed on DLBCL/OCI-LY3 cell-line using metronomic VNR and ETO and their combination. Both metronomic VNR and ETO had concentration-dependent antiproliferative (IC50 = 0.036 ± 0.01 nM and 7.9 ± 3.6 nM, respectively), and proapoptotic activities in DLBCL cells. Co-administration of the two drugs showed a strong synergism (combination index < 1 and dose reduction index > 1) against cell proliferation and survival. This low-dose schedule seems to compare favourably with intravenous-CHEMO protocols used in the same subset. Indeed, the high synergism shown by metronomic VRN+ETO in in vitro studies, explains the remarkable clinical responses and it allows significant dose reductions.

Keywords: metronomic chemotherapy; chemo-free; DLBCL; diffuse-large-b-cell-lymphoma; elderly; frail; comprehensive geriatric assessment

Citation: Bocci, G.; Pelliccia, S.; Orlandi, P.; Caridi, M.; Banchi, M.; Musuraca, G.; Di Napoli, A.; Bianchi, M.P.; Patti, C.; Anticoli-Borza, P.; et al. Remarkable Remission Rate and Long-Term Efficacy of Upfront Metronomic Chemotherapy in Elderly and Frail Patients, with Diffuse Large B-Cell Lymphoma. *J. Clin. Med.* 2022, *11*, 7162. https://doi.org/10.3390/jcm11237162

Academic Editors: Tadeusz Robak and Andrea Gallamini

Received: 22 October 2022
Accepted: 30 November 2022
Published: 1 December 2022

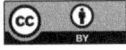

Copyright: © 2022 by the authors. Licensee MDPI, Basel, Switzerland. This article is an open access article distributed under the terms and conditions of the Creative Commons Attribution (CC BY) license (https://creativecommons.org/licenses/by/4.0/).

1. Introduction

Diffuse large B-cell lymphoma (DLBCL) is an aggressive and most common type of lymphoma, with an incidence of about 7 cases per 100.000 persons per year [1]. As up to 70% of patients, who are <80 years and fit, can be cured by the combination of Rituximab-CHOP [2] and the use of intravenous chemotherapy (iv-CHEMO), which remains a pillar of upfront treatment. However, in patients ≥80 years and in frail subjects, alternative approaches are urgently needed [3]. In fact, vulnerable elderly, currently represents a fast-growing subset of DLBCL [4] and their management, is a matter of concern in clinical practice. As none of the iv-CHEMO schedules so far experimented in this subset [5–7] have become the standard of care.

Conversely, ongoing clinical trials based on immunomodulators [8], new monoclonal antibodies [9] and small molecules targeting pathogenetic pathways [10] will hopefully help a shift towards therapeutic schedules defined as chemo-free, in vulnerable DLBCL. As a matter of fact, results from a few phase II trials, based on chemo-free combinations, have already reported encouraging data [11,12].

Worthy of note, in the changing landscape of DLBCL treatment, the potential of metronomic chemotherapy (mCHEMO), which is a different way of delivering and utilising well-known cytotoxic drugs, has been very little explored [13]. This lack of knowledge, compared with solid tumours [14], is presumably due to the high success rate of standard iv-CHEMO schedules in fit patients.

In 2011 we started to experiment in vulnerable non-Hodgkin lymphoma (NHL) patients, the DEVEC [Deltacortene®/Prednisolone (PDN), Etoposide (ETO), Vinorelbine (VNR), Cyclophosphamide (CTX)] schedule, which is an all-oral metronomic poli-chemotherapy combination. Herein, we report the updated results of this metronomic schedule used upfront in elderly/frail DLBCL patients. We also support the clinical results with data from in-vitro experiments, which assessed the activity of metronomic VNR and metronomic ETO combinations in DLBCL cells.

2. Methods and Patients

2.1. In Vitro Experiments

Cells, Drugs and Reagents

OCI-LY3, a DLBCL cell line, was purchased from DMSZ (Leibniz Institute DSMZ-German Collection of Microorganisms and Cell Cultures GmbH, Braunschweig, Germany; ACC 761) and grown in an 80% RPMI-1640 medium supplemented with 20% heat-inactivated FBS, antibiotics, and L-glutamine 2 mM. The cells grow singly or in clumps in suspension and were maintained in tissue culture flasks and kept in a humidified atmosphere of 5% CO_2 at 37 °C.

VNR and ETO were obtained from Selleckchem (DBA Italia, Milan, Italy) and were diluted from a 10 mM stock solution (in 100% dimethylsulfoxide) for in vitro studies. Vehicle-treated controls received the same concentration of dimethylsulfoxide in the media as cells of the highest concentration of VNR and ETO.

Sterile plastics for cell culture were from Costar (Cambridge, MA, USA), whereas L-glutamine, antibiotics, RPMI-1640 medium, foetal bovine serum (FBS) and all the other cited reagents were purchased from Sigma Aldrich SRL (Milan, Italy).

2.2. Antiproliferative Assay of Metronomic Vinorelbine and Etoposide

The assay was performed as previously described [15] with minor modifications. OCI-LY3 cells were exposed for 144 h with metronomic VNR (0.001–10 nM) and ETO (0.025–100 nM), or with vehicle alone. VNR or ETO were added every 48 h or 24 h, respectively, to mimic the clinical schedules. At the end of the treatment, the viable cells, assessed by trypan blue dye exclusion, were counted with a hemocytometer. The drug concentrations that inhibited cell proliferation by 50% (IC_{50}) versus vehicle-treated cells were determined by a nonlinear regression fit of the mean values obtained in triplicate experiments (at least 9 wells for each concentration).

2.3. Determination of Synergism between Metronomic Vinorelbine plus Etoposide on OCI-LY3 Cells

The determination of synergism between metronomic vinorelbine and metronomic etoposide on OCI-LY3 cells in vitro was performed to report the type of pharmacodynamic interaction between the drugs and the possible dose reduction in each drug when used in this combination schedule.

The concomitant combination of metronomic VNR and ETO was investigated at different concentrations with a fixed molar ratio of 1:100, respectively. Synergism was calculated by the combination index (CI) and the dose reduction index (DRI) method [16], where CI < 1, CI = 1, and CI > 1 indicate synergism, additive effect, and antagonism, respectively. The DRI represents the theoretical magnitude of concentration decrease that could be obtained for each drug in combination to obtain the same effect of each drug alone. Briefly, synergism, additivity, or antagonism for metronomic vinorelbine plus metronomic etoposide was calculated on the basis of the multiple drug-effect equations and quantitated by the combination index (CI). Based on the classic isobologram, the CI value was calculated as:

$$CI = [(D)_1/(D_x)_1] + [(D)_2/(D_x)_2]$$

As an example, at the 90% inhibition level, $(D_x)_1$ and $(D_x)_2$ are the concentrations of metronomic vinorelbine and metronomic etoposide, respectively, that induce a 90% inhibition of cell growth; $(D)_1$ and $(D)_2$ are the concentrations of metronomic vinorelbine and metronomic etoposide in combination that also inhibits cell growth by 90% (isoeffective as compared with the single drugs alone). The dose-reduction index (DRI) defines the degree of dose reduction that is possible in combination with a given degree of effect as compared with the concentration of each drug alone, and it was calculated as follows:

$$(DRI)_1 = (D_x)_1/(D)_1 \text{ and } (DRI)_2 = (D_x)_2/(D)_2$$

The CI and DRI indexes were estimated by the CalcuSyn v.2.0 software (Biosoft, Cambridge, UK). Furthermore, the synergistic, additive, and antagonistic effect of the drug combination was also mapped with the Loewe additivity model, using the Combenefit software (v.2.021) [15].

2.4. Apoptosis Assay

To quantify the extent of apoptosis, 3×10^5 OCI-LY3 cells were treated for 48 h with metronomic VNR, metronomic ETO, and their concomitant combination at the experimental IC_{50} or with vehicle alone as a control. At the end of the experiment, control and treated cells were analysed using the Cell Death Detection ELISA Plus Kit (Roche, Basel, Switzerland) as per the manufacturer's instructions. The optical density was measured using a Multiskan Spectrum microplate reader (Thermo Labsystems, Milan, Italy) set to a wavelength of 405 nm (with a wavelength of 490 nm correction). All the absorbance values were plotted as a percentage of apoptosis relative to vehicle-treated cells which are labelled as 100%. All experiments were repeated three times with at least three replicates per sample.

2.5. Statistical Analysis of In Vitro Studies

The investigators responsible for data analysis were blinded to which samples represented treatments and controls. The results (mean ± SEM) of all the experiments were analysed with ANOVA, followed by the Student-Newman-Keuls test. The statistical significance was set at $p < 0.05$. Statistical analyses were carried out by the GraphPad Prism software package version 5.0 (GraphPad Software, Inc., San Diego, CA, USA).

2.6. Clinical Study

This is a multicentre, observational study involving six clinical centres, which adopted the all-oral DEVEC mCHEMO schedule to treat vulnerable elderly NHL patients. From 25 October 2015 to 31 December 2017, data were retrospectively collected, while from

1 January 2018 to 30 September 2022 they were prospectively recorded. The schedule was offered to patients who were considered unfit for treatment with curative intent as an alternative to IV-CHEMO. The first patient described in this study started treatment on 16 October 2015, while the last follow-up was carried out on 30 September 2022. Rituximab (R) was added to DEVEC in B-cell NHL expressing the CD20-antigen. Only subjects with a confirmed diagnosis of DLBCL, who were treated up-front with the R-DEVEC schedule were considered for this report. This 28-days schedule (Supplementary Figure S1) was repeated for six cycles, as previously described [17]. The starting dose of ETO was empirically fixed to 14 days, with the intention to taper ETO doses within the first cycle of mCHEMO, and to allow haematological values within the established threshold. The first four Rituximab (R) infusions were administered weekly at a dose of 375 mg/m^2 starting from day +8 of cycle 1, while the last two doses (5th and 6th) were both given at an interval of 21–28 days. There was no need of pre-phase with 50 mg PDN [18]. The Hans algorithm [19] was used to classify DLBCL cases. In addition, when immunohistochemistry showed double expression of the genes: MYC (i.e., >40%) and BCL2 (i.e., >50%) or BCL6 (i.e., >40%), FISH analysis was performed to assess if these genes were split. Patients, who achieved at least a partial remission (PR), at the end of induction were offered to continue treatment with additional six maintenance cycles of 21-days and a post maintenance phase (Supplementary Figure S1). Also, it was explained to patients and their family that maintenance therapy was optional and the benefit of it uncertain. Each cycle was initiated if polymorphonuclear leukocytes (PMN) $\geq$ 1500, platelet (PLT) $\geq$ 50,000 and haemoglobin (Hb) $\geq$ 9.5 gr/dL. Granulocyte colony stimulating factor (G-CSF) and erythropoietin were allowed during the induction cycles. Low molecular weight heparin (LMWH) and low-dose aspirin were administered to patients at high and low-medium risk of thrombosis respectively, during the induction phase. Cotrimoxazole and acyclovir prophylaxis were suggested for all subjects, while ciprofloxacin prophylaxis was started if PMN < 1.0×10^9 Adverse events were coded following the CATCAE v4.03 (https://www.eortc.be/services/doc/ctc/CTCAE_4.03, accessed on 2 July 2022).

Statistical analysis was performed with GraphPad Prism 5 (GraphPad Software, San Diego, CA, USA). Overall (OS), progression-free (PFS) and event-free survival (EFS) analyses were carried out using Kaplan-Meier, and its significance was assessed by the log-rank (Mantel-Cox) test. Treatment stops, before six cycles of induction by any cause, progression, and deaths were all considered events for the EFS analysis. Fisher's exact test was used to evaluate the impact of significant co-variates on survival.

Caregivers were required to guarantee the proper administration of DEVEC in patients who were very old and frail. Restaging was scheduled by computerized-tomography (CT) scan between the 2nd and 3rd induction-cycles at the end of the induction phase by FDG positron-emission CT-scan (CT-PET) [20] and every six months in the following two years. Last follow-up data were retrieved as of 30 September 2022.

3. Results

3.1. In Vitro Results

The 144h treatment with metronomic VNR and metronomic ETO showed a significant concentration-dependent inhibitory activity on human OCI-LY3 cell proliferation. The calculated IC$_{50}$s at 144 h was obtained in these cells at 0.036 $\pm$ 0.01 nM with VNR, whereas the 50% of cell proliferation was inhibited at a concentration of 7.9 $\pm$ 3.6 nM with ETO (Figure 1A). Simultaneous exposure to metronomic VNR and ETO showed synergism (CI < 1) at effect levels exceeding 60% inhibition represented by the fraction of affected cells (Figure 1B). Synergism corresponding to CI < 1 always yielded a favourable DRI for both drugs (Table 1). Indeed, in the cases of metronomic VNR or ETO, it could be possible to reduce the concentration of the drug in vitro more than 15-fold or 217-fold, respectively, when the drug is combined to obtain the same 95% level of cytotoxic effects (Table 1). The Loewe analysis of synergism (Figure 1C) confirmed the findings obtained with the Chou method for high percentage of cell proliferation inhibition but also showed a wide area of additivity effect (light green and azure colours) between the 40 and 60% of cell proliferation decrease. Interestingly, synergism and related reductions of drug concentrations are favourable for high level of inhibition of cell proliferation (>90%) to obtain a clinical benefit such as the reduction in the number of tumour cells or the control of neoplastic disease. A representative 95% isobologram of OCI-LY3 cells exposed to concomitant metronomic VNR and ETO for 144 h has been drawn (Supplementary Figure S2). The IC_{95} values of each drug are plotted on the axes while the line represents the additive effect; the point, reported on the left of the connecting line, reproduces the concentrations of VNR and ETO resulting in 95% growth inhibition of the concomitant combination, indicating synergism.

The proapoptotic activity of the concomitant combination of metronomic VNR and ETO on DLBCL cells was quantified using an ELISA test. The extent of DNA fragmentation was dependent on the exposure of the experimental drug and on the combination. In particular, the Figure 2 shows a significant proapoptotic activity of both single drugs at the IC_{50} already after 48 h of exposure in OCI-LY3 cells, whereas the same drug concentration greatly and significantly enhances the apoptotic signal.

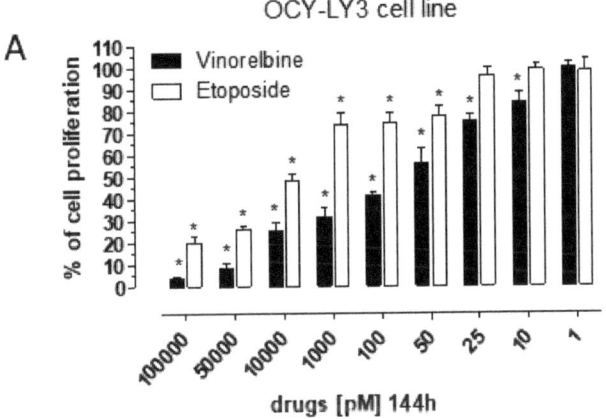

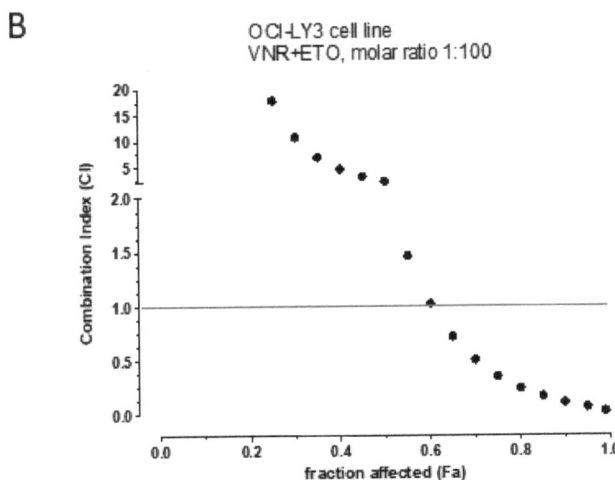

Figure 1. *Cont.*

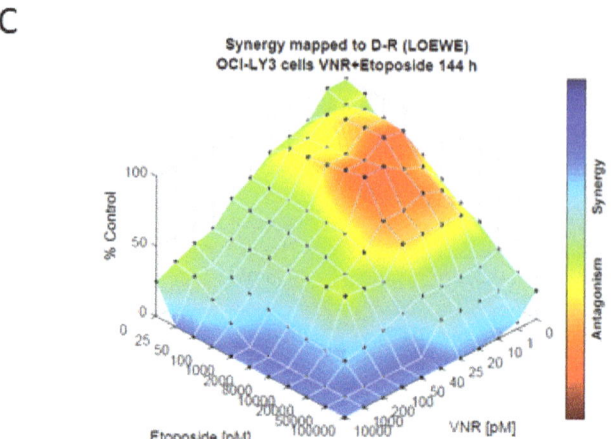

Figure 1. (**A**) Antiproliferative effects of metronomic vinorelbine and metronomic etoposide after 144 h of exposure. Columns and bars, mean values ± SEM, respectively. * $p < 0.05$ vs. vehicle-treated controls. (**B**) Combination index (CI)-fraction affected (Fa) plot of the metronomic vinorelbine (VNR) and etoposide (ETO) combination 144 h at the molar ratio of 1:100 in OCI-LY3 cell line; CI < 1, CI = 1 and CI > 1 indicate synergism, additive effect, and antagonism, respectively. (**C**) The 3-dimensional landscape of the dose matrix of combination responses for metronomic VNR and metronomic ETO based on the Loewe model, where blue reflects evidence of synergy and red represents evidence of antagonism. The model supported synergy of the combination in reducing OCI-LY3 cell line viability. Cell viability was plotted as % control.

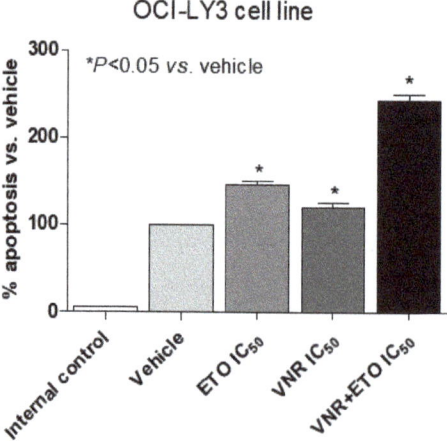

Figure 2. Apoptosis measurements using the Cell Death Detection ELISA Plus kit after 48 h of treatment. Absorbance values are representative of vehicle-treated and metronomic VNR, metronomic ETO and their combination cell cytosolic nucleosomes. All the absorbance values were plotted as a percentage of apoptosis relative to vehicle-treated cells which is labelled as 100%. The internal negative control was provided by the ELISA kit. Columns and bars, mean values ± SD, respectively. * $p < 0.05$ vs. vehicle-treated controls.

Table 1. Dose reduction index (DRI) values of Vinorelbine and Etoposide for fraction affected (Fa) of OCI-LY3 cell proliferation ranging from 0.60 to 0.99. The concomitant combination treatment of vinorelbine and etoposide was administered at the molar ratio of 1:100 for 144 h. The DRI defines the degree of dose reduction that is possible in combination for a given degree of effect as compared with the concentration of each drug alone.

Fraction Affected	Dose Reduction Index	
	Vinorelbine	Etoposide
0.60	4.795	1.232
0.65	5.304	1.903
0.70	5.908	3.030
0.75	6.653	5.056
0.80	7.621	9.087
0.85	8.984	18.478
0.90	11.177	47.431
0.95	15.907	217.423
0.99	34.687	6281.652

3.2. Clinical Results

Twenty-two DLBCL patients started R-DEVEC upfront (Table 2). All subjects were elderly and most were ≥80 years (n = 18/22, 82%). Comprehensive geriatric assessment (CGA), as published by Merli and co-workers [21], was carried out before starting treatment. All patients, but one who was unfit, scored Frail or Super-frail (n = 21/22, 95%) (Table 2). Fifteen patients out of 22 (57%) completed six induction cycles (median = 7 cycles, range 2–18). Only 8 out of 14 (57%) patients who achieved CR, started maintenance cycles (median = 6, range = 4–12). The remaining six patients did not, because of personal or medical choice.

Table 2. Clinical features and Response in 22 Elderly/Frail patients with DLBCL, treated upfront with R-DEVEC.

Factors	B-cell Lymphoma (n = 22) n (%)
Median Age (range)	84.5 (77–93)
Male	14 (64)
Stage III-IV	19 (86)
Ecog PS 1	5 (22)
PS 2	13 (59)
PS 3	4 (18)
Hemoglobin <12 g/dL	11 (50)
Albumin <3.5 g/dL	11 (50)
Bulky ≥7.5cm [21]	9 (41)
IPI 1–2	5 (22)
IPI 3	5 (22)
IPI 4–5	12 (54.5)
[a] CGA	Unfit = 1(4) Frail = 15 (68) Super-Frail = 6 (27)
[b] EPI	Int = 5 (22) High = 17 (78)
Histologic subtypes	DLBCL NOS = 2(9) Non-GC-type = 9 (41) GCB-type = 7 (32) Transformed-NHL = 3 (14) CHL/DLBCL = 1 (4)

Table 2. Cont.

Factors	B-cell Lymphoma (n = 22) n (%)
Interim Response	ORR = 17 (77) PR = 10 (45) CR/CRu = 7 (32) NR = 3 (14) NE = 2 (9)
Final Response	ORR = 14 (64) PR = 0 CR = 14 (64) NR = 4 (18) NE = 4 (18)

IPI 1–2; 3 and 4–5 international prognostic index score of 1–2; 3 and 4–5. [a] CGA: comprehensive geriatric assessment as defined by Merli and co-workers. [b] EPI: Elderly-IPI, from the Elderly Project of the Fondazione Italiana Linfomi by Merli and co-workers. DLBCL-NOS: diffuse large B-cell lymphoma without other specifications Non-GC type: non germinal center type; GC-type: germinal center type on the basis of the Hans' algorithm [19] CHL/DLBCL= histology with feature of both Hodgkin and non-Hodgkin lymphoma, ORR = Overall response PR = partial response; CRu = Complete remission undetermined; NR = non-respondent; NE = not evaluable.

After a median follow-up of 24 months (range 4–80 months), 15 patients had died seven (47%) for causes unrelated to DLBCL or its treatment (Supplementary Table S1), six (40%) for progression, and two (13%) for multiorgan failure. The latter two subjects had stopped treatment following cycles one and two, respectively, because of excessive toxicity. No patient's death was considered as directly related to treatment toxicity. The first 12 patients started R-DEVEC within 14 days of ETO administration [17]. However, 5/12 (42%) subjects required a reduction in ETO doses during cycles 1 or 2 because of the occurrence of grade ≥ 3 extra-hematologic toxicities. Therefore, the following 11 subjects started the schedule with only seven days of ETO, while the drug was omitted in all Super-Frail patients (i.e., R-DEVEC-light) from cycle one or two. Also, G-CSF prophylaxis from day 22, was thereafter recommended, in all subjects. Overall, treatment-related serious adverse events (TR-SAE) were recorded in 6/22 subjects (27%; 95% CI = 14–33): three febrile neutropenia, one urosepsis and two cases of pneumonia, respectively. Indeed, only one TR-SAE occurred after the upfront reduction in ETO. Neutropenia and anaemia of grade ≥ 3 were recorded in 9/22 (41%) and 5/22 (23%), respectively.

At the interim evaluation, the overall response (ORR) and the complete remission rate (CRR) were 77% and 32%, respectively, while at the end of induction the ORR and the CRR were both 64% (Table 3). Overall (OS) (Figure 3A) and event-free (EFS) survivals at 24 months were both 54% 95% CI = 32–72), while disease-free survival (DFS) was 74% (95% CI = 48–88%) (Figure 3B). Univariate analysis was also carried out to investigate the influence of several parameters on survival (Table 3). International prognostic index (IPI), Elderly-IPI (EPI) [22] and not achieving CR at the end of induction, negatively affected both EFS and OS (Table 3). In addition, there was a negative prognostic trend also for bulky mass ≥ 7.5 cm, which did not achieve statistical significance (Table 3). Noteworthy, there was no difference in outcome between patients, who following R-DEVEC received and who did not receive maintenance (Table 3). Conversely, the three super-frail subjects, who achieved CR, following R-DEVEC-light, received at least six cycles of maintenance.

Table 3. Univariate analysis for OS, EFS, and DFS of several risk factors.

Factors	EFS and OS			DFS		
	Odds Ratio	95% CI	p Value	Odds Ratio	95% CI	p Value
Hb < 12 g/dL	1.167	0.2475–5.276	1	1.125	0.2120–5.919	1
Bulky > 7.5 cm (n = 20) *	6.222	0.8219–31.78	0.0861	10	1.136–127.1	0.0635
DEVEC-light	1.429	0.2653–7.492	1	0.48	0.03458–4.368	1
No maintenance cycles following CR (n = 14)	2	0.08546–42.12	1	0	0.000–3.871	0.5055
EPI high	+∞	1.207–+∞	0.0457	+∞	0.4506–+∞	0.2725
Low albumin	0.6857	0.1427–3.442	1	0.9167	0.1423–6.078	1
Male sex	0.3673	0.07937–2.258	0.4015	0.1778	0.01380–1.408	0.179
IPI 3–5	+∞	1.207–+∞	0.0457	+∞	0.4506–+∞	0.2725
Not CR as Intermediate Response (n = 21)	6	0.7510–77.24	0.1736	+∞	1.015–+∞	0.0609
Not CR as Final Response (n = 18)	+∞	2.397–+∞	0.0049	+∞	2.397–+∞	0.0049
Super-frail	0.9643	0.1924–5.171	1	0.3667	0.02713–3.089	0.6214
Age ≥ 80	3	0.3652–42.70	0.594	0.2857	0.03816–2.418	0.2919
PS = 3	3.667	0.5689–22.33	0.3413	4.667	0.7269–26.94	0.2786

CI: Confidence interval; CR: complete response; EFS: event-free survival; EPI: elderly prognostic index; Hb: hemoglobin; IPI: international prognostic index; OS: overall survival; DFS: disease-free survival; PS: performance status. *: the number of patients for whom the factor was available is reported in parenthesis.

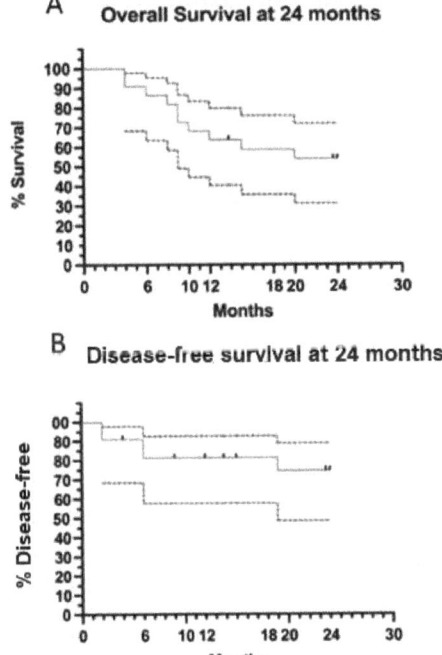

Figure 3. (**A**) Overall survival (OS) estimated at 24 months is 54%; (**B**) disease-free survival estimated at 24 months is 74%. The dotted black lines represent the 95% Confidence Intervals. Dots on survival curves are the events.

4. Discussion

This study confirmed our preliminary report regarding metronomic chemotherapy in DLBCL [17]. The main clinical result consists in the ability of upfront R-DEVEC, to achieve long-lasting remission in Elderly/Frail DLBCL. Moreover, based on this extended clinical experience, we were able to provide more accurate, practical suggestions about dosing, duration, and administration of R-DEVEC, in very elderly and frail subjects. More importantly, we report new pharmacological data about this schedule, which rationally supported the clinical results and could help to optimize its use in vulnerable elderly patients.

Indeed, our in vitro data on the human DLBCL cell line OCI-LY3 demonstrated that both metronomic VNR and ETO directly and remarkably inhibited the DLBCL cell proliferation and promoted the apoptotic process. The selection of the OCI-LY3 cell line was based on various characteristics: (i) the origin of the cell was not from a young patient but from a middle-aged man with a stage IV DLBCL that reflects more our population (64% elderly male; 86% stage III-IV); (ii) the cell line is CD20+, CD19+, CD37+ and CD80+ that opens the possibility to future in vitro combination of metronomic chemotherapy with target therapies such as rituximab, tafasitamab or antiCD37 antibodies; (iii) the cell line has been described to harbor 3–4 copies of cMYC and the rearrangements of BCL-2 and BCL-6 [23]. OCI-LY3 cells were extremely sensitive to both VNR and ETO given in vitro metronomically, with calculated IC_{50}s in the range of picomolar and nanomolar concentrations, respectively, if maintained constant for a protracted time (i.e., six days). However, more central for clinical translation of the results, their simultaneous metronomic association showed a robust synergistic effect—described with two different methodologies—on OCI-LY3 cells for high percentages of cell proliferation inhibition and exhibited a powerful proapoptotic effect (+142% vs. control). These characteristics suggest that the combination of the two drugs is far more effective than the single treatment. This observation opens to a strong reduction in the doses of both compounds when combined (as witnessed by the DRIs in Table 1) without losing any activity on cancer cells and further reducing the risk of dangerous toxicities. These low and effective concentrations can be easily reached in the plasma of patients administered with metronomic schedules, including DEVEC, as demonstrated by our group and other teams [24–26]. Of more interest, Gusella and colleagues reported that metronomic vinorelbine-treated patients who had long-term benefits without toxicity, showed lower VNR concentrations than those who had not [26].

In this series, the higher value of DFS versus OS reflects that a fair percentage of deaths occurred in CR patients; we would highlight that these subjects, due to their old age and burden of comorbidities, often had died for causes unrelated to DLBCL or its therapy. This observation further emphasizes the tolerability and activity of R-DEVEC. Based on our experience, we suggest elderly frail patients receive no more than 7 days of ETO. Alternatively, because of the synergistic activity of ETO and VNR, observed in our in vitro pharmacological experiments, elderly frail may: (1) be treated with a much lower daily dose of ETO for more days; or (2) receive 50 mg of ETO every two days. Conversely, to avoid excessive toxicity, ETO should be omitted in Super-frail subjects, who instead can be safely treated with Rituximab, VNR, CTX and PDN combination (i.e., R-DEVEC-light). Also, G-CSF should be scheduled in all patients from day 21. Worthy of note, peripheral neuropathy, which is an insidious long-term side effect of iv-CHEMO containing vinca-alkaloids, such as R-mini-CHOP, never occurred in patients treated with DEVEC [15,17]. Both high IPI and EPI scores, which were prevalent in this series, had a poor prognostic impact, while the presence of a bulky mass did not achieve statistical significance. Hence, we can speculate that impaired delivery of iv-CHEMO, due to vessels compression, which occurs in tumour mass [27–29], may not be an issue with mCHEMO. In fact, the lower and persistent plasma concentrations, allowed by mCHEMO, determine the tumour vascular normalization and the ability to better diffuse in tumour tissues [30]. Interestingly, 3/6 (50%) of Super-frail patients, who were treated with R-DEVEC-light (i.e., devoid of ETO), achieved CR and had a sustained remission following maintenance cycles. Conversely, maintenance, may not be necessary in treatment-naïve patients who achieve CR after six R-DEVEC cycles (i.e., containing ETO). In fact, PFS was not negatively affected by stopping mCHEMO after induction (Table 3). We acknowledge this study has several limitations: (1) not a controlled study; (2) a limited sample size and (3) the lack of information about the overall number of very elderly and frail subjects who started iv CHEMO.

Notwithstanding, our data seems to compare favourably with the seminal work of Peyrade and Co-workers [5]. In fact, following R-miniCHOP the 24-months disease free survival was reported to be slightly less than 60% (vs. 74% for R-DEVEC) [5]. Furthermore, two recent trials based on Rituximab-lenalidomide [11] and Rituximab-lenalidomide-ibrutinib(iR2) [12] combinations, respectively, reported a 12-months PFS of 55%, [11] and a 24-months PFS of 53%, respectively. We acknowledge these comparisons, although intriguing, remain speculative. A prospective, randomized clinical trial is needed to fully legitimize the use of all-oral, non-expensive mCHEMO as a first-line treatment for the vulnerable and elderly. Unfortunately, as no drug of the DEVEC combination is under patent, the making of a prospective trial is currently hampered by a lack of funding.

Indeed, lenalidomide is a cytotoxic compound. Nonetheless, because it is administered orally and at low doses, it is not properly classified as a chemo-free treatment. Hence, lenalidomide, as well as other chemotherapeutic drugs given at metronomic doses, should be more appropriately indicated as chemo-free-like schedules.

Despite low concentrations of cytotoxic drugs, our in vitro data and clinical results rationally supported the use of the metronomic schedule R-DEVEC in elderly, treatment-naïve DLBCL patients. Indeed, this therapeutic approach allows an effective pharmacological activity on cancer cells that translates into a remarkable remission rate and long-term efficacy, with acceptable toxicity and good tolerability.

Supplementary Materials: The following supporting information can be downloaded at: https://www.mdpi.com/article/10.3390/jcm11237162/s1, Supplementary Figure S1: DEVEC schedule; Supplementary Figure S2: Isobologram analysis of OCI-LY3 cell growth inhibition by the concomitant combination of metronomic vinorelbine (VNR) and etoposide (ETO); Supplementary Table S1: Causes of death of 15 patients treated with R-DEVEC.

Author Contributions: Conceptualization, G.B. and M.C.C.; methodology G.B., S.P., P.O., M.C., M.B., A.D.N., G.M., M.P.B., C.P., P.A.-B., R.B., I.C., T.L., A.T. and M.C.C.; statistical analysis, P.O., M.C. and S.P.; writing—original draft preparation, G.B. and M.C.C.; funding acquisition, G.B. and M.C.C. All authors have read and agreed to the published version of the manuscript.

Funding: This research was funded, in part, by the "Fondi di Ateneo" of the University of Pisa.

Institutional Review Board Statement: The study was conducted according to the guidelines of the Declaration of Helsinki and approved by the Sapienza ethics committee (EC approval n° 4640).

Informed Consent Statement: An informed consent for research aims was obtained from all participants at the time of enrolment.

Data Availability Statement: The data are available at the Department of Clinical and Experimental Medicine, University of Pisa (Prof. G. Bocci) and at the Hematology Unit, Fondazione Policlinico Tor Vergata (Dr. MC Cox).

Acknowledgments: The authors thank Rory Parker, the participating patients and their families.

Conflicts of Interest: The authors declare no conflict of interest.

References

1. Smith, A.; Howell, D.; Patmore, R.; Jack, A.; Roman, E. Incidence of haematological malignancy by sub-type: A report from the Haematological Malignancy Research Network. *Br. J. Cancer* **2011**, *105*, 1684–1692. [CrossRef] [PubMed]
2. Coiffier, B.; Lepage, E.; Brière, J.; Herbrecht, R.; Tilly, H.; Bouabdallah, R.; Morel, P.; Van Den Neste, E.; Salles, G.; Gaulard, P.; et al. CHOP Chemotherapy plus Rituximab Compared with CHOP Alone in Elderly Patients with Diffuse Large-B-Cell Lymphoma. *N. Engl. J. Med.* **2002**, *346*, 235–242. [CrossRef] [PubMed]
3. Thieblemont, C.; Grossoeuvre, A.; Houot, C.; Thieblemont, R.; Grossoeuvre, A.; Houot, R.; Broussais-Guillaumont, F.; Salles, G.; Traullé, C.; Espinouse, D.; et al. Non-Hodgkin's lymphoma in very elderly patients over 80 years. A descriptive analysis of clinical presentation and outcome. *Ann. Oncol.* **2008**, *19*, 774–779. [CrossRef] [PubMed]
4. National Cancer Institute. Cancer Stat Facts: NHL—Diffuse Large B-Cell Lymphoma (DLBCL). Available online: https://seer.cancer.gov/statfacts/html/dlbcl.html (accessed on 6 August 2020).
5. Peyrade, F.; Jardin, F.; Thieblemont, C.; Thyss, A.; Emile, J.F.; Castaigne, S.; Coiffier, B.; Haioun, C.; Bologna, S.; Fitoussi, O.; et al. Attenuated immunochemotherapy regimen (R-miniCHOP) in elderly patients older than 80 years with diffuse large B-cell lymphoma: A multicentre, single-arm, phase 2 trial. *Lancet Oncol.* **2011**, *12*, 460–468. [CrossRef]

6. Shen, Q.D.; Hua-Yuan Zhu, H.Y.; Wang, L.; Fan, L.; Liang, J.H.; Cao, L.; Wu, W.; Xia, Y.; Li, J.Y.; Xu, W. Gemcitabine-oxaliplatin plus rituximab (R-GemOx) as first-line treatment in elderly patients with diffuse large B-cell lymphoma: A single-arm, open-label phase 2 trial. *Lancet Haematol.* **2018**, *5*, e261–e269. [CrossRef]
7. Storti, S.; Spina, M.; Pesce, E.A.; Salvi, F.; Merli, M.; Ruffini, A.; Cabras, G.; Chiappella, A.; Angelucci, E.; Fabbri, A.; et al. Rituximab plus bendamustine as front-line treatment in frail elderly (>70 years) patients with diffuse large B-cell non-Hodgkin lymphoma: A phase II multicenter study of the Fondazione Italiana Linfomi. *Haematologica* **2018**, *103*, 1345–1350. [CrossRef]
8. Thieblemont, C.; Delfau-Larue, M.-H.; Coiffier, B. Lenalidomide in Diffuse Large B-Cell Lymphoma. *Adv. Hematol.* **2012** *2012*, 861060. [CrossRef]
9. Tilly, H.; Morschhauser, F.; Sehn, L.H.; Friedberg, J.W.; Trněný, M.; Sharman, J.P.; Herbaux, C.; Burke, J.M.; Matasar, M. Rai, S.; et al. Polatuzumab Vedotin in Previously Untreated Diffuse Large B-Cell Lymphoma. *N. Engl. J. Med.* **2022**, *386*, 351–363 [CrossRef]
10. Wilson, W.H.; Young, R.M.; Schmitz, R.; Yang, Y.; Pittaluga, S.; Wright, G.; Lih, C.-J.; Williams, P.M.; Shaffer, A.L. Gerecitano, J.; et al. Targeting B cell receptor signaling with ibrutinib in diffuse large B cell lymphoma. *Nat. Med.* **2015**, *21* 922–926. [CrossRef]
11. Gini, G.; Tani, M.; Bassan, R.; Tucci, A.; Ballerini, F.; Sampaolo, M.; Merli, F.; Re, F.; Olivieri, A.; Petrini, M.; et al. Lenalidomide and Rituximab (ReRi) As Front-Line Chemo-Free Therapy for Elderly Frail Patients with Diffuse Large B-Cell Lymphoma. a Phase II Study of the Fondazione Italiana Linfomi (FIL). *Blood* **2021**, *138*, 305. [CrossRef]
12. Xu, P.-P.; Shi, Z.-Y.; Qian, Y.; Cheng, S.; Zhu, Y.; Jiang, L.; Li, J.-F.; Fang, H.; Huang, H.-Y.; Yi, H.-M.; et al. Ibrutinib, rituximab, and lenalidomide in unfit or frail patients aged 75 years or older with de novo diffuse large B-cell lymphoma: A phase 2, single-arm study. *Lancet Healthy Longev.* **2022**, *3*, e481–e490. [CrossRef] [PubMed]
13. Cox, M.C.; Bocci, G. Metronomic chemotherapy regimens and targeted therapies in non-Hodgkin lymphoma: The best of two worlds. *Cancer Lett.* **2021**, *524*, 144–150. [CrossRef] [PubMed]
14. André, N.; Carré, M.; Pasquier, E. Metronomics: Towards personalized chemotherapy? *Nat. Rev. Clin. Oncol.* **2014**, *11*, 413–431 [CrossRef] [PubMed]
15. Cox, M.C.; Banchi, M.; Pelliccia, S.; Di Napoli, A.; Marcheselli, L.; Patti, C.; Borza, P.A.; Battistini, R.; Di Gregorio, F. Orlandi, P.; et al. All-oral metronomic DEVEC schedule in elderly patients with peripheral T cell lymphoma. *Cancer Chemother. Pharmacol.* **2020**, *86*, 841–846. [CrossRef]
16. Di Desidero, T.; Orlandi, P.; Gentile, D.; Banchi, M.; Alì, G.; Kusmic, C.; Armanetti, P.; Cayme, G.J.; Menichetti, L.; Fontanini, G.; et al. Pharmacological effects of vinorelbine in combination with lenvatinib in anaplastic thyroid cancer. *Pharmacol. Res.* **2020** *158*, 104920. [CrossRef]
17. Cox, M.C.; Pelliccia, S.; Marcheselli, L.; Battistini, R.; Arcari, A.; Borza, P.A.; Patti, C.; Casaroli, I.; di Landro, F.; Di Napoli, A.; et al The metronomic all-oral DEVEC is an effective schedule in elderly patients with diffuse large b-cell lymphoma. *Investig. New Drugs* **2019**, *37*, 548–558. [CrossRef]
18. Pfreundschuh, M. How I treat elderly patients with diffuse large B-cell lymphoma. *Blood* **2010**, *116*, 5103–5110. [CrossRef]
19. Hans, C.P.; Weisenburger, D.D.; Greiner, T.C.; Gascoyne, R.D.; Delabie, J.; Ott, G.; Müller-Hermelink, H.K.; Campo, E.; Braziel, R.M.; Jaffe, E.S.; et al. Confirmation of the molecular classification of diffuse large B-cell lymphoma by immunohistochemistry using a tissue microarray. *Blood* **2004**, *103*, 275–282. [CrossRef] [PubMed]
20. Cheson, B.D.; Pfistner, B.; Juweid, M.E.; Gascoyne, R.D.; Specht, L.; Horning, S.J.; Coiffier, B.; Fisher, R.I.; Hagenbeek, A.; Zucca, E.; et al. Revised Response Criteria for Malignant Lymphoma. *J. Clin. Oncol.* **2007**, *25*, 579–586. [CrossRef]
21. Merli, F.; Luminari, S.; Rossi, G.; Mammi, C.; Marcheselli, L.; Ferrari, A.; Spina, M.; Tucci, A.; Stelitano, C.; Capodanno, I.; et al. Outcome of frail elderly patients with diffuse large B-cell lymphoma prospectively identified by Comprehensive Geriatric Assessment: Results from a study of the Fondazione Italiana Linfomi. *Leuk. Lymphoma* **2013**, *55*, 38–43. [CrossRef]
22. Merli, F.; Luminari, S.; Tucci, A.; Arcari, A.; Rigacci, L.; Hawkes, E.; Chiattone, C.S.; Cavallo, F.; Cabras, G.; Alvarez, I.; et al. Simplified Geriatric Assessment in Older Patients With Diffuse Large B-Cell Lymphoma: The Prospective Elderly Project of the Fondazione Italiana Linfomi. *J. Clin. Oncol.* **2021**, *39*, 1214–1222. [CrossRef] [PubMed]
23. Li, Y.; Gupta, S.K.; Han, W.; Kundson, R.A.; Nelson, S.; Knutson, D.; Greipp, P.T.; Elsawa, S.F.; Sotomayor, E.M.; Gupta, M. Targeting MYC activity in double-hit lymphoma with MYC and BCL2 and/or BCL6 rearrangements with epigenetic bromodomain inhibitors. *J. Hematol. Oncol.* **2019**, *12*, 73. [CrossRef] [PubMed]
24. Di Desidero, T.; Derosa, L.; Galli, L.; Orlandi, P.; Fontana, A.; Fioravanti, A.; Marconcini, R.; Giorgi, M.; Campi, B.; Saba, A.; et al. Clinical, pharmacodynamic and pharmacokinetic results of a prospective phase II study on oral metronomic vinorelbine and dexamethasone in castration-resistant prostate cancer patients. *Investig. New Drugs* **2016**, *34*, 760–770. [CrossRef] [PubMed]
25. Yong, W.P.; Desai, A.A.; Innocenti, F.; Ramirez, J.; Shepard, D.; Kobayashi, K.; House, L.; Fleming, G.F.; Vogelzang, N.J.; Schilsky, R.L.; et al. Pharmacokinetic modulation of oral etoposide by ketoconazole in patients with advanced cancer. *Cancer Chemother. Pharmacol.* **2007**, *60*, 811–819. [CrossRef]
26. Gusella, M.; Pasini, F.; Caruso, D.; Barile, C.; Modena, Y.; Fraccon, A.P.; Bertolaso, L.; Menon, D.; Crepaldi, G.; Bononi, A.; et al. Clinical outcomes of oral metronomic vinorelbine in advanced non-small cell lung cancer: Correlations with pharmacokinetics and MDR1 polymorphisms. *Cancer Chemother. Pharmacol.* **2019**, *83*, 493–500. [CrossRef]
27. Padera, T.P.; Stoll, B.R.; Tooredman, J.B.; Capen, D.; di Tomaso, E.; Jain, R.K. Pathology: Cancer cells compress intratumour vessels. *Nature* **2004**, *427*, 695. [CrossRef]

28. Lane, R.J.; Khin, N.Y.; Pavlakis, N.; Hugh, T.J.; Clarke, S.J.; Magnussen, J.; Rogan, C.; Flekser, R.L. Challenges in chemotherapy delivery: Comparison of standard chemotherapy delivery to locoregional vascular mass fluid transfer. *Futur. Oncol.* **2018**, *14*, 647–663. [CrossRef]
29. Choi, I.-K.; Strauss, R.; Richter, M.; Yun, C.-O.; Lieber, A. Strategies to Increase Drug Penetration in Solid Tumors. *Front. Oncol.* **2013**, *3*, 193. [CrossRef]
30. Mpekris, F.; Baish, J.W.; Stylianopoulos, T.; Jain, R.K. Role of vascular normalization in benefit from metronomic chemotherapy. *Proc. Natl. Acad. Sci. USA* **2017**, *114*, 1994–1999. [CrossRef]

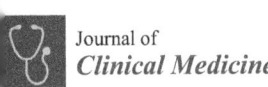

Review

Metronomic Chemotherapy in Pediatric Oncology: From Preclinical Evidence to Clinical Studies

Marta Banchi, Elisabetta Fini, Stefania Crucitta and Guido Bocci *

Department of Clinical and Experimental Medicine, University of Pisa, Via Roma 55, 56126 Pisa, Italy
* Correspondence: guido.bocci@unipi.it; Tel.: +39-0502218756

Abstract: Metronomic chemotherapy (MC) is the frequent, regular administration of drug doses designed to maintain a low, but active, range of concentrations of chemotherapeutic drugs, during prolonged periods of time without inducing excessive toxicities. To date, more than 400,000 children and adolescents under the age of 20 are diagnosed with cancer, per year, with 80% survival in most high-income countries, but less than 30% in low- and middle-income ones. In this review, we summarized the principal preclinical and clinical studies involving the use of MC in the most common pediatric tumors, with an overview of efficacy, toxicity, pharmacokinetic profile, and biomarkers. The best advantages of MC are low toxicity, oral administration and, thus, the feasibility of a more comfortable, home-based treatment, therefore improving the quality of life of the children themselves and of their parents and caregivers. Moreover, MC could represent a valid method to reduce the economic burden of anticancer therapy in the pediatric setting.

Keywords: metronomic chemotherapy; pediatric tumors; preclinical studies; clinical studies; pharmacokinetic studies; biomarkers

Citation: Banchi, M.; Fini, E.; Crucitta, S.; Bocci, G. Metronomic Chemotherapy in Pediatric Oncology: From Preclinical Evidence to Clinical Studies. *J. Clin. Med.* **2022**, *11*, 6254. https://doi.org/10.3390/jcm11216254

Academic Editors: Nikolas Herold and Julie C. Fanburg-Smith

Received: 29 September 2022
Accepted: 21 October 2022
Published: 24 October 2022

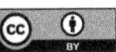

Copyright: © 2022 by the authors. Licensee MDPI, Basel, Switzerland. This article is an open access article distributed under the terms and conditions of the Creative Commons Attribution (CC BY) license (https://creativecommons.org/licenses/by/4.0/).

1. Introduction

Metronomic chemotherapy (MC) is the frequent, regular administration of drug doses designed to maintain a low, but active, range of concentrations of chemotherapeutic drugs, during prolonged periods of time without inducing excessive toxicities. MC regimens were developed to optimize the antitumor efficacy of cytotoxic agents, thus avoiding recurrent issues of standard maximum tolerated dose (MTD) chemotherapy [1]. MC acts through different mechanisms, depending on doses and schedules: the inhibition of tumor angiogenesis with a privileged activity against endothelial cells [2,3]; induction of tumor dormancy [4]; direct cytotoxic effect on cancer stem cells [5]; activation of anticancer immune response by depletion of T regulatory (Treg) cells [6] (Figure 1).

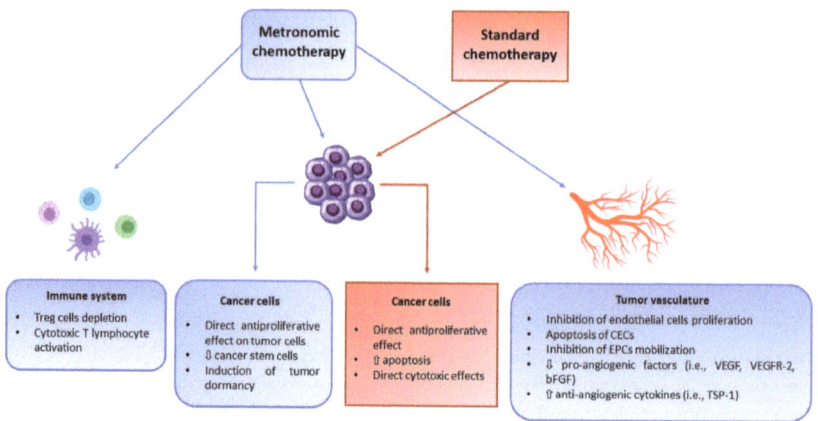

Figure 1. Main mechanisms of action of metronomic chemotherapy vs. standard chemotherapy bFGF, basic fibroblast growth factor; CEC, circulating endothelial cell; EPC, endothelial progenitor cell; TSP-1, thrombospondin-1; T_{reg}, regulatory T cell; VEGF, vascular endothelial growth factor.

Despite major improvements in treatment and cure rates, childhood cancer incidence tends to increase with time worldwide [7]. To date, more than 400,000 children and adolescents under the age of 20 are diagnosed with cancer, per year, with 80% survival in most high-income countries, but less than 30% in low- and middle-income ones [8].

The implementation of MC in pediatric oncology, alone or in combination with other approaches such as radiotherapy, MTD chemotherapy, immunotherapy, and targeted agents, has mostly adjuvant, palliative, and maintenance purposes [9].

The main goal of administering a metronomic regimen to this specific patient population is about improving the quality of life of the children themselves and of their parents and caregivers. In fact, the best advantages of MC are low toxicity, oral administration and, thus, the feasibility of a more comfortable, home-based treatment. MC avoids the need for central venous access, contributing to a reduced risk of infection. Hematological, hepatic, or renal adverse events, after metronomic therapy, are rare and thus minimal monitoring and supportive care are necessary [10]. The lower costs, wide availability, and less need for hospitalization due to MC represent additional benefits, especially in resource-limited countries, where the majority of children with cancer live. As a result, a well-tolerated and easy-to-take metronomic treatment represents a valid strategy as maintenance or adjuvant therapy, when tumor masses are limited, or also in case of advanced disease with minimal chance of survival [10].

In this review, we summarized the major preclinical and clinical studies involving the use of MC in the most common pediatric tumors, with an overview of efficacy, toxicity, pharmacokinetic profile, and biomarkers.

2. Methodology

The methodology search was conducted in the PubMed database using the terms listed in Table 1, including both original articles and reviews written in the English language, published from January 2000 to September 2022. Pivotal papers published before January 2000 were also included.

Table 1. Main and secondary keywords used for the literary search.

Main Key Words	Secondary [a] Key Words
Metronomic	Preclinical study
Low dose	Cell culture
Chemotherapy	Animal model
Pediatric	Clinical study
Childhood	Randomized controlled trial
Cancer	Observational study
Tumor	Efficacy
Neoplasia	Toxicity
	Angiogenesis
	Biomarkers

[a] Secondary key words were utilized in combination (by using "AND") with the main key words. Main keywords were combined by using "OR", reported in left column.

3. Preclinical Activity of Metronomic Chemotherapy in Pediatric Tumor Models

All the described preclinical studies are summarized in Table 2.

3.1. Preclinical Models of Neuroblastoma

Neuroblastoma (NB) is an embryonic cancer arising from neural crest stem cells. It is the most common malignancy in infants and the most common extracranial solid tumor in children [11].

The first attempt to apply metronomic chemotherapy in these pediatric cancers was from the group guided by Robert Kerbel at the University of Toronto [12]. The xenografts of poor prognosis-related human neuroepithelioma (SK-N-MC, expressing multidrug resistance-associated protein) and neuroblastoma (SK-N-AS, highly tumorigenic) cell lines, implanted subcutaneously in CB-17 SCID mice, were continuously exposed to low doses of vinblastine (1.5 mg/m^2 i.p. every 3 days; about 1/4 of the MTD in humans and 1/16–1/20 of the MTD in mice), DC101 (a monoclonal neutralizing antibody targeting the VEGFR-2; 800 µg/mouse, i.p. every 3 days), or their combination. Either single treatment caused a significant but short-term tumor regression, reduced tumor vascularization, and directly inhibited the angiogenic process. Interestingly, the combination induced complete and sustained tumor regression, without marked toxicity or appearance of drug resistance during more than 6 months of treatment [12]. Indeed, blocking VEGF sensitized endothelial cells to the cytotoxic effects of chemotherapy, especially when given at low doses, owing to the downregulation of various antiapoptotic proteins typically induced by VEGF itself (i.e., Bcl-2, XIAP, survivin) [13–15]. The microtubule-targeting agent vinblastine, given at very low doses, has been found to damage specific functions of endothelial cells, and thus angiogenesis, inducing a slight perturbance of the cytoskeleton, without evident apoptosis [16]. Rapamycin is an mTOR inhibitor with immune-suppressor activities, which directly inhibits tumor cell proliferation by arresting the cell cycle, and angiogenesis through a decrease in the production of VEGF [17]. Moreover, it inhibits the in vitro proliferation of human NB cells [18]. Marimpietri and colleagues [19] demonstrated the synergistic antiangiogenic effect of the frequent, low-dose delivery of vinblastine and rapamycin. Vinblastine (0.625–250 pM) and rapamycin (1.56–1000 pM), administered for 144 h (6 days) thrice a week, led to an in vitro antiproliferative effect on endothelial cells, starting from a concentration of 1.25 pM and 3 pM, respectively. Interaction indices showed a synergistic effect after the combination of these two agents at low doses in endothelial cells. The inhibition of proliferation was also observed in endothelial cells previously incubated with a conditioned medium from the human NB cell line HTLA-230. In the chick embryo chorioallantoic membrane (CAM) in vivo assay, each drug administered alone and, in particular, their combination inhibited the angiogenic effects induced by HTLA-230-derived conditioned media, NB cell line-derived tumor xenografts, and human NB biopsy specimens [19].

Another interesting experimental approach to neuroblastoma was performed with the camptothecin topotecan, a topoisomerase-I inhibitor. Metronomic topotecan (0.36 mg/kg, i.p. 5 times a week) was administered either alone or in combination with a humanized monoclonal anti-VEGF antibody (A4.6.1, 100 µg, i.p. twice a week) [20]. After 5 weeks of treatment, metronomic topotecan significantly suppressed the growth of human NGP-GFP neuroblastoma xenograft in athymic mice, compared with anti-VEGF treatment alone or control animals. All treated mice showed reduced tumor vascularization as opposed to the untreated ones at 6 weeks. However, tumor regrowth was observed in all treated mice at 9 weeks (3 weeks after treatment withdrawal), and it was associated with pronounced neo-angiogenesis. Interestingly, only the combination treatment was able to significantly stop the regrowth, if compared to single anti-VEGF therapy. The cooperation of low-dose chemotherapy with antiangiogenic drugs improved the efficacy and the extent of neuroblastoma tumor suppression [20].

Topotecan at low, not cytotoxic, doses has been previously shown to block the upregulation of hypoxia-inducible factor (HIF) -1α and -2α in NB cells in vitro [21]. Neuroblastoma xenografts, established by Hartwich and colleagues [22] through the injection of unmodified (CHLA-20 or NB-1691) or HIF-1α knockdown (SKNAS or NB-1691 shHIF-1α) NB cells into the retroperitoneal space of CB-17 SCID mice, were treated for 2 weeks with bevacizumab (5 mg/kg daily i.p.) or sunitinib (40 mg/kg daily by oral gavage) and low-dose topotecan (0.5 mg/kg daily i.p.) alone or in combination. Interestingly, as previously established, the introduction of low-dose topotecan to the bevacizumab and sunitinib-based antiangiogenic therapy elicited a significant reduction in tumor growth compared to either treatment alone. A similar outcome was detected in mice with HIF-1α knockdown tumors exposed to either bevacizumab or sunitinib alone, demonstrating that metronomic topotecan acted mostly via HIF-1α inhibition. Moreover, both antiangiogenic drugs caused a strong overexpression of HIF-1α-dependent growth factors, such as VEGF and GLUT3, while the addition of metronomic topotecan downregulated these two proteins [22].

MYCN amplification is the major genetic aberration which correlates with high-risk NB disease and poor clinical outcome [23]. This aggressive phenotype has been also associated with increased tumor neovascularization [24,25]. Taschner-Mandl and collaborators [26] found that metronomic topotecan in vitro (5 nM for 3 weeks) selectively promoted DNA damage and a tumor-inhibiting favorable senescence-associated secretory phenotype (SASP) in aggressive MYCN-amplified neuroblastoma cells (i.e., STA-NB-10 and CLB-Ma). In MYCN-amplified STA-NB-10 xenografts established in CD1:Foxn1$^{nu/nu}$ mice, continuous low-dose topotecan (0.1 mg/kg/day i.p. for 6 or 15 weeks) led to tumor regression and prolonged survival, with no evident toxicity. MYCN mRNA and protein expression was significantly reduced both in vitro and in vivo by metronomic topotecan, which also decreased VEGF-A expression and tumor vascularization [26]. Indeed, it has been demonstrated that hypoxia halts senescence in normal and cancer cell lines [27]; thus, the downregulation of HIF-1α by topotecan [28] may also contribute to the induction of senescence.

Kumar and colleagues [29] established both subcutaneous (s.c.) NB xenografts (i.e., SK-N-BE2 and SH-SY5Y) and metastatic NB models (BE2-c and NUB-7) in NOD/SCID mice. In both in vivo modalities, the mice were treated with daily oral gavage of the antiangiogenic tyrosine kinase inhibitor (TKI) pazopanib (150 mg/kg), metronomic topotecan (1.0 mg/kg), or their combination. Low-dose topotecan plus pazopanib slowed tumor growth in subcutaneous SK-N-BE2 and SH-SY5Y tumors and limited micro-metastases in BE2-c and NUB-7 models. The in vitro proliferation assay showed no synergism between topotecan and pazopanib after 72 h of exposure; therefore, the mechanism underlying the effectiveness of the combination is probably related to the antiangiogenic activity. In fact, a significant reduction in viable CECs and CEPs and tumor microvessel density has been observed compared with control and single agents in SH-SY5Y xenografts [29].

In a following study of the same group, SK-N-BE2 xenograft–bearing mice were treated with the same aforementioned treatment schedules for 28, 56, and 80 days. Only the animals receiving metronomic topotecan plus pazopanib survived up to 80 days. Combined treatment significantly reduced microvessel density compared to control and monotherapy groups. However, enriched pericyte coverage was evident only in tumors exposed to the combination for 56 and 80 days. Additionally, the concomitant treatment upregulated the expression of hypoxia and pro-angiogenic factors (i.e., HIF-1α and VEGF), as well as that of Glut-1 and hexokinase II, which are markers of enhanced aerobic glycolysis [30].

Differently from the abovementioned combination studies, Zhang and colleagues revealed a direct synergistic antiproliferative effect in ALK^{F1174L}-mutated SH-SY5Y cells when exposed for 6 days to increasing concentration of crizotinib, a double inhibitor of c-MET and ALK receptor tyrosine kinases, in combination with metronomic topotecan [31]. Interestingly, the same authors did not observe any synergism in the *MYCN*-amplified SK-N-BE2, KELLY, and LAN-5 cells, suggesting that *MYCN* is potentially involved in the emergence of resistance to ALK inhibitors. In vivo, crizotinib (50 mg/kg) and metronomic topotecan (1 mg/kg) were administered daily for 9 days by oral gavage, alone or in combination, in ALK^{F1174L}-mutated SH-SY5Y and KELLY mouse xenografts. The combined treatment significantly delayed tumor growth derived from KELLY cells, whereas it induced the complete regression of SH-SY5Y tumors [31].

Although metronomic topotecan and vinblastine are the chemotherapeutic drugs that have been most frequently used in preclinical models of neuroblastoma, other metronomic therapeutic approaches have been tested with metronomic cyclophosphamide (mCTX) at the dose of 40 mg/kg/day p.o. in SH-SY5Y (chemotherapy-sensitive, non-*MYCN*-amplified) and SK-N-BE2 (chemotherapy-resistant, *MYCN*-amplified) tumor xenografts. Morscher and colleagues [32] observed a greater inhibition of tumor expansion in *MYCN*-amplified mCTX-treated xenografts, as well as a considerable diminution of blood vessel density and intratumoral bleeding. Moreover, they detected a decreased Bcl-2 expression and elevated caspase-3 cleavage. In contrast, non-*MYCN*-amplified tumors showed up-regulation of Bcl-2 and developed resistance [32]. Intriguingly, combining mCTX with a calorie-restricted ketogenic diet [33] significantly enhanced the antitumor effects of this therapeutic approach, resulting in tumor regression and the complete growth arrest of both NB xenografts [32]. However, calorie restriction would not be recommended in most young oncologic patients. Optimization of KD with 25% of 8-carbon medium-chain triglycerides proved to increase the efficacy of mCTX therapy (oral dose of 40 and 13 mg/kg/day given to SH-SY5Y- and SK-N-BE2-bearing mice, respectively), similarly to that achieved with calorie-restricted KD. This combination induced a significant suppression of tumor growth and prolonged survival, especially in SH-SY5Y xenografts. Furthermore, it caused an obvious inhibition of angiogenesis in vivo and activation of AMPK in NB cells. These data highlight that the metabolic stress, induced by dietary manipulation, selectively sensitized the NB cells to low-dose chemotherapy [33].

3.2. Pediatric Brain Tumor Models

Pediatric cancers of the central nervous system (CNS) are the most common solid tumors in children and the second most recurrent childhood malignancies. Medulloblastoma is an embryonal tumor of the posterior fossa, and it accounts for nearly 20% of all pediatric brain tumors, making it the most common malignant brain tumor in children. Almost 20% of all childhood gliomas are high-grade gliomas, and include anaplastic astrocytoma (AA), diffuse intrinsic pontine glioma (DIPG), and glioblastoma multiforme (GBM). Ependymoma, representing around 8% to 10% of all childhood CNS tumors, is the third most frequent brain tumor in children. Unlike adult patients with GBM, where the standard of care is represented by the combination of temozolomide and radiotherapy [34], there is currently no similar recommendation for chemotherapy in the management of pediatric high-grade glioma [35].

PEX is a fragment of human metalloproteases-2 that has significant antimitotic, anti-invasive, and antiangiogenic activities against human glioblastoma cells in vitro and glioblastoma models in vivo [36]. The research of Bello and collaborators [37] suggested that combining low and semicontinuous chemotherapeutic drugs for more than 120 days, such as carboplatin and etoposide (bolus at day 1 with 6 mg/kg carboplatin i.p. and 4 mg/kg etoposide i.p., followed by 2 mg/kg carboplatin + 2 mg/kg etoposide), with PEX (2 mg/kg of PEX i.p. for 2 days, every 3 days) was more effective than chemotherapy alone at a low dose, in the treatment of nude mice bearing intracranial human U87 glioblastoma xenografts. This regimen was accountable for better survival, substantial reduction in tumor volume, vascularization and proliferation index, increased apoptosis and no complications [37].

Folkins and colleagues [5] focused their investigations on the effect of antiangiogenic therapy on glioma tumor stem-like cells (TSLCs). Actually, there is evidence that brain TSLCs are preserved, such as a neural stem cell, by a vascular niche, and consequently have the possibility to stimulate tumor growth. The researchers treated athymic nude mice bearing s.c. rat C6 glioma xenografts, with either anti-VEGFR-2 antibody DC101 (800 µg/mouse i.p. every 3 days), low dose metronomic (LDM) cyclophosphamide (20 mg/kg/day p.o via the drinking water), MTD cyclophosphamide (100 mg/kg i.p. on days 1, 3, and 5 of a 21-day cycle), or combinatorial regimes. Antiangiogenic or cytotoxic therapy alone was not sufficient to reduce the amount of glioma TSLCs. Interestingly, the combination of LDM cyclophosphamide with the potent inhibition of angiogenesis by DC101 was the best therapeutic option for the significant and selective elimination of TSLCs from glioma Therefore, antiangiogenic therapy acquires a potential new role in chemo-sensitizing TSLCs in order to improve the effectiveness of chemotherapy [5].

Topotecan has shown to inhibit HIF-1α protein amassing in human cancer cell lines [28] independently of replication-mediated DNA damage, suggesting the existence of an alternative mechanism of action to the cytotoxic one. In their study, Rapisarda and colleagues showed that low concentrations of topotecan delivered on a daily, but not intermittent, schedule (1 mg/kg, 10 total doses) caused a sustained inhibition of tumor progression in human U251-HRE glioblastoma xenografts. Topotecan exerted its antitumor activity through the prominent diminution of the HIF-1α protein amount, angiogenesis, and expression of genes targeted by HIF-1 in the tumor mass, compared to untreated controls [38].

In a subsequent work, the same investigators found that combining a very low dose of topotecan (0.5 mg/kg once a day, for 10 days) with bevacizumab significantly suppressed glioblastoma growth, as opposed to either agent alone. Whereas bevacizumab alone induced the expression of HIF-1-dependent genes, the addition of topotecan clearly abrogated HIF-1 transcriptional activity in the tumor microenvironment, and significantly inhibited proliferation and induced apoptosis of tumor cells [39].

The alkylating agent temozolomide is one of the most successful chemotherapeutic drugs against glioblastoma, but its antitumor activity is often limited by the onset of resistance. Kim and collaborators showed that C6/LacZ rat glioma cells were more resistant to LDM temozolomide (1–100 µM daily for 144 h), with a ~10-fold greater IC$_{50}$ value than U-87MG human glioblastoma cells. In an orthotopic SD rat model of C6/LacZ glioma, LDM temozolomide (2 mg/kg p.o. daily for 16 days) significantly hampered tumor growth and angiogenesis and promoted apoptosis, compared to the conventional schedule (7 mg/kg for 5 days). In an orthotopic nude mouse xenograft of U-87MG glioblastoma, despite no significant changes in tumor volume between conventional and metronomic regimens, the periodic administration of temozolomide even at a very low dose (0.25 mg/kg daily for 25 days) markedly reduced the microvessel density. In summary, LDM temozolomide demonstrated a striking antiangiogenic effect, either in resistant or sensitive glioma models, suggesting the possibility to overcome resistance in standard temozolomide chemotherapy [40].

Banissi and colleagues studied the impact of LDM versus standard temozolomide regimens on the regulatory T cell (Treg) fraction in Fischer rats bearing an s.c. temozolomide-resistant RG2 glioma tumor. Temozolomide significantly decreased the Treg/CD4+ T cell proportion when given at very low doses (0.5 or 2 mg/kg/die, 5 days per week for 21 days), but not at high doses (30 mg/kg/die for 5 days, or 10 mg/kg/die, 5 days per week for 21 days). Such Treg exhaustion was marked among the splenic lymphocyte population, and it was almost significant among the tumor-infiltrating lymphocytes. However, Treg depletion alone, detected in LDM temozolomide-treated rats, was not sufficient to significantly inhibit tumor progression as well, in comparison with control animals. In conclusion, LDM, but not conventional, schedules of temozolomide showed selective cytotoxicity to the circulating Tregs population [6].

Morphine is the most used drug for pain management in oncological patients. The preclinical studies investigating the effect of opioid receptor agonists on the proliferation, migration, and invasion of cancer cells, as well as their immunosuppressive and proangiogenic activities, show conflicting results. It is presumed that the activation of μ-opioid receptor (MOP) and Toll-like receptor 4 receptors may contribute to tumor growth and progression, while the activation of κ-opioid receptor may promote anticancer and antiangiogenic effects [41]. It has been highlighted that methadone, an agonist of MOP, increased the sensitivity of wild-type leukemic cells, but not MOP-depleted cells, to L-asparaginase treatment. Therefore, MOP was necessary for the synergistic action of L-asparaginase and methadone, and MOP loss promoted leukemic cell survival likely through the downregulation of the MOP-mediated apoptotic pathway [42]. For the first time, Iorio and colleagues demonstrated that morphine acts as an inhibitor of P-glycoprotein, an ATP-binding cassette transporter overexpressed in the endothelial cells of the blood brain barrier and involved in resistance to many chemotherapeutic drugs (i.e., temozolomide). Therefore, morphine might increase the effects of chemotherapy on brain tissue. The authors showed that LDM temozolomide (1.77 mg/kg/day) was effective, from the beginning of the treatment, in hampering the growth of an orthotopic human U87MG-luc2 glioblastoma xenograft, implanted intracranially in Foxn1 nude mice. Noteworthy, combining temozolomide (1.77 and 0.9 mg/kg/day, for a total of 5 weeks) with weekly morphine enhanced the antitumor efficacy and the long-term response to the metronomic regimens in this glioblastoma model [43].

Chen and colleagues described a peculiar metronomic schedule, named MEDIC (medium-dose intermittent chemotherapy), consisting of an immunogenic chemotherapeutic agent (i.e., cyclophosphamide), given at a concentration between a daily low dose (i.e., 20–25 mg/kg) and an MTD dose (i.e., 150–170 mg/kg × 2 or 3 consecutive days, every 21 days), with a medium-term drug-free break and low systemic toxicity. The MEDIC regimen, in addition to the direct cytotoxic effect on tumor cells, can trigger a prolonged antitumor immune response [44].

In murine s.c. models of rat 9L gliosarcoma, mouse GL261 glioma, and human U251 glioblastoma, cyclophosphamide (140 mg/kg i.p.), given on an intermittent metronomic schedule (every 6 days), activated robust and persistent immune responses, as well as induced a striking and extended tumor regression, even with the lack of an evident antiangiogenic effect. Conversely, the MTD regimen caused temporary immune responses, concurrently with appreciable tumor re-growth [44–46]. Interestingly, the MEDIC protocol was also more effective than the corresponding daily low-dose metronomic regimen [44]. In addition, it stimulated a strong CD8+ T cell response leading to tumor disappearance and the gain of immune memory in an immunocompetent, syngeneic s.c. GL261 glioma [47]. Suppression of immune activity occurred if the drug-free interval lasted more than 6 days, as indicated by a significant increase in Foxp3+ Treg cells within the tumor and decreased expression of the cytotoxic immune mediator perforin [47].

Ferrer-Font and collaborators [48] aimed to assess if the every 6-day metronomic regimens of cyclophosphamide (140 mg/kg) or temozolomide (140, 200, and 240 mg/kg) were also effective in an immunocompetent orthotopic GL261 mouse model. They found a longer survival rate in mice treated with both regimes than in control animals. The best results were obtained with 140 mg/kg temozolomide, which resulted in the best dosing in the reduction in tumor volume and improved survival, and in comparison with a previously tested non-metronomic schedule of this drug (60 mg/kg for three cycles on days 11–15, 19–20, and 24–25) [49]. However, in contrast with the results described by Wu and Waxman, no tumor eradication was achieved in this model, highlighting the existence of relevant differences in the tumor environment between ectopic and orthotopic glioblastoma xenografts, which may influence the response to metronomic chemotherapy [47].

It has been demonstrated that there is an immunomodulatory—dosing dependent—effect of temozolomide, which could impact the response to immunotherapy. In GL261 and KR158 murine intracranial glioma models, the standard (50 mg/kg × 5 days), but not metronomic (25 mg/kg × 10 days), regimen of temozolomide led to overexpression of exhaustion markers (i.e., TIM-3 and LAG-3) on peripheral and tumor-infiltrating T cells and to an increase in immunosuppressive cells. Interestingly, the addition of metronomic temozolomide to PD-1 immune checkpoint inhibition preserved the survival benefit gained with anti-PD-1 therapy alone in the GL261 model, while it was abolished by standard temozolomide. Therefore, these findings suggest metronomic dosing of temozolomide as a preferential strategy in chemoimmunotherapy regimens for the management of glioblastoma [50].

3.3. Soft Tissue and Bone Sarcoma Models

Soft tissue sarcomas represent 7.4% of cancer cases in children younger than 20 years of age. Rhabdomyosarcoma is the most common (50%) soft tissue sarcoma among children less than 14 years old [51]. Ewing sarcoma and osteosarcoma are the two most commonly diagnosed bone cancers in pediatric patients [52].

Continuous low-dose doxorubicin (1.2 mg/kg, twice weekly for 4 weeks) was found to modestly inhibit the tumor growth of human rhabdomyosarcoma RD s.c. xenografts, well-established in SCID mice, corresponding to 46.5% of that achieved with the standard treatment (6 mg/kg once every 2 weeks). Moreover, the development of human leiomyosarcoma SKLMS-1 s.c. tumors was not halted by metronomic doxorubicin. However, the combination of low-dose doxorubicin and DC101 at a lower concentration (400 µg/dose every 3 days for a total of seven times) markedly reduced the volume of both SKLMS-1 and RD tumors, compared to either agent alone. Microvessel counts were significantly lower in combination-treated mice, compared to either agent alone, and no further toxicity was detected as opposed to low-dose doxorubicin alone. Moreover, DC101 plus doxorubicin exerted a direct additive inhibitory effect on endothelial cell functions (i.e., migration, proliferation, tube-like formation) in vitro and enhanced apoptosis of endothelial cells, through caspase-3 activation. These results support antiangiogenic activity as one of the main mechanisms for the antitumor effect of combined low-dose treatment with DC101 and doxorubicin [53].

Osteosarcoma UMR 106-bearing SD rats were treated, for a period of 8 weeks, with: (i) a conventional schedule including a high dosage of methotrexate (1.35 g/kg i.v., 6 h infusion, once weekly, at week 0, 1, 5 and 6), adriamycin and cisplatin (10 mg/kg and 20 mg/kg, respectively; once weekly, at week 2 and 7); (ii) a metronomic schedule of low-dose methotrexate (1.2 mg/kg i.v., bolus, twice a week); and (iii) a combination schedule of metronomic and conventional chemotherapy, with low-dose methotrexate administered at week 3, 4, and 8 of the conventional scheduling. After the first 6 weeks of treatment, in which the rate of tumor inhibition was similar for all three regimens, only the combination showed a protracted inhibitory effect on tumor growth. Anyway, the metronomic protocol had a better effect compared to the conventional one. Furthermore, both metronomic and combination schedules showed a much lower VEGF-A expression than the conventional group, which may support a greater antiangiogenic effect [54].

3.4. Pediatric Retinoblastoma Models

The standard chemotherapy for retinoblastoma, the most common intraocular cancer of childhood [55], includes intravenous or local intravitreal injections of melphalan, carboplatin, and topotecan, which unfortunately induce retinal toxicity [56].

Both commercial (Y79 and WERI-RB1) and patient-derived retinoblastoma cell lines (HSJD-RBT-7 and HSJD-RBT-8) together with human vascular endothelial cells (HUVEC and EPC) were exposed to increasing concentrations of melphalan or topotecan in a conventional (0.001–1000 µM or 0.001–10.000 nM, respectively, single 72 h exposure) or metronomic

(0.0001–100 µM or 0.0001–1000 nM, respectively, 7-day continuous exposure) treatment protocol. The continuous administration of melphalan and topotecan increased the sensitivity of retinoblastoma and endothelial cell lines with significant lower IC_{50} values (i.e., 18.4- and 12.3-fold for topotecan and 8.3- and 13.5-fold for melphalan in Y79 and WERI-RB1, respectively) compared to conventional treatment. The cytotoxic effect of metronomic chemotherapy was more evident in commercial cell lines compared to the patient-derived HSJD-RBT-8 cells. Furthermore, the heavily pretreated HSJD-RBT-8 cells had enhanced chemosensitivity to the metronomic schedule (3 to 4-fold decreased IC_{50}) compared to conventional dosing, while no change was evident for naïve HSJD-RBT-7 cells, suggesting a possible mechanism to overcome resistance. Both treatment regimens led to cell death through apoptosis and/or necrosis in all cell lines. Moreover, metronomic topotecan or melphalan significantly inhibited in vitro tube formation in HUVEC and EPC compared to control cells. In athymic nude mice harboring a Y79 retinoblastoma xenograft, low-dose topotecan (0.6 mg/kg i.p., 5 days a week for 2 weeks) determined significantly lower tumor volumes compared to the MTD protocol (3 mg/kg i.p., once a week for 2 weeks) and the control group after 14 days of treatment, with a similar toxicity profile and no weight loss. These results highlighted the dual cytotoxic/antiangiogenic, schedule-dependent effect of chemotherapy in retinoblastoma preclinical models. [57].

3.5. Acute Lymphoblastic Leukemia Models

Acute lymphoblastic leukemia (ALL) is the most common pediatric malignancy, representing 75%–80% of acute leukemias among children, with a median age at diagnosis of 15 years [58]. Glucocorticoid (GC) resistance represents a crucial challenge in treating ALL; therefore, there is an urgent need for new therapeutic strategies to enhance chemosensitivity, which may also allow for reduction in the intensity and toxicity of standard chemotherapy [59].

It has been demonstrated that a low, subtoxic concentration of arsenic trioxide (0.25 µM) significantly increased in vitro dexamethasone sensitivity of 3 different GC-resistant ALL cell lines (CEM-C1-15, Jurkat, and MOLT-4), as well as T-ALL and precursor B-ALL cells from pediatric patients with poor response to prednisone. The effect of this combination was explained in part by a reduction in Akt phosphorylation and following alteration of downstream Akt targets such as an increase in Bad, a proapoptotic Bcl-2 family member, and a decrease in the X-linked inhibitor of apoptosis protein (XIAP). These results indicate that a combination of low-dose arsenic trioxide with glucocorticoids may be a valuable approach to reverse GC resistance and improve prognosis in ALL pediatric patients [60].

Next, 2-deoxy-D-glucose (2-DG) is a glucose analogue that inhibits the proliferation of cancer cells through the inhibition of glycolysis and N-linked glycosylation [61]. Recently, Gu and co-workers showed that a low, nontoxic dose of 2-DG (1 mM for 48 h) was able to induce apoptosis and cell-cycle arrest and to overcome GC resistance in ALL cells under normoxia. In fact, low-dose 2-DG combined with dexamethasone (1 µM) recovered the sensitivity of GC and produced a strong synergistic cytotoxic effect in GC-resistant Molt-4 (T lineage) and Raji (B lineage) cells. Interestingly, these effects were achieved mainly by blocking N-Linked glycosylation and inducing endoplasmic reticulum stress [62].

L-asparaginase (L-ASNase) is a critical anticancer agent used in the treatment of ALL and some types of non-Hodgkin's lymphoma, including natural killer (NK)-cell lymphoma [63]. Many leukemia or lymphoma cells rely on the supply of the amino acid asparagine (Asn) from plasma, due to a deficiency of l-asparagine synthetase [64]. L-ASNase hydrolyzes L-Asn to L-aspartic acid, therefore, lowering the level of plasma Asn, which leads leukemic cells to apoptosis [65]. L-ASNase also shows some glutaminase (GLS) activity, that converts the circulating glutamine (Gln) to glutamate and ammonia, thus reducing Gln intracellular uptake. Interestingly, low doses (0.01 U/mL for 24 h) of L-ASNase induced Asn depletion and effectively killed Asn-dependent NK-YS cells, whereas clinically achievable intermediate doses (1 U/mL for 24 h) caused Gln depletion and robust apoptosis in Gln-dependent ALL Jurkat and mantle cell lymphoma Jeko cell lines. In addition, the high expression of glutaminase GLS1 was found to be related to increased sensitivity to L-ASNase in pediatric B lineage ALL [66].

3.6. Metronomic Combined Schedules in Multiple Pediatric Tumor Models

Zhang and collaborators revealed that low-dose topotecan (20 nmol/L) significantly enhanced the cytotoxic effect of the hypoxia-activated prodrug (HAP) evofosfamide on a wide range of neuroblastoma and rhabdomyosarcoma cell lines, in in vitro 72 h exposure experiments. Aggressive neuroblastoma (CHLA-20 and SK-N-BE(2)), rhabdomyosarcoma (RH4 and RD) s.c. xenografts, and the neuroblastoma SK-N-BE(2) metastatic model were subsequently treated with evofosfamide, (50 mg/kg daily i.p., 5 days/week), LDM topotecan (1 mg/kg daily by oral gavage, 5 days/week), and their combination. In every neuroblastoma and rhabdomyosarcoma xenograft, the combined treatment resulted in a better antitumor effect than both monotherapies and induced complete tumor regression after 2 weeks of treatment. The combination also improved survival in the SK-N-BE(2) metastatic model (median survival of 46 days), compared to either agent alone. There was no serious toxicity related to therapy in any of the experimental models. Interestingly, in RH4 xenografts, evofosfamide induced apoptosis of tumor cells localized mostly in hypoxic regions, while topotecan targeted tumor cells mainly within normoxic areas. Thus, administering evofosfamide with LDM topotecan allowed it to kill tumor cells in both normoxic and hypoxic regions, explaining the higher efficacy of the combination regimen in all tumor models [67].

Talazoparib is a potent, selective PARP1/2 inhibitor and shows strong PARP trapping activity, which means it firmly traps PARP1 to the sites of DNA single-strand breaks [68,69]. Methylating agents (i.e., temozolomide) are extremely useful at prompting single-strand breaks that could become substrates for PARP trapping [70]. Thus, Smith and collaborators evaluated the in vitro 96 h exposure of temozolomide (0.3–1000 µmol/L) in the presence of talazoparib (10 nmol/L), which resulted in a marked potentiation of temozolomide toxicity in Ewing sarcoma (50-fold) and ALL (30-fold) cell lines. In vivo, several pediatric s.c. xenograft models (including Ewing sarcoma, Wilms tumor, rhabdomyosarcoma, osteosarcoma, neuroblastoma, brain tumors) were treated with temozolomide (30 mg/kg/day for 5 days) and talazoparib (0.25 mg/kg twice daily for 5 days) alone or in two different combinations: high-dose temozolomide (30 mg/kg/day for 5 days) + talazoparib (0.1 mg/kg twice daily for 5 days), or low-dose temozolomide (12 mg/kg/day for 5 days) + talazoparib (0.25 mg/kg twice daily for 5 days). Toxicity was comparable for both combinations. Unlike single treatments, both combinations exhibited significant antitumor effects and induced total tumor regression in 5 out 10 Ewing xenografts tested (TC-71, CHLA-258, SKNEP-1, ES-4, and ES-7), within 6 weeks of treatment. Combined treatments were also successful against pediatric preclinical models with low MGMT expression (i.e., GBM2 glioblastoma and Rh28 rhabdomyosarcoma), responsive to temozolomide, and those with a defective homologous recombination, responsive to talazoparib (i.e., KT-10 Wilms tumor). In conclusion, administering an efficacious PARP trapping concentration of talazoparib plus low-dose temozolomide is a promising strategy for translation to the pediatric clinical setting [71].

Pawlik and co-workers [72] found IC$_{50}$ values (~2 nM) for medulloblastoma Daoy cells exposed to topotecan for a total of 6 days, in three different ways of delivering: continuous, for 8 h daily, or for 8 h every other day. In contrast, topotecan IC$_{50}$ increased with extending the drug-free time in Rh30 rhabdomyosarcoma cells (3.9, 8.7, and 12.4 nM, respectively). In vivo experiments confirmed in vitro results. Rh30 xenografts regressed completely when treated with topotecan 0.6 mg/kg i.v. daily (dx5), whereas no growth delay was observed with 1.0 mg/kg every other day (for 2 weeks, repeated every 21 days for 3 cycles). Increased doses of topotecan 2 mg/kg daily and 3.3 mg/kg every other day, which produced comparable antitumor activity, were needed to obtain complete tumor regression of the less sensitive in vivo Daoy models. These results clearly show that the antitumor effect of topotecan was extremely schedule-dependent in Rh30, but not in Daoy cells and xenograft models.

Table 2. Preclinical studies of metronomic chemotherapy in pediatric tumor models.

Metronomic Regimen	Preclinical Tumor Model	Results	Reference
Neuroblastoma			
Vinblastine (1.5 mg/m^2 i.p. every 3 days), anti-VEGFR-2 antibody DC101 (800 µg/mouse, i.p. every 3 days), or combination, for >6 months	Human SK-N-MC neuroepithelioma and SK-N-AS neuroblastoma cell lines implanted s.c. in CB-17 SCID mice, aged 4 to 6 weeks	Combined treatment induced complete and sustained tumor regression, without marked toxicity or appearance of drug resistance.	Klement et al. [12]
Topotecan (0.36 mg/kg, i.p. 5x/week), anti-VEGF antibody A4.6.1 (100 µg, i.p. twice a week), or combination for a total of 5 weeks	Human NGP-GFP neuroblastoma xenograft in female NCR athymic mice, aged 4 to 6 weeks	LDM topotecan either with or without anti-VEGF antibody significantly suppresses NB xenograft growth. All treated mice showed reduced tumor vascularization. Only combined treatment significantly stopped the regrowth. LDM topotecan increased apoptosis of neuroblastoma cells.	Kim et al. [20]
Vinblastine (0.625–250 pM) and rapamycin (1.56–1000 pM), administered for 144 h, thrice a week	In vitro ECs (HUVEC and EA.hy926) and ECs preincubated with CM from the human NB cell line HTLA-230. In vivo CAM assay with HTLA-230-derived CM, HTLA-230-derived tumor xenografts, and human NB biopsy specimens	Significant antiproliferative effect in ECs preincubated with HTLA-230 CM after combination at low doses. Combination of 50 pM vinblastine and 0.5 nM rapamycin was synergistic in arresting the cell cycle and increased apoptosis of ECs. The combination markedly inhibited the angiogenic effects induced in vivo in the CAM assay.	Marimpietri et al. [19]
Topotecan (0.5 mg/kg daily i.p.), bevacizumab (5 mg/kg daily i.p.) or sunitinib (40 mg/kg daily p.o.), or combination, for 2 weeks	Unmodified CHLA-20 and NB-1691, and shHIF-1α-modified NB-1691 and SKNAS neuroblastoma cell lines injected into the retroperitoneal space of CB-17 SCID mice	Combined LDM treatment significantly reduced tumor growth and downregulated the expression of VEGF and GLUT3.	Hartwich et al. [22]
In vitro: topotecan (5 nM, 2×/week for 3 weeks) In vivo: topotecan (0.1 mg/kg/day i.p. for 6 or 15 weeks)	In vitro WT or *MYCN*-amplified neuroblastoma cell lines (i.e., STA-NB-10 and CLB-Ma). In vivo STA-NB-10 xenografts established in female CD1: *Foxn1$^{nu/nu}$* mice, 6 to 10 weeks old	Induction of DNA-damage and a tumor-inhibiting favorable SASP selectively in *MYCN*-amplified cells in vitro. Tumor regression and prolonged survival, with no evident toxicity in vivo. Significant reduction of MYCN mRNA and protein expression both in vitro and in vivo Decreased VEGF-A expression and tumor vascularization in vivo.	Taschner-Mandl et al. [26]

Table 2. Cont.

Metronomic Regimen	Preclinical Tumor Model	Results	Reference
Cyclophosphamide (mCTX, 40 mg/kg/day, p.o. through the drinking water), calorie restricted KD, optimized KD, or combination	Non-MYCN-amplified SH-SY5Y and MYCN-amplified SK-N-BE(2) NB cell lines injected s.c. in female CD1 nude mice, aged 5 to 6 weeks	mCTX induced greater tumor inhibition in MYCN-amplified xenografts, diminution of blood vessel density, and intratumoral bleeding, decreased Bcl-2 expression, and increased caspase-3 cleavage. Combining mCTX with calorie restricted KD resulted in tumor regression and complete growth arrest of both NB xenografts. Combining mCTX with optimized KD resulted in significant tumor growth suppression and prolonged survival, especially in SH-SY5Y xenografts, and inhibition of angiogenesis.	Morscher et al. [32] Aminzadeh-Gohari et al. [33]
Topotecan (1.0 mg/kg/day p.o.), pazopanib (150 mg/kg/day p.o.), or combination	SK-N-BE(2) and SH-SY5Y s.c. (into inguinal fat pad) NB xenografts, BE(2)-c and NUB-72 metastatic (into lateral tail vein) NB xenografts in NOD/SCID mice	Combined treatment slowed tumor growth in SK-N-BE(2) and SH-SY5Y models, and limited micrometastasis in BE(2)-c and NUB-7 models. Significant reduction in viable CECs and CEPs and tumor microvessel density in SH-SY5Y xenografts.	Kumar et al. [29]
Topotecan (1.0 mg/kg/day p.o.), pazopanib (150 mg/kg/day p.o.), or combination for 28, 56, and 80 days	SK-N-BE(2) s.c. xenograft–bearing NOD/SCID mice, 4 to 8 weeks old	Only the animals receiving the combination survived up to 80 days. All three durations of combined treatment significantly reduced microvessel density. Higher proliferative and mitotic indices after 28 days of combined treatment.	Kumar et al. [30]
In vitro: crizotinib, LDM topotecan, or combination (ratio 20:1, 0,01–10 µM) continuously for 6 days In vivo: topotecan (1 mg/kg/day p.o.), crizotinib (50 mg/kg/day p.o.) for 9 days	In vitro ALK^{F1174L}-mutated SH-SY5Y cell line and MYCN-amplified SK-N-BE(2), KELLY, and LAN-5 cell lines. In vivo ALK^{F1174L}-mutated SH-SY5Y and KELLY xenografts in female NOD/SCID mice, 4 to 6 weeks old.	Combined treatment resulted in a synergistic antiproliferative effect only in SH-SY5Y cells in vitro and a significantly delayed tumor growth of KELLY xenografts, and complete regression of SH-SY5Y tumors in vivo.	Zhang et al. [31]
Brain tumor			
Bolus at day 1 with 6 mg/kg carboplatin i.p. and 4 mg/kg etoposide i.p., followed by 2 mg/kg carboplatin + 2 mg/kg etoposide and 2 mg/kg of PEX i.p. for 2 days, every 3 days. Treatment duration ≥ 120 days	Intracranial human U87 glioblastoma xenografts in 5-week-old Swiss male nude mice	This combination was more effective than chemotherapy alone and induced better survival, substantial reduction in tumor volume, vascularization and proliferation index, increased apoptosis, and no complications.	Bello et al. [37]

Table 2. Cont.

Metronomic Regimen	Preclinical Tumor Model	Results	Reference
DC101 (800 µg/mouse i.p. every 3 days), LDM cyclophosphamide (20 mg/kg/day p.o. via the drinking water), MTD cyclophosphamide (100 mg/kg i.p. on days 1, 3, and 5 of a 21-day cycle), and their combinations	Athymic nude mice bearing s.c. rat C6 glioma xenografts	The combination of LDM cyclophosphamide with potent inhibition of angiogenesis by DC101 caused a significant and selective elimination of TSLCs from the glioma.	Folkins et al. [5]
Low-dose topotecan (1 mg/kg daily, 10 total doses)	Female athymic nude (NCr/nu) mice bearing human U251-HRE glioblastoma xenografts	Sustained inhibition of xenograft tumor progression, with prominent diminution of HIF-1α protein amount, angiogenesis, and expression of genes targeted by HIF-1 in tumor mass	Rapisarda et al. [38]
Very low-dose topotecan (0.5 mg/kg daily, for 10 days) + bevacizumab	Female athymic nude (NCr/nu) mice bearing human U251-HRE glioblastoma xenografts	The combination significantly suppressed glioblastoma growth. Addition of topotecan clearly abrogated HIF-1 transcriptional activity in the tumor microenvironment, significantly inhibited proliferation, and induced apoptosis.	Rapisarda et al. [39]
In vitro: LDM TMZ (1–100 µM daily for 144 h) In vivo rat model: conventional TMZ (7 mg/kg p.o. for 5 days) vs. LDM TMZ (1 or 2 mg/kg p.o., every day for 16 days) In vivo mouse model: conventional TMZ (2.5 or 1.25 mg/kg p.o., for 5 days) vs. LDM TMZ (0.5 and 0.25 mg/kg p.o., daily for 25 days)	In vitro C6/LacZ rat glioma cells and U-87MG human glioblastoma cells. In vivo male Sprague-Dawley (SD) rats (200–250 g) bearing intracranial C6/LacZ glioma and male Balb/c-nu mice (6 weeks) bearing intracranial U-87MG glioblastoma	In vitro C6/LacZ rat glioma cells were more resistant to LDM TMZ than U-87MG human glioblastoma cells. In the orthotopic C6/LacZ glioma model, LDM TMZ significantly hampered tumor growth and angiogenesis and promoted apoptosis, compared to the conventional schedule. In the orthotopic U-87MG xenograft, TMZ even at a very low dose (0.25 mg/kg daily for 25 days) markedly reduced the microvessel density.	Kim et al. [40]
LDM TMZ (0.5 or 2 mg/kg/die p.o., 5 days per week for 21 days) vs. standard TMZ (30 mg/kg/die p.o. for 5 days, or 10 mg/kg/die, 5 days per week for 21 days)	TMZ-resistant RG2 glioma cells implanted s.c. in Fischer rats	TMZ significantly decreased the Treg/CD4+ T cell proportion when given at very low doses but not at high standard doses. Treg depletion alone, detected in LDM TMZ-treated rats, was not sufficient to significantly inhibit tumor progression, compared to control.	Banissi et al. [6]
LDM TMZ (1.77 and 0.9 mg/kg/day, for a total of 5 weeks) + weekly morphine	Orthotopic human U87MG-luc2 glioblastoma xenograft, implanted intracranially in Foxn1 nude mice	Addition of morphine enhanced the antitumor efficacy and the long-term response to the TMZ metronomic regimens.	Iorio et al. [43]

Table 2. Cont.

Metronomic Regimen	Preclinical Tumor Model	Results	Reference
MEDIC (medium-dose intermittent chemotherapy) Cyclophosphamide (140 mg/kg i.p., every 6 day)	SCID mice bearing s.c. xenografts of rat 9L gliosarcoma, mouse GL261 glioma, and human U251 glioblastoma	The MEDIC schedule activated robust and persistent immune responses, as well as induced a striking and extended tumor regression. More effective than the corresponding daily low-dose metronomic regimen. Induction of a strong CD8+ T cell response leading to tumor disappearance and gain of immune memory in the GL261 glioma xenograft.	Chen et al. [44] Doloff et al. [45] Wu et al. [46,47]
Every 6-day metronomic cyclophosphamide (140 mg/kg) or temozolomide (140, 200, and 240 mg/kg)	Orthotopic GL261 glioma model in immunocompetent C57BL/6 mice	Longer survival rate in mice treated with both regimes than in control animals. In total, 140 mg/kg temozolomide was the best dosing in reduction of tumor volume and improving survival. No tumor eradication was achieved.	Ferrer-font et al. [48]
Metronomic TMZ (25 mg/kg × 10 days) vs. standard TMZ (50 mg/kg × 5 days) + immunotherapy	GL261 and KR158 intracranial glioma models in C57BL/6 mice	Addition of metronomic TMZ to PD-1 immune checkpoint inhibition preserved the survival benefit gained with anti-PD-1 therapy alone in the GL261 model, while it was abolished by standard temozolomide.	Karachi et al. [50]
Soft tissue sarcoma			
MTD doxorubicin (6 mg/kg once every 2 weeks), LDM doxorubicin (1.2 mg/kg, twice weekly for 4 weeks), DC101 (400 µg/dose every 3 days for a total of seven times), or combination	Female SCID mice (weight 18–22 g) harboring human RD rhabdomyosarcoma and SKLMS-1 leiomyosarcoma s.c. tumors	LDM doxorubicin alone was less effective than MTD doxorubicin. The combination of LDM doxorubicin and DC101 markedly reduced the volume of both SKLMS-1 and RD tumors, and the microvessel count, without overt toxicity.	Zhang et al. [53]
Bone sarcoma			
MTD methotrexate (1.35 g/kg i.v., 6 h infusion, once weekly, at week 0, 1, 5, and 6), adriamycin and cisplatin (10 mg/kg and 20 mg/kg, respectively; once weekly, at week 2 and 7), LDM methotrexate (1.2 mg/kg i.v., bolus, twice a week), combination of MTD and LDM schedules, for a total of 8 weeks	5-week-old SD rats bearing s.c. UMR 106 tumors	After the first 6 weeks of treatment, only the combination showed a protracted inhibition of tumor growth. Both MTD and combination schedules showed a much lower VEGF-A expression.	Zhu et al. [54]

Table 2. Cont.

Metronomic Regimen	Preclinical Tumor Model	Results	Reference
Retinoblastoma			
In vitro: melphalan or topotecan in a conventional (0.001–1000 µM or 0.001–10.000 nM, respectively) single 72 h exposure vs. metronomic (0.0001–100 µM or 0.0001–1000 nM, respectively) 7-day continuous exposure. In vivo: topotecan LDM topotecan (0.6 mg/kg i.p., 5 days a week) for 2 weeks vs. MTD (3 mg/kg i.p., once a week) for 2 weeks	In vitro: commercial Y79 and WERI-RB1 and patient-derived HSJD-RBT-7 and HSJD-RBT-8 retinoblastoma cell lines. HUVEC and EPC human vascular endothelial cells. In vivo: Y79 retinoblastoma s.c. xenografts in female athymic nude mice, weighing 18–22 g	Continuous administration increased the sensitivity to chemotherapy of retinoblastoma and endothelial cells. The heavily pretreated HSJD-RBT-8 cells had enhanced chemosensitivity to the metronomic schedule compared to the conventional one. Both treatment regimens led to cell death through apoptosis and/or necrosis in all cell lines. Metronomic schedules significantly inhibited in vitro tube formation in endothelial cells. LDM topotecan significantly lowered tumor volumes compared to the MTD protocol and control group, with a similar toxicity profile and no weight loss.	Winter et al. [57]
Acute lymphoblastic leukemia			
Dexamethasone (0.1, 1, and 7.6 µM) alone or in combination with low-dose arsenic trioxide (0.25 µM) for 72 h	GC-resistant ALL cell lines (CEM-C1-15, Jurkat, and MOLT-4), T-ALL, and precursor B-ALL cells from pediatric patients with poor response to prednisone	Low-dose arsenic trioxide significantly increased in vitro dexamethasone sensitivity. This combination reduced Akt phosphorylation, which is associated with an increase in Bad and decrease in XIAP protein.	Bornhauser et al. [60]
The 2-DG (0.2 to 10 mM) alone and in combination with dexamethasone (1 µM) for 24 h and 48 h	T-ALL cell lines: Molt-4 (GC resistance), Jurkat (GC resistance); CEM-C1-15 (GC resistance), CEM-C7-14(GC sensitive) B-ALL cell lines: Nalm-6 (GC sensitive), RS4:11 (GC sensitive) Burkitt lymphoma cell line: Raji (B-lineage, GC resistance)	Low-dose of 2-DG (1 mM) for 48 h induced apoptosis and cell-cycle arrest. Its combination with dexamethasone recovered the sensitivity of GC and produced a strong synergistic cytotoxic effect in GC-resistant Molt-4 and Raji cells.	Gu et al. [62]
L-ASNase 0.01 U/mL vs. 1 U/mL for 24 h	Cell lines: Jurkat and Reh (ALL), Jeko (mantle cell lymphoma), NK-YS (nasal-type NK-cell lymphoma)	Low-dose L-ASNase (0.01 U/mL) effectively killed Asn-dependent NK-YS cells, whereas clinically achievable intermediate doses (1 U/mL) induced robust apoptosis in Gln-dependent Jurkat and Jeko cell lines.	Sugimoto et al. [66]

Table 2. Cont.

Metronomic Regimen	Preclinical Tumor Model	Results	Reference
Miscellaneous			
In vitro: increasing concentrations of evofosfamide with or without the presence of low-dose topotecan (20 nmol/L) In vivo: evofosfamide, (50 mg/kg daily i.p., 5 days/week), LDM topotecan (1 mg/kg daily by oral gavage, 5 days/week), and their combination	In total, 5 different neuroblastoma cell lines (CHLA-15, CHLA-20, CHLA-90, SK-N-BE(2), and SH-SY5Y) and 3 rhabdomyosarcoma cell lines (RH4, RH30, and RD) in vitro. Aggressive s.c. xenografts using two neuroblastoma cell lines [CHLA-20 and SK-N-BE(2)] and two rhabdomyosarcoma cell lines (RH4 and RD); metastatic (intravenous) SK-N-BE(2) neuroblastoma model in NOD/SCID mice	Low-dose topotecan enhanced the cytotoxic effect of evofosfamide in all cell lines in vitro. Combined treatment resulted in a better antitumor effect than both monotherapies and induced complete tumor regression after 2 weeks of treatment in each s.c. xenograft. It also improved survival in the SK-N-BE(2) metastatic model.	Zhang et al. [67]
In vitro: 96 h exposure of temozolomide (0.3–1000 µmol/L) with or without talazoparib (10 nmol/L) In vivo: temozolomide (30 mg/kg/day × 5 days) and talazoparib (0.25 mg/kg twice daily × 5 days) alone or in two different combinations: high-dose temozolomide (30 mg/kg/day × 5) + talazoparib (0.1 mg/kg twice daily × 5) or low-dose temozolomide (12 mg/kg/day × 5) + talazoparib (0.25 mg/kg twice daily × 5)	Pediatric Preclinical Testing Program (PPTP) cell line panel including a total of 23 cell lines of rhabdomyosarcoma, rhabdoid, Ewing sarcoma, neuroblastoma, glioblastoma, ALL, AML, ALCL, and NHL origin, for cytotoxic in vitro assays. In vivo pediatric xenografts: C.B-17 $scid^{-/-}$ female mice for s.c. implantation of Wilms tumor, rhabdoid tumor, Ewing sarcoma, osteosarcoma, rhabdomyosarcoma, neuroblastoma, and non-glioblastoma brain tumors; BALB/c nu/nu mice for glioma models; female NOD.CB17-Prkdcscid/J mice for intravenous inoculation of human leukemia cells	In vitro, the combination resulted in a marked potentiation of temozolomide toxicity in Ewing sarcoma (50-fold) and ALL (30-fold) cell lines. In vivo, toxicity was comparable for both combinations. Both exhibited significant antitumor effects and induced total tumor regression in 5 of 10 Ewing xenografts, within 6 weeks of treatment. It was successful against xenografts with low MGMT expression (i.e., GBM2 glioblastoma and Rh28 rhabdomyosarcoma) and those with defective homologous recombination (i.e., KT-10 Wilms tumor).	Smith et al. [71]
In vitro: Topotecan for a total of 6 days, on three different ways of administration: continuous, for 8 h daily, or for 8 h every other day. In vivo: low-dose topotecan 0.6 mg/kg i.v. daily ×5 and 1.0 mg/kg every other day; increased dose 2 mg/kg daily ×5 and 3.3 mg/kg every other day (for 2 weeks, repeated every 21 days for 3 cycles)	In vitro: Daoy pediatric medulloblastoma and Rh30 pediatric rhabdomyosarcoma cells In vivo: Daoy and Rh30 s.c. xenografts in 4-week-old CBA/Caj tyhmectomized female mice	Topotecan IC_{50} values of ~2 nM for Daoy cells, while they increased with extending drug-free time in Rh30 cells. Rh30 xenografts regressed completely when treated with topotecan 0.6 mg/kg i.v. daily ×5. Increased doses of 2 mg/kg daily and 3.3 mg/kg every other day to obtain complete tumor regression of the less sensitive in vivo Daoy models.	Pawlik et al. [72]

2-DG, 2-deoxy-D-glucose; Akt, Protein kinase B; ALK, anaplastic lymphoma kinase; ALCL, Anaplastic large cell lymphoma; ALL, acute lymphoblastic leukemia; ALM, Acute myeloid leukemia; Bad, BCL2 associated agonist of cell death; Bcl-2, B-cell lymphoma 2; CAM, chorioallantoic-membrane; CEC, circulating endothelial cell; CEP, circulating endothelial progenitor; CM, conditioned medium; EC, endothelial cells; GC, glucocorticoid; GLUT3, Glucose transporter 3; HIF, hypoxia-inducible factor; IC50, half maximal inhibitory concentration; i.p., intraperitoneal; i.v., intravenous; KD, ketogenic diet; L-ASNase, L-asparaginase; LDM, low dose metronomic; mCTX, metronomic cyclophosphamide; MEDIC, medium-dose intermittent chemotherapy; MGMT, O-6-methylguanine-DNA methyltransferase; MTD, maximum tolerated dose; MYCN, Proto-Oncogene BHLH Transcription Factor; NB, neuroblastoma; NHL, Non-Hodgkin lymphoma; PD-1, programmed cell death protein 1; PEX, a fragment of human metalloproteases-2; p.o., per os; SASP, senescence-associated secretory phenotype; s.c., subcutaneous; TMZ, temozolomide; Treg; T regulatory cells; TSLC, tumor stem-like cells; VEGF, vascular endothelial growth factor; VEGFR-2, VEGF receptor 2; WT, wild type; XIAP, X-linked inhibitor of apoptosis protein.

4. Pharmacokinetic Studies on Metronomic Chemotherapy in Preclinical, Pediatric Tumor Models

The first preclinical pharmacokinetic (PK) study was performed by Zhou and colleagues [73] in SF188V+ glioma-bearing athymic rats receiving multiple i.v. administrations of temozolomide at a metronomic (3.23 mg/kg/day for 28 days) or standard (18 mg/kg/day for 5 days) dosing. The pharmacokinetic profile of temozolomide was linear, and dose- and time-independent. Indeed, the main PK parameters such as half-life ($t_{1/2}$), volume of distribution (Vd), and systemic clearance of the drug were superimposable at the beginning and at the end of either metronomic or standard treatment. Moreover, a marked and similar decrease in tumor volume was observed in mice treated with both regimens, but the peak plasma concentration (C_{max}) of metronomic temozolomide was considerably lower (7–8-fold) than that obtained after administration of the standard schedule, and it was maintained for a longer period of time [73].

Kumar and colleagues [29] have also investigated the pharmacokinetic interactions of metronomic topotecan in combination with pazopanib in a preclinical model of aggressive pediatric solid tumors. Pazopanib is a substrate of cytochrome P450 3A4 (CYP3A4) [74], whereas topotecan is an inhibitor of CYP3A4 [75]. However, no substantial difference was reported in the plasma concentration of topotecan or pazopanib among the group of animals treated with the drug combination and those treated with either agent alone. Therefore, interestingly, no relevant drug concentration alteration was detected between topotecan and pazopanib despite a theoretical metabolic drug interaction.

Interestingly, Chen and co-workers [44] carried out a pharmacokinetic analysis of plasma 4-OH-cyclophosphamide (active metabolite) levels in 9L glioma cell tumor-bearing mice administered with cyclophosphamide at 11.65 mg/kg p.o. daily, 70 mg/kg i.p. every 3 days, and 140 mg/kg i.p. every 6 days. The highest intermittent i.p. amount resulted in a C_{max} of 4-OH-cyclophosphamide almost 20-fold higher than that detected in mice treated with the lowest daily oral dose, although the total exposure was the same, and it was accountable for the activation of the strongest, broad-spectrum, antitumor innate immunity and tumor regression.

5. Clinical Studies on Metronomic Chemotherapy in Pediatric Patients

All the described clinical studies are summarized in Table 3.

Table 3. Clinical studies on metronomic chemotherapy in pediatric patients.

Disease	N° of Patients	Type of Study	Metronomic Regimen	Main Results	Reference
Low-grade glioma (pLGG)	18	Retrospective	Bevacizumab with or without irinotecan + vinblastine/vinorelbine	2-year OS: 94%	Roux et al. [76]
Progressive or relapsed solid tumors	74	Retrospective	COMBAT I, COMBAT II, COMBAT IIS, COMBAT III	43.1% (median: 15.4 months) was 2-year OS	Zapletalova et al. [77]
Rhabdoid tumor	6	Case series	Etoposide + cyclophosphamide + celecoxib + valproic acid	SD (death from bone marrow transplant-related infectious complications)	Carcamo B. and Francia G. [78]
Anaplastic ependymoma			Etoposide + cyclophosphamide + celecoxib + valproic acid	CR	
Medulloblastoma			Etoposide + valproic acid	CR	
Medulloblastoma			Temozolomide + cyclophosphamide + celecoxib + valproic acid	PD	

Table 3. Cont.

Disease	N° of Patients	Type of Study	Metronomic Regimen	Main Results	Reference
Neuroblastoma	6	Case series	Etoposide + cyclophosphamide + sulindac/celecoxib	Relapse	Carcamo B. and Francia G. [78]
Cervicomedullary tumor			Temozolomide + cyclophosphamide + valproic acid + celecoxib + bevacizumab	SD	
Poor prognosis brain tumors	8	Pilot	Temozolomide 90 mg/m^2/day for 42 days	Six patients responded to treatment	Sterba et al. [79]
Refractory solid tumors	12	Pilot, prospective	Vincristine, cyclophosphamide, and methotrexate	Disease stabilization occurred in 7 patients (58%)	Fousseyni et al. [80]
Recurrent or progressive solid tumor	33	Pilot	Celecoxib + vinorelbine or cyclophosphamide	Median time to progression was 8.5 weeks (range: 3 to 62.5 week) Four (13%) patients had a stable disease with durations of 28 to 76 weeks	Stempak et al. [81]
Refractory cancer	7	Pilot, prospective	Vincristine, cyclophosphamide, methotrexate	Mean duration treatment: 34 ± 31 weeks PR: 2 patients	Traore et al. [82]
Recurrent or progressive poor prognosis solid tumors	20	Feasibility trial	Four-drug regimen: thalidomide + celecoxib + alternating cyclophosphamide/VP16 every 21 days for 6 months	Eight patients completed the six-month therapy	Kieran et al. [83]
Relapsed or refractory solid tumors	30	Phase I	Topotecan + pazopanib	The recommended dose was topotecan 0.22 mg/m^2/day and pazopanib PfOS 160 mg/m^2/day In total, 10 patients (4 neuroblastoma, 3 osteosarcoma, 2 Ewing sarcoma/PNET, and 1 medulloblastoma) had stable disease with median duration of 6.4 months (1.7–45.1) The longest stable disease was 45 months	Manji et al. [84]
Relapsed or refractory solid tumors	64	Prospective	Celecoxib, cyclophosphamide, vinblastine, and methotrexate	Forty-nine patients (77%) had a favorable response (PR and SD) 1-year OS: 62.3%	Ali A.M. and El-Sayed M.I. [85]
High-grade glioma, neuroblastoma, desmoplastic small round cell tumor-DSRCT, alveolar rhabdomyosarcoma, ependymoma, melanoma	13	Phase II	Nivolumab + cyclophosphamide +/- radiotherapy at discretion of physician	None of patients had confirmed objective response Stable disease occurred in 5 subjects Median PFS = 1.7 months (95% CI: 1.3–3.4) Median OS = 3.4 months (95% CI: 2.2–13.5)	Pasqualini et al. [86]
Recurrent or progressive tumors	101	Phase II, prospective	Five drugs: cyclophosphamide, etoposide, thalidomide, celecoxib, and fenofibrate	Twenty-four patients (25%) completed 27 weeks therapy	Robison et al. [87]

Table 3. Cont.

Disease	N° of Patients	Type of Study	Metronomic Regimen	Main Results	Reference
Relapsed/refractory pediatric brain tumors	29	Phase II	Four drugs: celecoxib, vinblastine, cyclophosphamide, and methotrexate	Median number of cycles was 6.8 (range 1–12) Good response in LGG patients	Verschuur et al. [88]
Refractory or relapsing tumors	16	Pilot	Vinblastine, cyclophosphamide, methotrexate, and celecoxib	Disease stabilizations (25%) that lasted 24 weeks or more	André at al. [89]
Neuroblastoma, soft-tissue sarcoma, bone sarcoma, miscellaneous	50	Phase II, prospective	Vinblastine, cyclophosphamide/methotrexate, celecoxib	1-year PFS = 6.8% 1-year OS = 55.3%	Heng-Maillard et al. [90]
Refractory/relapsing solid tumors, or advanced disease	98	Phase II, prospective	Cyclophosphamide + etoposide + valproic acid	6-month OS = 40% (95% CI) 1-year OS = 22% 1-year PFS = 19%	El Kababri et al. [91]
Rhabdomyosarcoma at high-risk of relapse	371	Phase III	G1: vinorelbine and cyclophosphamide G2: placebo	In G1 group: 86.5% (95% CI 80.2–90.9) was 5-year overall survival 77.8% (70.8–83.4) was 5-year disease-free survival	Bisogno et al. [92]
Non-hematopoietic primarily extracranial solid tumor progressive after treatment with at least 2 lines of chemotherapy	108 G1: 56 patients G2: 52 patients	Phase III	G1: thalidomide, celecoxib, and etoposide/cyclophosphamide G2: placebo	In the G1 group: 49 days (95% CI, 43–59 days) was the median PFS 85 days was the OS SD = 8 patients PR = 2 patients Good response in patients without a bone tumor	Pramanik et al. [93]

COMBAT I (celecoxib, etoposide, temozolomide, isotretinoin); COMBAT II (celecoxib, etoposide, temozolomide, fenofibrate, cholecalciferol for the first year and celecoxib, cyclophosphamide, isotretinoin, fenofibrate, cholecalciferol for the second year); COMBAT IIS (celecoxib, vinorelbine, cyclophosphamide, cis-retinoic acid, fenofibrate, cholecalciferol); COMBAT III (celecoxib, etoposide, temozolomide, fenofibrate, cholecalciferol, vitamin D3, bevacizumab for the first year and celecoxib, cyclophosphamide, isotretinoin, fenofibrate, cholecalciferol for the second year), CR, complete response; DSRCT, desmoplastic small round cell tumor; G1, group1; G2, group 2; OS, overall survival; PfOS, powder for oral suspension; PFS, progression-free survival; PD, progressive disease; pLGG, pediatric low-grade glioma; PNET, Primitive Neuro-Ectodermal Tumors; PR, partial response; SD, stable disease; VP16, etoposide.

5.1. Retrospective Studies

Roux and collaborators [76] conducted a monocentric retrospective study in 18 pediatric patients (7 males and 11 females) with pediatric low-grade glioma (pLGG). Induction treatment involved bevacizumab (10 mg/kg) alone or in combination with irinotecan (125 mg/m^2) on days 1 and 15 of 2-week cycles for 6 months, or until the best clinical or radiological response was obtained; later, the patients received metronomic vinblastine (6 mg/m^2 per week; in case of hematological toxicity, the dose could be reduced to 2 mg/m^2 per week). Two patients had disease progression; therefore, it was not possible to include them in the analysis. Metastases were present in 2 out of 16 children, while 2 patients had undergone other treatments (1 line and 6 lines). Bevacizumab and irinotecan were given to 13 children, while bevacizumab alone was given to 3 children. After induction, 5 of 16 partial radiological responses and 11 of 16 stable diseases occurred. Induction lasted an average of 6.2 months, while maintenance lasted 12 months. Maintenance treatment had to be stopped in one patient due to grade 3 gastrointestinal toxicity with vomiting and abdominal pain. After 3.9 years (range 11 months–7.2 years) from the end of induction, 15/16 children were alive and 9/16 were progression-free. Disease progression occurred in 7 of 16 patients with a median time of 23 months: 3 children progressed during vinblastine maintenance, and 4 children after. The 2-year OS was 94%. Treatment tolerance was good overall. No patient experienced renal toxicity or hypertension during induction. Vinblastine was discontinued in one child after 3 months due to persistent grade 2 gastrointestinal toxicity (vomiting/nausea) during maintenance. Vinblastine dosage was decreased in 7 patients (n = 4, 4 mg/m^2; n = 2, 3 mg/m^2; n = 1, 2 mg/m^2) due to hematological toxicities (grade 3 neutropenia). There were no peripheral neurotoxicity or long-term toxicities [76].

Seventy-four children with progressive, relapsed solid tumors, were treated by one of four different COMBAT chemotherapy regimens: COMBAT I (celecoxib, etoposide, temozolomide, isotretinoin) lasting 1 year; COMBAT II (celecoxib, etoposide, temozolomide, fenofibrate, cholecalciferol for the first year and celecoxib, cyclophosphamide, isotretinoin, fenofibrate, cholecalciferol for the second year) lasting 2 years; COMBAT IIS (celecoxib, vinorelbine, cyclophosphamide, cis-retinoic acid, fenofibrate, cholecalciferol) during 2 years for patients with soft tissue sarcomas and Ewing sarcomas; and COMBAT III (celecoxib, etoposide, temozolomide, fenofibrate, cholecalciferol, vitamin D3, bevacizumab for the first year and celecoxib, cyclophosphamide, isotretinoin, fenofibrate, cholecalciferol for the second year) lasting 2 years. Seventy-seven complete treatments were administered to 74 patients because 3 of them were re-challenged with a high-dose schedule. The investigators used these treatment schedules in a consecutive manner, displaying the progressive evolution of treatment protocols. The first 28 patients enrolled were treated with COMBAT I. Forty-four patients received COMBAT II and five patients COMBAT III. Overall, 43.1% of patients (median: 15.4 months) survived 2 years. The authors observed 62 patients with initially measurable diseases, 25 of whom progressed, but did not worsen during the follow-up period. The number of patients with measurable diseases who attained CR, PR, or SD after 6 months of COMBAT treatment had been defined as a clinical benefit, was 23%. Nine subjects showed a response 6 months after initiating COMBAT. During the follow-up, there were 50 (68%) deaths. In total, 24 patients survived: 6 (8%) patients had PD, 7 (9%) patients had PR/SD, and 11 (15%) had CR. Patients had a median time to response (CR/PR) of 6 months. Twelve children were affected by medulloblastoma (MBL)/primitive neuroectodermal tumors (PNET) and had the worst prognosis. They had a two-year OS of 33%; two children survived for a long time: 64 and 54 months. Twelve patients suffered from neuroblastoma, of which only two showed durable responses: one patient had a PR and progression-free survival (PFS) of 63 months, and one patient had a second very good PR at the last 12-month follow-up. Transient responses or stable disease with striking reduction in the dimension of the soft tissue mass have been shown by 8 patients. The patients with relapsed or progressive high-grade sarcoma did not have any long-term responses but had a palliative effect. Therapy led to response in 8 of 10 children with progressive LG tumors (LG glioma, giant bone cell tumors with lung metastasis, and LG sarcomas): tumor progression determined death, whereas a median PFS of 33 months was obtained in the remaining children. The treatment was administered on an outpatient basis and the tolerability was excellent. No therapy-related death or grade 3/4 non-hematological toxicity (except skin or hepatic toxicity) occurred. Grade 3 hepatic toxicities happened in only 8 children (11%). Grade 3 cheilitis occurred in 16 children (22%), when treated with cis-retinoic acid [77].

5.2. Case Series

Carcamo B. and Francia G. [78] reported a retrospective case series. Six children received metronomic treatment as a palliative cure because they had exhausted all therapeutic alternatives. Patient 1 was a male child diagnosed with metastatic rhabdoid tumor of the left kidney at about 3 years of age. At diagnosis, the metastases were located at the retroperitoneal level, in the lungs and bone marrow, as well as involving the renal vein and the inferior vena cava. The child, after courses of neoadjuvant chemotherapy and radiotherapy, had a progression of the disease in the lung and in bone marrow. At this point, the patient was treated with MC (etoposide 37.5 mg/m^2/day orally on days 1–21, followed by cyclophosphamide 50 mg/m^2/day orally on days 22–42, celecoxib 250 mg/m^2 orally twice per day, and valproic acid 15 mg/kg/day divided into two doses): the rhabdoid tumor did not recur, and the pulmonary nodules remained stable. Subsequently, the child died from transplant-related infectious complications without showing, on imaging, signs of recurrent rhabdoid tumor, which therefore responded effectively for 3 years due to treatment. Patient 2 (male) had anaplastic ependymoma from the age of 6. The tumor was partially removed by surgery, and later treated with radiotherapy. After 6 months, there was a relapse in the brain and metastases to the leptomeninges and thoracic spine. Metronomic therapy was therefore initiated with oral etoposide (50 mg/m^2/day for 21 days) alternating with oral CTX (50 mg/m^2/day for 21 days), valproic acid, and continuous celecoxib (120 mg/m^2 2 times/day), subsequently modified with sulindac (8 mg/kg/day). The patient had a CR and no evidence of residual disease after 2 years of therapy; he received another 18 months of MC and was lost to follow-up after 8 years of diagnosis and 4 years of metronomic treatment without recurrence. Patient 3 (female) was diagnosed with medulloblastoma at the age of 10 months, and surgically treated in a definitive manner. Upon examination of the ventricular liquor, the presence of microscopic disease was detected; therefore, the girl was treated with chemotherapy and radiotherapy. Six months after the completion of the therapy, she had a microscopic recurrence in the cerebrospinal fluid. She was then given MC and after 5 months she achieved complete remission. After 5 years, the MC was discontinued. Patient 4 (female), age 5, had medulloblastoma localized to the fourth ventricle without desmoplastic or anaplastic features. She was treated with surgical resection, radiotherapy, and vincristine for adjuvant purposes. After 3 months, she had a first relapse, treated with temozolomide, irradiation, and surgical resection on the residual nodule. After another 3 months, a second relapse occurred. She was administered with MC (temozolomide alternating with CTX, celecoxib, and valproic acid), to which the patient partially responded. Ten months after the start of the metronomic treatment, an infiltrative brain tumor formed which led to the patient's death 2 months later. Patient 5 (male) was diagnosed with metastatic neuroblastoma at age 9 and was treated with neoadjuvant chemotherapy, surgical resection, and finally with radiotherapy and isotretinoin. There was no evidence of residual disease at the end of treatment, but after 6 months there was a relapse treated with MC (etoposide alternating with CTX and continuous sulindac). Due to major hematological toxicities, it was necessary to reduce the dosage of etoposide and CTX, but the patient still showed a partial response at months 5 and 8. At the 11th month of treatment, there was a progression of the disease; thus, sulindac was replaced with celecoxib. After 2 months, the patient died. At 3 years of age, patient 6 (female) was diagnosed with type 2 neurocytoma of the spine. The tumor was treated surgically and later by irradiation, but a residual nodule remained. After 5 months, there was a progression of the disease with an increase in the size of the nodule and the formation of a second lesion; therefore, she received high-dose chemotherapy, developing important hematological toxicity and infectious complications, without obtaining any clinical benefit after 9 cycles. MC was then introduced (temozolomide alternating with CTX, valproic acid, celecoxib, and bevacizumab), and 3 months after the start of treatment there was a reduction in the size of the lesions. The metronomic treatment was gradually discontinued, but 10 months later it was necessary to resume it due to PD. It was possible to interrupt the treatment again, given that a stabilization of the disease was obtained; in the following 4 years of follow-up, the disease remained stable [78].

5.3. Phase I and Pilot Studies

Sterba and colleagues evaluated eight children with poor prognosis brain tumors treated by concomitant radiotherapy given 1×170 cGy, 5d/wk, for a total dose of 55/56 Gy, and temozolomide 90 mg/m^2/day for 42 days. The primary toxicity, recorded around day 21, was myelosuppression. Vomiting was the most common non-hematologic toxicity, but these were rare, and no cases of dose-limiting toxicity occurred. Six patients responded to treatment. Two patients with high-risk medulloblastoma had the best responses. Furthermore, there were one more complete and three partial responses at the end of temozolomide treatment [79]. This study reported promising responses in children with medulloblastomas, which progress soon after the first surgery.

A prospective, pilot, single-center study conducted in Mali evaluated the efficacy and safety of a metronomic combination schedule based on vincristine, cyclophosphamide, and methotrexate in 12 children with refractory cancer (Wilms tumor and retinoblastoma were the most frequent diagnoses). There was no objective response, but a disease stabilization occurred in 7 patients (58%). They continued therapy for 15 to 24 weeks. In total, 6 subjects (50%) were still living after 39 weeks of median follow-up. For at least six months after the end of treatment, 3 patients (25%) showed stable disease. One patient developed grade 4 anemia, and one patient grade 4 non febrile neutropenia. No other grade 3 or 4 toxicities were detected [80].

An open label, nonrandomized, multi-center pilot study was designed to assess the safety of celecoxib (250 mg/m^2 p.o. twice daily) combined with metronomic vinblastine (1 mg/m^2 i.v. thrice weekly) or cyclophosphamide (30 mg/m^2 p.o. daily) in patients under 21 years with a recurrent, refractory solid tumor. Patients with access were treated with vinblastine, and patients without access with cyclophosphamide. For the first week, the investigators administered only celecoxib to estimate safety and pharmacokinetics. In the second week, they added either vinblastine or cyclophosphamide. Thirty-three patients were enrolled, seventeen of whom were treated with vinblastine, and sixteen of whom with cyclophosphamide. Three patients of the vinblastine arm had a rapid disease progression, so were not evaluable and dropped out. The authors reported a small number of serious adverse events, none of which were likely associated with celecoxib, and observed no complete or partial responses. The median time to progression for the study was 8.5 weeks. Within 12 weeks, the progression of two-thirds of treated patients was observed, while 21% of patients received treatment for 12–24 weeks. In only 4 (13%) patients, a stable disease, lasting for 28 to 76 weeks, occurred. One patient presented a stable disease for over 15 months [81].

In a prospective, pilot, single-center study, 7 children from 3 to 21 years old with refractory cancer were administered with weekly vincristine (1.5 mg/m^2, days 1, 8, 15, and 22), daily cyclophosphamide (25 mg/m^2, days 1–21), twice-weekly methotrexate (15 mg/m^2, days 21–42), and daily valproic acid (30 mg/kg) followed by one week rest. In the succeeding cycles, vincristine was given only on weeks 1 and 5. The authors obtained a mean duration treatment of 34 ± 31 weeks at the end of the observation period; two patients were alive with a mean follow-up of 9 ± 11 weeks. Two patients had partial responses, which lasted more than 2 years. One death after a quick progression occurred in a patient with metastatic osteosarcoma; he received treatment for more than a year. Two progressions and one loss of follow-up happened during the treatment. Regarding adverse events, there were 1 grade 4 anemia and 1 grade 4 non-febrile neutropenia [82].

Another study enrolled 20 patients under the age of 22 with recurrent or progressive poor prognosis tumors without other therapeutic options. The treatment scheme provided continuous oral thalidomide and celecoxib with an alternation of oral etoposide and cyclophosphamide every 21 days for 6 months at antiangiogenic doses. Rapid disease progression occurred in seven patients exposed to therapy for less than 3 months. One more patient had less than 3 months of therapy because of toxicity (i.e., thrombosis). Three patients continued treatment for 3–6 months before disease progression. Eight patients underwent the 6-month treatment, three of whom exhibited a radiographic partial response (1 glioma, 2 ependymomas). Seven out of eight patients decided to prolong the therapy beyond 6 months, supporting its good tolerability. Some transitory grade 1 and 2 toxicities were observed, but none of these led to discontinuation of treatment. Instead, only one patient with a grade 3 toxicity (i.e., deep venous thrombosis related to thalidomide) interrupted therapy. A longer-term toxicities assessment was performed through a growth and development evaluation. Only one of three menstruating female patients at study enrollment experienced amenorrhea. No growth retardation was identified. For example, a patient continued treatment for over 2 consecutive years and maintained a protracted partial response. At the beginning of treatment, he was 94.1 cm tall (50th percentile) and achieved a height of 106 cm (50th percentile) two years later [83]. These data support the low toxicity of the metronomic scheme.

Manji and colleagues [84] conducted a phase I clinical trial with the aim of establishing the maximum tolerated doses of metronomic topotecan and pazopanib, detecting the toxicities of the combined schedule, and describing the pharmacokinetics of oral metronomic topotecan and pazopanib prepared as a powder for oral suspension (PfOS) in 30 patients (age 2–21 years) with relapsed or refractory solid tumors. The initial doses of topotecan and pazopanib PfOS were 0.12 mg/m^2 e 125 mg/m^2, respectively. To increase the doses, the Rolling Six design was used to reach the doses of 0.4 mg/m^2 and 160 mg/m^2 of topotecan and pazopanib PfOS, respectively. At the end of the study, the recommended dose was topotecan 0.22 mg/m^2/day and pazopanib PfOS 160 mg/m^2/day. The median duration of treatment was 1.9 months (0.1–44.2). For the response, it was possible to evaluate 25 patients. Ten patients (4 neuroblastoma, 3 osteosarcoma, 2 Ewing sarcoma/PNET, and 1 medulloblastoma) had stable disease with a median duration of 6.4 months (1.7–45.1). The longest stable disease was 45 months, and the therapy was continued as compassionate use even after the study ended [84].

Ali and El-Sayed performed a prospective study, enrolling 64 subjects aged ≤18 with relapsed or refractory solid tumors. The patients were treated with at least 3 cycles of metronomic chemotherapy, each for 6 weeks plus a 1-week break (total 21 weeks), including celecoxib, cyclophosphamide, vinblastine, and methotrexate. In case of partial response or stable disease, the treatment was prolonged beyond 21 weeks. The patients with isolated local relapse or distant metastasis received radiotherapy in combination with metronomic chemotherapy. In total, 49 patients (77%) had a favorable response: 22 (34%) exhibited a partial response and 27 (42%) showed a stable disease. In contrast, 15 (23%) patients developed a progressive disease. Acute toxicities were mild: 26 (41%) patients experienced grade 1 hematologic toxicities, 10 (16%) non-hematologic toxicities, and 5 (8%) suffered a combination of toxicities. No toxicities were found in 23 patients (36%). The most common hematological toxicity was anemia (n = 16), and the most frequent non-hematological toxicity was neuropathy (n = 6). The 1-year overall survival (OS) rate was 62.3% after a median follow-up of 14 months. The 1-year OS was lower for patients who exhibited a progressive disease (17%) than for patients who achieved a stable disease (70%) or a partial response (82%) [85].

5.4. Phase II Studies

Thirteen subjects (ten male and three female) were included in a European multi-center, proof-of-concept, multi-arm phase I/II platform study in pediatric patients with relapsed/refractory cancer. The children were treated with nivolumab 3 mg/kg intravenously twice (day 1 and day 15) in each 28-day cycle, and with metronomic cyclophosphamide 25 mg/m^2 orally twice daily, 1 week on and 1 week off. Patients were diagnosed from high-grade glioma (n = 3), neuroblastoma (n = 3), desmoplastic small round cell tumor-DSRCT (n = 3), alveolar rhabdomyosarcoma (n = 2), ependymoma (n = 1), and melanoma (n = 1). Metastases were present in 77% of patients (10/13). Previously, subjects were treated with a median of 3.5 treatment lines (range 1–5). During the study, 8 patients were irradiated at a dose of 20–40 Gy for locoregional metastases. There were 194 adverse events, but only 72 (37%) were probably drug-related: of these, 17 were grade 3 (15 of hematological type), whereas 5 were hematological grade 4. The 12 evaluable patients did not have a confirmed objective response. Stable disease occurred in 5 subjects. In the patient with DSRCT, there was a reduction in lesions observed at cycle 4 and confirmed at cycle 6, while in the patient with ependymoma the reduction in lesions observed at cycle 4 was not detectable at cycle 6. PD was the drop-out cause of all patients. The median PFS was 1.7 months (95% CI: 1.3–3.4), and the median OS was 3.4 months (95% CI: 2.2–13.5) [86].

In a multi-center, open-label, prospective two-stage phase II study, Robinson and colleagues evaluated an oral metronomic 5-drug regimen for children (age ≤ 21 years) with recurrent or progressive cancer. Cyclophosphamide and etoposide were administered in 21-day cycles and thalidomide, celecoxib, and fenofibrate were administered continuously. A total of 101 patients were enrolled in this study, and 97 began the treatment. Twenty-four patients (25%) appropriately performed 27 weeks of treatment without progressive disease (PD) or significant toxicity. Sixty-five (67%) interrupted therapy after PD, including three subjects who died of the disease. One death occurred because of complications of acute infection. Two subjects (2%) suspended therapy owing to toxicity. Five patients (5%) withdrew consent. Seven patients with ependymoma concluded therapy with stable disease (SD) or better. Twelve patients had low-grade glioma: three patients (25%) experienced PD within the first 9 weeks of the study, and nine patients (75%) experienced SD or better. One patient with an anaplastic glioneuronal tumor had an SD and proved an upcoming sustained complete response (CR). One subject with neurocytoma and chordoma had a PR. One patient with mixed malignant germ cell tumor, meningioma, hepatocellular carcinoma, and lymphangioma demonstrated an SD. Furthermore, one subject with choroid plexus carcinoma experienced PR. High-grade glioma and bone tumors had an unfavorable response rate. Three out of four patients affected by leukemia progressed soon after starting therapy. Six patients had medulloblastoma: three of them experienced the best response of SD or better, comprising one who showed a CR. One in three subjects with neuroblastoma ended therapy with SD. Most patients tolerated the treatment well. Hematological toxicities were the most common. One treatment-related death occurred for a patient with recurrent Ewing sarcoma who evolved Enterococcus faecalis bacteremia and neutropenia in week 4 of therapy. Two other patients dropped out of the study after the onset of toxicity: one with neutropenia and transaminase elevation, and one with a skin rash. The discontinuation of therapy led to the resolution of toxicities in both cases. Acute myelogenous leukemia (AML) was developed by an ependymoma patient exposed to the 5-drug regimen for 21 months. No other second malignancies have been reported [87].

A phase II clinical trial aimed to investigate the antitumor efficacy and the toxicity of metronomic weekly vinblastine (3 mg/m^2, weeks 1–7), daily cyclophosphamide (30 mg/m^2, days 1–21), twice weekly methotrexate (10 mg/m^2, days 21–42), and twice daily celecoxib (100–200–400 mg, body weight <20 kg, 20–50 kg, >50 kg, respectively, days 1–56) in relapsed/refractory pediatric brain tumors. This schedule was followed by 13 days of rest from chemotherapy. The authors enrolled 29 patients: 8 patients with ependymoma in the first cohort; and 3 patients with medulloblastoma, 5 with high-grade glioma, 11 with low-grade glioma, and 2 patients with other tumors in the second cohort. An SD for 4 months was observed in one patient with progressive ependymoma. Instead, a tumor progression occurred in the other seven ependymoma patients after two cycles. In the second cohort, the authors enrolled 21 patients: 1 subject dopped out for early progression, and 1 for osteomyelitis. In the low-grade glioma (LGG) group, there were 2 partial responses, 6 stable diseases, and 2 progressive diseases. In the high-grade glioma (HGG) group, there were 1 stable disease, and 4 progressive diseases. In the group of other tumors, there were 4 progressive diseases. The median number of cycles was 6.8 (range 1–12). The authors deduced that this metronomic regimen was effective, especially in the LGG group. The hematologic toxicity, in particular neutropenia, was the most usual (n = 11 patients). Overall, 11 patients presented grade 3/4 neutropenia. Grade 4 febrile neutropenia occurred in two patients (1 ependymoma, 1 LGG). Five patients exhibited grade 3/4 lymphopenia. The investigators did not observe any grade 4 thrombocytopenia and non-hematological adverse events. The most common non-hematologic AE (n = 8 grade 2/3) was hepatic enzyme increase. Three patients presented grade 2/3 mucositis. Other non-hematological AEs included grade 2 rhinitis/pharyngitis, fatigue, keratitis/conjunctivitis, diarrhea, anal fissure, dizziness, paresthesia, and grade 3 hypophosphatemia and constipation. Five patients interrupted, temporarily, treatment for grade 3/4 toxicity (hepatic and/or hematological), leading to provisional lowering of the dose [88].

This clinical trial was the development of a previous study by André and collaborators, where 16 children (age 3–21) with refractory or relapsing tumors without other therapeutic options were treated with the above-described scheme of treatment. However, the protocol was mildly changed from the initial schedule because of toxicity and clinical outcome observed in the first 3 patients treated. In fact, when the tumor progressed, evidencing active neo-angiogenesis in the course of chemotherapy break, celecoxib administration was continued between two cycles. Moreover, the investigators added a seventh vinblastine dose on day 42. While patients were taking methotrexate, they developed mucositis; therefore, the dosage was reduced from 15 mg/m^2 to 10 mg/m^2. Overall, the last implemented version of the protocol was administered to 10 out of 16 patients. At the end of the observation period, 1 patient was still on treatment, and 7 patients were alive. A child with Hodgkin's disease had the best response observed. The authors observed four stable diseases (25%), lasting 24 weeks or more, and four rapid tumor progressions (25%) in patients who had not completed the first cycle of treatment. Interestingly, they noted a rapid decline in pain and analgesic drug administration in 11 patients after the beginning of the metronomic therapy. Of greatest importance, tolerability was good. The toxicities were mostly hematological (83%). No child had alopecia and the investigators did not observe grade 3 or 4 nausea or vomiting. Toxicities did not lead to the treatment's end. Three patients reduced vinblastine dosage by 30% because of one peripheral neurotoxicity case and two severe hematological toxicity cases. Two patients discontinued celecoxib, one because of renal insufficiency, and the other for hemoptysis related to lung metastasis. Grade 2 or 3 mucositis led to a reduction in the methotrexate dose in 4 patients [89].

Fifty patients from 4 to 25 years of age were enrolled in a prospective, multi-center, nonrandomized, noncomparative, open-label combination phase II study, but only 44 were evaluated [90]. Patients were divided into 4 groups based on the type of tumor they were suffering from: (i) neuroblastoma group (NBL) consisting of 18 subjects; (ii) soft-tissue sarcoma group (STS) composed of 7 patients; (iii) bone sarcoma group (BS) including 10 subjects; (iv) miscellaneous group (Misc.) involving 9 patients. The therapeutic scheme included 6-week cycles of MC and two treatment-free weeks for a total of 56 days. The drugs used were: twice daily celecoxib 100–200–400 mg (< 20 kg, 20–50 kg, > 50 kg, respectively) for 56 days, weekly intravenous vinblastine at a dose of 3 mg/m^2 (days 1–8–15–22–29–36–43), and daily oral cyclophosphamide at a dose of 30 mg/m^2/day during three weeks (days 1–21) alternating with oral methotrexate at a dose of 10 mg/m^2 twice a week for three weeks (days 22–25–29–32–36–39–43). In 54% (24 out of 44) of patients, after 2 cycles of MC, no clinical signs of disease progression were detected, while in 46% (20 out of 44) of the subjects, it was necessary to interrupt the therapy due to a tangible PD. In total, 7 (4 NBL, 2 STS, 1 Misc.) out of 44 subjects (16%) clinically achieved a CR, PR, and SD from 2 cycles of treatment, whereas all BS patients (8 osteosarcoma and 2 Ewing sarcoma) had disease progression. The one-year PFS and the one-year OS of the whole cohort were 6.8% and 55.3%, respectively. In all, 33 out of 44 patients had 99 times grade 3/4 toxicity (24 events were grade 4). The most common toxicities were the hematological ones, in particular neutropenia: in fact, grade 3/4 neutropenia occurred 37 times in 24 subjects, while grade 3/4 thrombocytopenia occurred 6 times in 6 patients. Among the non-hematological toxicities, the most common was the elevation of transaminases: there was a grade 3 increase in liver enzymes in 6 subjects [90].

El Kababri and colleagues [91] performed a multi-center, prospective phase II study involving 98 pediatric patients with refractory/relapsing solid tumors or advanced disease. Patients were treated with 28-day cycles of oral cyclophosphamide (30 mg/m^2) and oral etoposide (25 mg/m^2) daily from day 1 to day 21, followed by 1 week off, and daily valproic acid (20 mg/kg) from day 1 to day 28. The subjects were suffering from neuroblastoma (n = 24), Ewing sarcoma (n = 18), osteosarcoma (n = 14), rhabdomyosarcoma (n = 14), and other miscellaneous diseases (n = 28). Metastases at diagnosis were present in 62 patients (63%). Patients received a median of 6 cycles (range 1–18) and, overall, tolerated the treatment well (no toxicity or maximum grade 1 toxicities in 95% of MC cycles). The only grade 3 or 4 toxicities observed were the hematological ones which occurred in 39 of 529 cycles. Toxicities did not necessitate a dose reduction. The 6-month OS was 40%; 1-year PFS was 19% and 1-year OS was 22%. Three children experienced a CR, 11 patients a PR, and

11 subjects had SD for more than 6 months. No relapses were observed 18 months after the end of treatment. Interestingly, 4 patients were relapse-free for 54 months. Ewing sarcoma, rhabdomyosarcoma, neuroblastoma, and Hodgkin lymphoma were most likely to respond to treatment, whereas osteosarcoma and Wilms' tumor did not respond to treatment even in terms of disease stabilization. Quality of life, according to Karnofsky/Lansky scores increased from 50% to 70% following MC [91].

5.5. Phase III Studies

In a multi-center, open label, randomized, controlled, phase III study, enrolling 371 patients aged 6 months to 21 years with rhabdomyosarcoma at high-risk of relapse standard treatment (9 cycles of ifosfamide, vincristine, dactinomycin alone or in combination with doxorubicin, and surgery or radiotherapy or both) led to remission. After remission, patients were randomized 1:1 to discontinue treatment or proceed with maintenance chemotherapy (6 cycles of vinorelbine 25 mg/m^2 i.v. on days 1, 8, and 15, and daily cyclophosphamide 25 mg/m^2 p.o. on days 1–28, for 24 weeks), given on an outpatient basis. Overall, 5.75 months was the median time from randomization to the end of maintenance chemotherapy. Seven children interrupted treatment on parents' request. At least one cycle modification occurred in 144 (80%) of 181 patients: the doses were lowered in the cases of neutropenia or thrombocytopenia in 74 (51%) patients, toxicity in 63 (44%), and other reasons in 7 patients (5%). Totally, 86.5% was 5-year overall survival in patients who received metronomic chemotherapy and 73.7% was 5-year overall survival in patients who discontinued treatment (HR 0.52 [95% CI 0.32–0.86]; $p = 0.0097$). Overall, 69.9% was 5-year disease-free survival in the group without further treatment, and 77.8% was 5-year disease-free survival in the group given maintenance chemotherapy. A relapse event occurred in 94 (25%) of 371 patients with similar distribution in the two groups. In particular, 6.9 months and 10.1 were the median times to relapse determined from the randomization date to the event in the arm given no further treatment, and in the arm with maintenance chemotherapy, respectively. There were 66 (18%) deaths: 42 (23%) of 186 in the subjects who stopped treatment, and 24 (13%) of 185 in the subjects still on chemotherapy. The patients died of relapse except for two patients in the group given no further treatment (one patient died of a surgical complication after a local relapse, and one was suicide) and two patients in the maintenance chemotherapy group (one patient with lung metastasis died of H1N1 infection, and one patient died of high-grade glioma, a second tumor appeared 69.7 months after rhabdomyosarcoma). The most common adverse event was grade 4 neutropenia, which occurred in 82 patients (45%). Fifty-six patients (31%) had grade 3 infection. Grade 3–4 leukopenia was reported in 136 (75%) of 181 patients, grade 3–4 neutropenia in 148 (82%) patients, anemia in 19 (10%) patients, and thrombocytopenia (1%) in 2 patients. One case (1%) of grade 4 non-hematological toxicity occurred. There were two treatment-related serious adverse events: one case of inappropriate antidiuretic hormone secretion, and one severe steppage gait with limb pain. The resolution of the events was reached, but in the patient with inappropriate antidiuretic hormone secretion, the treatment was permanently discontinued [92].

In a double-blinded, placebo-controlled, randomized clinical trial, 108 children aged from 5 to 15 years old were enrolled, affected by non-hematopoietic primarily extracranial solid tumors which progressed after at least 2 lines of chemotherapy. They were randomized 1:1 to receive placebo and best supportive care or metronomic chemotherapy and best supportive care. The eventual disease progression led to treatment stop. Metronomic chemotherapy consisted of two different alternating cycles; each cycle lasted 3 weeks. Cycle A was characterized by thalidomide, celecoxib, and etoposide administered daily; cycle B was characterized by thalidomide, celecoxib, and cyclophosphamide administered daily too. The placebo arm consisted of 52 patients; the metronomic chemotherapy arm consisted of 56 patients. At the cut-off date for data collection, the progression occurred in 107 patients (52 placebo; 55 metronomic chemotherapy), and death occurred in 107 patients (52 placebo; 55 metronomic chemotherapy). Overall, 2.9 months was the median follow-up for all the patients. Totally, 46 days and 49 days were the median PFS in the placebo group and in the metronomic chemotherapy group, respectively. In particular, 85 days was the OS in both groups. No complete responses occurred in either group. Eight patients had a stable disease and two patients had partial responses in the metronomic chemotherapy group. In a post hoc subgroup analysis, more than 3 cycles were administered to 40 patients and the PFS significantly increased (HR, 0.46; 95% CI, 0.23–0.93; p = 0.03). Furthermore, patients without a bone tumor benefited from metronomic chemotherapy for PFS (HR, 0.39; 95% CI, 0.18–0.81; p = 0.01) and OS (HR, 0.44; 95% CI, 0.21–0.90; p = 0.02). Grade 3–4 hematologic adverse events were the most common: anemia (7.1% vs. 11.7%), neutropenia (0% vs. 10.7%), thrombocytopenia (0% vs. 10.7%), and febrile neutropenia (0% vs. 8.8%) found in the placebo vs. metronomic chemotherapy group. The most common non-hematologic adverse event was mucositis (grade 1–2, 8.8%; grade 3–4, 5.3%) in the metronomic chemotherapy group. Eight patients (14.2%) needed a lowering of the dose, and nine patients had a delay in administration (metronomic chemotherapy group) [93]. The results obtained from the analysis of the subgroups showed an encouraging perspective in order to select the pediatric patients who can really have an advantage from the low-dose schedule.

In the same study, HRQoL (Health-Related Quality of Life) was also evaluated, using the PedsQOL Cancer module V.3, at baseline (A1), A2 (9 weeks or earlier if progressed), or A3 (18 weeks or earlier if progressed). No significant difference was observed in the change in the quality of life induced by each group from A1 to A2 in either mean total scores or individual domain scores. Moreover, no significant difference, defined as a 4.5-point improvement, was found either between bone sarcomas, other cancers, responders ($\geq$9 weeks of treatment), or non-responders. This is in line with the survival outcomes observed in the study [94].

6. Biomarkers of Metronomic Chemotherapy in Pediatric Patients

Diagnostic, predictive, and prognostic biomarkers are urgently needed to select which pediatric patients could benefit most from metronomic therapy and to monitor treatment activity. These therapies are slow acting and may not induce tumor regression. Moreover, diverse biomarkers may be needed according to the treatment and disease type.

Conflicting results have been published on cytokines as biomarkers of metronomic in the pediatric setting, some in favor and others opposing their role in predicting the effectiveness of metronomic therapies [81,83,87,95]. Driven biomarkers, as cytokines, may not be the best parameters, as there are different upstream and downstream pathways involved, and a single parameter (i.e., VEGF) may not be representative of all.

First, the previously described study of Kieran and colleagues [83] also evaluated serum, plasma, and urine levels of VEGF; basic fibroblast growth factor (bFGF); thrombospondin-1 (THBS1); and endostatin. Baseline THBS1 levels in serum above 75 µg/mL were associated with extended disease-free survival (>1 year) in three patients, while VEGF, bFGF, and endostatin levels during therapy did not show a change relative to baseline values. On the contrary, four subjects with baseline levels below 75 µg/mL demonstrated early progression. Nevertheless, THBS1 levels did not increase further during therapy, independently of radiographic response, stable disease, or rapid tumor progression [83].

Similarly, Stempak and collaborators assessed several circulating plasma proteins (i.e., VEGF, bFGF, THBS1, endostatin, soluble vascular and intercellular cell adhesion molecule) as surrogate markers of angiogenic activity in children with recurrent, refractory solid tumors continuously exposed to celecoxib and either low-dose vinblastine or cyclophosphamide. However, these markers were highly variable and showed no significant correlation with disease progression or stable disease [81].

André and colleagues monitored the influence of the maintenance of metronomic-like chemotherapy on angiogenic cytokines (i.e., VEGF, VEGFR-1, Ang-2), THBS1, Treg, and endothelial biomarkers (i.e., CEC, EPC, EMP), in 47 children with ALL. Along with a remarkable increase in THBS1 levels, a statistically significant reduction in EPC and EMP counts was detected during this stage. No appreciable variation was observed in other angiogenic markers or in the Treg fraction [95].

Furthermore, biomarkers of angiogenesis were evaluated in a pediatric population treated with sirolimus in combination with metronomic oral topotecan and cyclophosphamide. A statistically significant reduction has been observed in THBS1 and soluble VEGFR-2 plasma levels at 21 days if compared to baseline, demonstrating that this regimen can regulate angiogenic pathways [96].

Robinson and co-workers [87] conducted a surrogate marker analysis evaluating VEGF, bFGF, endostatin, and THBS1 levels in blood and urine samples at baseline and every ninth week, in children with recurrent or progressive cancer administered with the aforementioned 5-drug oral regimen. Interestingly, patients who completed therapy showed significantly higher baseline serum THBS1 levels than patients who discontinued treatment (median 9163 vs. 4299 ng/mL), suggesting an association with tumor susceptibility to antiangiogenic therapy. No statistical differences between completer and non-completer patients have been reported concerning the other biomarkers analyzed (VEGF, bFGF, and endostatin) [87].

Recently, Pramanik and colleagues evaluated serum VEGF and THBS1 concentrations in 108 pediatric patients with progressive malignancies who randomly received metronomic chemotherapy or placebo [97]. They found no differences for both these biomarkers at baseline and two other time points (week-9 (A2) and week-18 (A3) or earlier if progressed) between the two arms, as well as at the change from baseline to A2 in each group. Responders to metronomic chemotherapy, who completed at least 3 cycles, displayed significantly inferior levels of mean baseline VEGF [659.7 vs. 1143.9 µg/mL] and a substantial decrease in THBS1 from baseline to A2 [−4.43 vs. 1.7 µg/mL], as opposed to non-responders. Responders in the placebo group did not show such alterations [97].

Based on these conflicting results, VEGF and THBS1 cannot yet be considered valid biomarkers of the response to metronomic chemotherapy in pediatric patients.

Moreover, studies have investigated the role of other potential biomarkers such as HIF-1α expression [98], and factors implied in resistance to metronomic chemotherapy (i.e., cathepsin B, ANXA3) [99].

In particular, Tho and collaborators demonstrated that among the clinically used topoisomerase II (TOP2)–targeting drugs evaluated in their study (i.e., mitoxantrone, doxorubicin, and etoposide), only mitoxantrone induced a potent, dose- and time-dependent, inhibition of HIF-1α expression under hypoxic conditions, similar to that caused by cycloheximide. In vitro experiments using HIF-1α mRNA corroborated that mitoxantrone inhibited the HIF-1α translation step. Noteworthy, mitoxantrone treatment was associated with increased polysome-bound HIF-1α and decreased VEGF-A mRNA levels [98].

Immune cells such as Treg cells and myeloid-derived suppressor cells may also be considered as potential biomarkers.

However, the studies mentioned above have several limitations. First, the small groups of proteins evaluated in these studies do not represent the total effect of all the regulators of angiogenesis. Furthermore, the absence of standard reference ranges to detect circulating proteins could lead to a problematic interpretation of the results.

It is also difficult to identify potential biomarkers for metronomic chemotherapy because of the various mechanisms of action, multiple drug combinations, and many clinical settings used. However, the search for new potential biomarkers may be plausible in the future thanks to the broad accessibility of next-generation sequencing. Further biomarkers could be considered for measuring the efficacy of metronomic chemotherapy such as circulating cell-free DNA, circulating endothelial cells, and circulating endothelial precursor cells and micro-particles. Future studies including homogenous patient populations and focusing on validating surrogate markers to monitor treatment activity are needed.

7. Conclusions and Future Perspective

The costs of cancer treatment have increased worldwide over the years, especially with the advent of immunotherapy and targeted therapy. Within the USA, the overall national costs of cancer care are predicted to rise by over 30% from 2015 to 2030, corresponding to over $245 billion, based on population growth [100].

Metronomic chemotherapy could represent a valid method to reduce the economic burden of anticancer therapy in the pediatric setting. In fact, most metronomic regimens involve the use of inexpensive, old drugs available for oral administration (Figure 2), thus reducing costs for hospitalization, intravenous injections, risk of infection, and travel or accommodation outlay for patients and their families who must visit well-equipped health centers in large and distant cities. Side effects associated with low-dose metronomic chemotherapy are usually limited compared with MTD therapy. Therefore, treatment complications and the frequency of monitoring tests could be reduced, resulting in improved quality of life, both for patients and caregivers, and further lowering of costs for cancer treatment without impairing clinical outcomes [10].

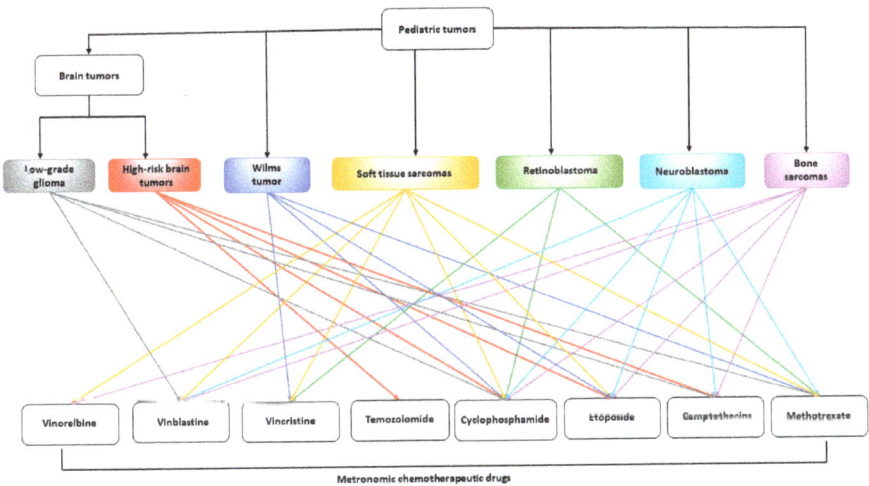

Figure 2. Chemotherapeutic drugs metronomically administered in pediatric clinical trials in different tumor types.

Maintenance therapy in pediatric patients is administered to hamper cancer progression and/or relapse after successful initial therapy. It aims at extending survival while preserving the quality of life [101]. Metronomic chemotherapy represents a good option for maintenance therapy because it is usually well-tolerated, and it can be given orally and at a relatively low cost. Moreover, its activity on angiogenesis, cancer stem cells, and the regulation of the immune system allows the possibility to overcome resistance and delay tumor progression [99].

However, long-term morbidities such as the development of secondary tumors have become a relevant issue for pediatric patients. Chemotherapy use including alkylating agents has been correlated with the increased risk of hematologic malignancies [102]. Therefore, it will be of interest to deeply evaluate the impact of the total dose of a metronomic cyclophosphamide-based schedule, which may expose pediatric individuals to the risk of developing secondary tumors. Moreover, intensive surveillance and counselling of these patients are necessary to monitor and anticipate secondary tumor diagnosis and treatment [102].

All metronomic phase I and II studies published in the last decade reveal good tolerance and acceptable side effect profiles in outpatient care without affecting the normal growth of children [83]. Most of the evidence comes from preclinical studies or phase I and phase II clinical studies performed in the relapse/refractory setting. Unfortunately, the lack of large, randomized phase III trials and of reliable biomarkers made the clinicians question using a low-dose, continuous regimen as the standard of care in pediatric oncology. Therefore, further phase III studies are urgently needed to validate the role of metronomic chemotherapy in the present and future disease control [9]. As metronomic chemotherapy is assumed to display its effect also by immunomodulation, we might expect interesting results from a combination of immunotherapies. Furthermore, a proper combination with radiotherapy, MTD chemotherapy, and novel targeted drugs should be tested in future research [9].

The most plausible approach may be to proceed with investigations and gradually integrate metronomic treatments into the current clinical practice, taking advantage of their low toxicity, oral administration and, therefore, the feasibility of a more comfortable home-based treatment.

Author Contributions: Conceptualization, G.B.; writing—original draft preparation, M.B., E.F. and S.C.; writing—review and editing, G.B. and M.B.; supervision, G.B. All authors have read and agreed to the published version of the manuscript.

Funding: This research received no external funding.

Institutional Review Board Statement: Not applicable.

Informed Consent Statement: Not applicable.

Acknowledgments: The authors thank Giulia Gianfilippo for her suggestions to the manuscript preparation.

Conflicts of Interest: The authors declare no conflict of interest.

References

1. Bocci, G.; Kerbel, R.S. Pharmacokinetics of metronomic chemotherapy: A neglected but crucial aspect. *Nat. Rev. Clin. Oncol.* **2016**, *13*, 659–673. [CrossRef]
2. Bocci, G.; Francia, G.; Man, S.; Lawler, J.; Kerbel, R.S. Thrombospondin 1, a mediator of the antiangiogenic effects of low-dose metronomic chemotherapy. *Proc. Natl. Acad. Sci. USA* **2003**, *100*, 12917–12922. [CrossRef]
3. Bocci, G.; Nicolaou, K.C.; Kerbel, R.S. Protracted low-dose effects on human endothelial cell proliferation and survival in vitro reveal a selective antiangiogenic window for various chemotherapeutic drugs. *Cancer Res.* **2002**, *62*, 6938–6943.
4. Natale, G.; Bocci, G. Does metronomic chemotherapy induce tumor angiogenic dormancy? A review of available preclinical and clinical data. *Cancer Lett.* **2018**, *432*, 28–37. [CrossRef]
5. Folkins, C.; Man, S.; Xu, P.; Shaked, Y.; Hicklin, D.J.; Kerbel, R.S. Anticancer therapies combining antiangiogenic and tumor cell cytotoxic effects reduce the tumor stem-like cell fraction in glioma xenograft tumors. *Cancer Res.* **2007**, *67*, 3560–3564. [CrossRef] [PubMed]
6. Banissi, C.; Ghiringhelli, F.; Chen, L.; Carpentier, A.F. Treg depletion with a low-dose metronomic temozolomide regimen in a rat glioma model. *Cancer Immunol. Immunother.* **2009**, *58*, 1627–1634. [CrossRef]
7. Steliarova-Foucher, E.; Colombet, M.; Ries, L.A.G.; Moreno, F.; Dolya, A.; Bray, F.; Hesseling, P.; Shin, H.Y.; Stiller, C.A. International incidence of childhood cancer, 2001-10: A population-based registry study. *Lancet. Oncol.* **2017**, *18*, 719–731. [CrossRef]
8. World Health Organization. *Framework: WHO Global Initiative for Childhood Cancer*; WHO: Geneva, Switzerland, 2020; ISBN 9789240025271.
9. Pramanik, R.; Bakhshi, S. Metronomic therapy in pediatric oncology: A snapshot. *Pediatr. Blood Cancer* **2019**, *66*, e27811. [CrossRef] [PubMed]
10. André, N.; Banavali, S.; Snihur, Y.; Pasquier, E. Has the time come for metronomics in low-income and middle-income countries? *Lancet. Oncol.* **2013**, *14*, e239–e248. [CrossRef]
11. Newman, E.A.; Abdessalam, S.; Aldrink, J.H.; Austin, M.; Heaton, T.E.; Bruny, J.; Ehrlich, P.; Dasgupta, R.; Baertschiger, R.M.; Lautz, T.B.; et al. Update on neuroblastoma. *J. Pediatr. Surg.* **2019**, *54*, 383–389. [CrossRef] [PubMed]
12. Klement, G.; Baruchel, S.; Rak, J.; Man, S.; Clark, K.; Hicklin, D.J.; Bohlen, P.; Kerbel, R.S. Continuous low-dose therapy with vinblastine and VEGF receptor-2 antibody induces sustained tumor regression without overt toxicity. *J. Clin. Investig.* **2000**, *105*, R15–R24. [CrossRef] [PubMed]
13. Nör, J.E.; Christensen, J.; Mooney, D.J.; Polverini, P.J. Vascular endothelial growth factor (VEGF)-mediated angiogenesis is associated with enhanced endothelial cell survival and induction of Bcl-2 expression. *Am. J. Pathol.* **1999**, *154*, 375–384. [CrossRef]

4. Tran, J.; Rak, J.; Sheehan, C.; Saibil, S.D.; LaCasse, E.; Korneluk, R.G.; Kerbel, R.S. Marked induction of the IAP family antiapoptotic proteins survivin and XIAP by VEGF in vascular endothelial cells. *Biochem. Biophys. Res. Commun.* **1999**, *264*, 781–788. [CrossRef] [PubMed]
5. O'Connor, D.S.; Schechner, J.S.; Adida, C.; Mesri, M.; Rothermel, A.L.; Li, F.; Nath, A.K.; Pober, J.S.; Altieri, D.C. Control of apoptosis during angiogenesis by survivin expression in endothelial cells. *Am. J. Pathol.* **2000**, *156*, 393–398. [CrossRef]
6. Vacca, A.; Iurlaro, M.; Ribatti, D.; Minischetti, M.; Nico, B.; Ria, R.; Pellegrino, A.; Dammacco, F. Antiangiogenesis is produced by nontoxic doses of vinblastine. *Blood* **1999**, *94*, 4143–4155. [CrossRef] [PubMed]
7. Guba, M.; von Breitenbuch, P.; Steinbauer, M.; Koehl, G.; Flegel, S.; Hornung, M.; Bruns, C.J.; Zuelke, C.; Farkas, S.; Anthuber, M.; et al. Rapamycin inhibits primary and metastatic tumor growth by antiangiogenesis: Involvement of vascular endothelial growth factor. *Nat. Med.* **2002**, *8*, 128–135. [CrossRef]
8. Misawa, A.; Hosoi, H.; Tsuchiya, K.; Sugimoto, T. Rapamycin inhibits proliferation of human neuroblastoma cells without suppression of MycN. *Int. J. cancer* **2003**, *104*, 233–237. [CrossRef] [PubMed]
9. Marimpietri, D.; Nico, B.; Vacca, A.; Mangieri, D.; Catarsi, P.; Ponzoni, M.; Ribatti, D. Synergistic inhibition of human neuroblastoma-related angiogenesis by vinblastine and rapamycin. *Oncogene* **2005**, *24*, 6785–6795. [CrossRef]
10. Kim, E.S.; Soffer, S.Z.; Huang, J.; McCrudden, K.W.; Yokoi, A.; Manley, C.A.; Middlesworth, W.; Kandel, J.J.; Yamashiro, D.J. Distinct response of experimental neuroblastoma to combination antiangiogenic strategies. *J. Pediatr. Surg.* **2002**, *37*, 518–522. [CrossRef]
11. Puppo, M.; Battaglia, F.; Ottaviano, C.; Delfino, S.; Ribatti, D.; Varesio, L.; Bosco, M.C. Topotecan inhibits vascular endothelial growth factor production and angiogenic activity induced by hypoxia in human neuroblastoma by targeting hypoxia-inducible factor-1alpha and -2alpha. *Mol. Cancer Ther.* **2008**, *7*, 1974–1984. [CrossRef] [PubMed]
12. Hartwich, J.; Orr, W.S.; Ng, C.Y.; Spence, Y.; Morton, C.; Davidoff, A.M. HIF-1α activation mediates resistance to anti-angiogenic therapy in neuroblastoma xenografts. *J. Pediatr. Surg.* **2013**, *48*, 39–46. [CrossRef] [PubMed]
13. Seeger, R.C.; Brodeur, G.M.; Sather, H.; Dalton, A.; Siegel, S.E.; Wong, K.Y.; Hammond, D. Association of multiple copies of the N-myc oncogene with rapid progression of neuroblastomas. *N. Engl. J. Med.* **1985**, *313*, 1111–1116. [CrossRef] [PubMed]
14. Meitar, D.; Crawford, S.E.; Rademaker, A.W.; Cohn, S.L. Tumor angiogenesis correlates with metastatic disease, N-myc amplification, and poor outcome in human neuroblastoma. *J. Clin. Oncol. Off. J. Am. Soc. Clin. Oncol.* **1996**, *14*, 405–414. [CrossRef] [PubMed]
15. Sköldenberg, E.G.; Larsson, A.; Jakobson, A.; Hedborg, F.; Kogner, P.; Christofferson, R.H.; Azarbayjani, F. The angiogenic growth factors HGF and VEGF in serum and plasma from neuroblastoma patients. *Anticancer Res.* **2009**, *29*, 3311–3319.
16. Taschner-Mandl, S.; Schwarz, M.; Blaha, J.; Kauer, M.; Kromp, F.; Frank, N.; Rifatbegovic, F.; Weiss, T.; Ladenstein, R.; Hohenegger, M.; et al. Metronomic topotecan impedes tumor growth of MYCN amplified neuroblastoma cells in vitro and in vivo by therapy induced senescence. *Oncotarget* **2016**, *7*, 3571–3586. [CrossRef]
17. Leontieva, O.V.; Natarajan, V.; Demidenko, Z.N.; Burdelya, L.G.; Gudkov, A.V.; Blagosklonny, M.V. Hypoxia suppresses conversion from proliferative arrest to cellular senescence. *Proc. Natl. Acad. Sci. USA* **2012**, *109*, 13314–13318. [CrossRef]
18. Rapisarda, A.; Uranchimeg, B.; Sordet, O.; Pommier, Y.; Shoemaker, R.H.; Melillo, G. Topoisomerase I-mediated inhibition of hypoxia-inducible factor 1: Mechanism and therapeutic implications. *Cancer Res.* **2004**, *64*, 1475–1482. [CrossRef]
19. Kumar, S.; Mokhtari, R.B.; Sheikh, R.; Wu, B.; Zhang, L.; Xu, P.; Man, S.; Oliveira, I.D.; Yeger, H.; Kerbel, R.S.; et al. Metronomic oral topotecan with pazopanib is an active antiangiogenic regimen in mouse models of aggressive pediatric solid tumor. *Clin. Cancer Res. Off. J. Am. Assoc. Cancer Res.* **2011**, *17*, 5656–5667. [CrossRef] [PubMed]
20. Kumar, S.; Mokhtari, R.B.; Oliveira, I.D.; Islam, S.; Toledo, S.R.C.; Yeger, H.; Baruchel, S. Tumor dynamics in response to antiangiogenic therapy with oral metronomic topotecan and pazopanib in neuroblastoma xenografts. *Transl. Oncol.* **2013**, *6*, 493–503. [CrossRef]
21. Zhang, L.; Wu, B.; Baruchel, S. Oral Metronomic Topotecan Sensitizes Crizotinib Antitumor Activity in ALKF1174L Drug-Resistant Neuroblastoma Preclinical Models. *Transl. Oncol.* **2017**, *10*, 604–611. [CrossRef] [PubMed]
22. Morscher, R.J.; Aminzadeh-Gohari, S.; Hauser-Kronberger, C.; Feichtinger, R.G.; Sperl, W.; Kofler, B. Combination of metronomic cyclophosphamide and dietary intervention inhibits neuroblastoma growth in a CD1-nu mouse model. *Oncotarget* **2016**, *7*, 17060–17073. [CrossRef]
23. Aminzadeh-Gohari, S.; Feichtinger, R.G.; Vidali, S.; Locker, F.; Rutherford, T.; O'Donnel, M.; Stöger-Kleiber, A.; Mayr, J.A.; Sperl, W.; Kofler, B. A ketogenic diet supplemented with medium-chain triglycerides enhances the anti-tumor and anti-angiogenic efficacy of chemotherapy on neuroblastoma xenografts in a CD1-nu mouse model. *Oncotarget* **2017**, *8*, 64728–64744. [CrossRef]
24. Stupp, R.; Hegi, M.E.; Mason, W.P.; van den Bent, M.J.; Taphoorn, M.J.B.; Janzer, R.C.; Ludwin, S.K.; Allgeier, A.; Fisher, B.; Belanger, K.; et al. Effects of radiotherapy with concomitant and adjuvant temozolomide versus radiotherapy alone on survival in glioblastoma in a randomised phase III study: 5-year analysis of the EORTC-NCIC trial. *Lancet. Oncol.* **2009**, *10*, 459–466. [CrossRef]
25. Udaka, Y.T.; Packer, R.J. Pediatric Brain Tumors. *Neurol. Clin.* **2018**, *36*, 533–556. [CrossRef]
26. Bello, L.; Lucini, V.; Carrabba, G.; Giussani, C.; Machluf, M.; Pluderi, M.; Nikas, D.; Zhang, J.; Tomei, G.; Villani, R.M.; et al. Simultaneous inhibition of glioma angiogenesis, cell proliferation, and invasion by a naturally occurring fragment of human metalloproteinase-2. *Cancer Res.* **2001**, *61*, 8730–8736.

37. Bello, L.; Carrabba, G.; Giussani, C.; Lucini, V.; Cerutti, F.; Scaglione, F.; Landré, J.; Pluderi, M.; Tomei, G.; Villani, R.; et al. Low-dose chemotherapy combined with an antiangiogenic drug reduces human glioma growth in vivo. *Cancer Res.* **2001**, *61*, 7501–7506.
38. Rapisarda, A.; Zalek, J.; Hollingshead, M.; Braunschweig, T.; Uranchimeg, B.; Bonomi, C.A.; Borgel, S.D.; Carter, J.P.; Hewitt, S.M.; Shoemaker, R.H.; et al. Schedule-dependent inhibition of hypoxia-inducible factor-1alpha protein accumulation, angiogenesis, and tumor growth by topotecan in U251-HRE glioblastoma xenografts. *Cancer Res.* **2004**, *64*, 6845–6848. [CrossRef]
39. Rapisarda, A.; Hollingshead, M.; Uranchimeg, B.; Bonomi, C.A.; Borgel, S.D.; Carter, J.P.; Gehrs, B.; Raffeld, M.; Kinders, R.J.; Parchment, R.; et al. Increased antitumor activity of bevacizumab in combination with hypoxia inducible factor-1 inhibition. *Mol. Cancer Ther.* **2009**, *8*, 1867–1877. [CrossRef]
40. Kim, J.T.; Kim, J.-S.; Ko, K.W.; Kong, D.-S.; Kang, C.-M.; Kim, M.H.; Son, M.J.; Song, H.S.; Shin, H.-J.; Lee, D.-S.; et al. Metronomic treatment of temozolomide inhibits tumor cell growth through reduction of angiogenesis and augmentation of apoptosis in orthotopic models of gliomas. *Oncol. Rep.* **2006**, *16*, 33–39. [CrossRef]
41. Carli, M.; Donnini, S.; Pellegrini, C.; Coppi, E.; Bocci, G. Opioid receptors beyond pain control: The role in cancer pathology and the debated importance of their pharmacological modulation. *Pharmacol. Res.* **2020**, *159*, 104938. [CrossRef]
42. Kang, S.M.; Rosales, J.L.; Meier-Stephenson, V.; Kim, S.; Lee, K.Y.; Narendran, A. Genome-wide loss-of-function genetic screening identifies opioid receptor µ1 as a key regulator of L-asparaginase resistance in pediatric acute lymphoblastic leukemia. *Oncogene* **2017**, *36*, 5910–5913. [CrossRef] [PubMed]
43. Iorio, A.L.; da Ros, M.; Genitori, L.; Lucchesi, M.; Colelli, F.; Signorino, G.; Cardile, F.; Laffi, G.; de Martino, M.; Pisano, C.; et al. Tumor response of temozolomide in combination with morphine in a xenograft model of human glioblastoma. *Oncotarget* **2017**, *8*, 89595–89606. [CrossRef] [PubMed]
44. Chen, C.S.; Doloff, J.C.; Waxman, D.J. Intermittent metronomic drug schedule is essential for activating antitumor innate immunity and tumor xenograft regression. *Neoplasia* **2014**, *16*, 84–96. [CrossRef] [PubMed]
45. Doloff, J.C.; Waxman, D.J. VEGF receptor inhibitors block the ability of metronomically dosed cyclophosphamide to activate innate immunity-induced tumor regression. *Cancer Res.* **2012**, *72*, 1103–1115. [CrossRef] [PubMed]
46. Wu, J.; Waxman, D.J. Metronomic cyclophosphamide schedule-dependence of innate immune cell recruitment and tumor regression in an implanted glioma model. *Cancer Lett.* **2014**, *353*, 272–280. [CrossRef]
47. Wu, J.; Waxman, D.J. Metronomic cyclophosphamide eradicates large implanted GL261 gliomas by activating antitumor Cd8(+) T-cell responses and immune memory. *Oncoimmunology* **2015**, *4*, e1005521. [CrossRef]
48. Ferrer-Font, L.; Arias-Ramos, N.; Lope-Piedrafita, S.; Julià-Sapé, M.; Pumarola, M.; Arús, C.; Candiota, A.P. Metronomic treatment in immunocompetent preclinical GL261 glioblastoma: Effects of cyclophosphamide and temozolomide. *NMR Biomed.* **2017**, *30*, e3748. [CrossRef]
49. Delgado-Goñi, T.; Julià-Sapé, M.; Candiota, A.P.; Pumarola, M.; Arús, C. Molecular imaging coupled to pattern recognition distinguishes response to temozolomide in preclinical glioblastoma. *NMR Biomed.* **2014**, *27*, 1333–1345. [CrossRef]
50. Karachi, A.; Yang, C.; Dastmalchi, F.; Sayour, E.J.; Huang, J.; Azari, H.; Long, Y.; Flores, C.; Mitchell, D.A.; Rahman, M. Modulation of temozolomide dose differentially affects T-cell response to immune checkpoint inhibition. *Neuro. Oncol.* **2019**, *21*, 730–741. [CrossRef]
51. Loeb, D.M.; Thornton, K.; Shokek, O. Pediatric soft tissue sarcomas. *Surg. Clin. N. Am.* **2008**, *88*, 615–627. [CrossRef]
52. Grohar, P.J.; Janeway, K.A.; Mase, L.D.; Schiffman, J.D. Advances in the Treatment of Pediatric Bone Sarcomas. *Am. Soc. Clin. Oncol. Educ. book. Am. Soc. Clin. Oncol. Annu. Meet.* **2017**, *37*, 725–735. [CrossRef] [PubMed]
53. Zhang, L.; Yu, D.; Hicklin, D.J.; Hannay, J.A.F.; Ellis, L.M.; Pollock, R.E. Combined anti-fetal liver kinase 1 monoclonal antibody and continuous low-dose doxorubicin inhibits angiogenesis and growth of human soft tissue sarcoma xenografts by induction of endothelial cell apoptosis. *Cancer Res.* **2002**, *62*, 2034–2042. [PubMed]
54. Zhu, X.; Yin, H.; Mei, J. Inhibition of tumors cell growth in osteosarcoma-bearing SD rats through a combination of conventional and metronomic scheduling of neoadjuvant chemotherapy. *Acta Pharmacol. Sin.* **2010**, *31*, 970–976. [CrossRef]
55. Dimaras, H.; Kimani, K.; Dimba, E.A.O.; Gronsdahl, P.; White, A.; Chan, H.S.L.; Gallie, B.L. Retinoblastoma. *Lancet* **2012**, *379*, 1436–1446. [CrossRef]
56. Abramson, D.H.; Shields, C.L.; Munier, F.L.; Chantada, G.L. Treatment of Retinoblastoma in 2015: Agreement and Disagreement. *JAMA Ophthalmol.* **2015**, *133*, 1341–1347. [CrossRef]
57. Winter, U.; Mena, H.A.; Negrotto, S.; Arana, E.; Pascual-Pasto, G.; Laurent, V.; Suñol, M.; Chantada, G.L.; Carcaboso, A.M.; Schaiquevich, P. Schedule-Dependent Antiangiogenic and Cytotoxic Effects of Chemotherapy on Vascular Endothelial and Retinoblastoma Cells. *PLoS ONE* **2016**, *11*, e0160094. [CrossRef] [PubMed]
58. Brown, P.; Inaba, H.; Annesley, C.; Beck, J.; Colace, S.; Dallas, M.; DeSantes, K.; Kelly, K.; Kitko, C.; Lacayo, N.; et al. Pediatric Acute Lymphoblastic Leukemia, Version 2.2020, NCCN Clinical Practice Guidelines in Oncology. *J. Natl. Compr. Canc. Netw.* **2020**, *18*, 81–112. [CrossRef] [PubMed]
59. Tissing, W.J.E.; Meijerink, J.P.P.; den Boer, M.L.; Pieters, R. Molecular determinants of glucocorticoid sensitivity and resistance in acute lymphoblastic leukemia. *Leukemia* **2003**, *17*, 17–25. [CrossRef]
60. Bornhauser, B.C.; Bonapace, L.; Lindholm, D.; Martinez, R.; Cario, G.; Schrappe, M.; Niggli, F.K.; Schäfer, B.W.; Bourquin, J.P. Low-dose arsenic trioxide sensitizes glucocorticoid-resistant acute lymphoblastic leukemia cells to dexamethasone via an Akt-dependent pathway. *Blood* **2007**, *110*, 2084–2091. [CrossRef]

1. Pelicano, H.; Martin, D.S.; Xu, R.-H.; Huang, P. Glycolysis inhibition for anticancer treatment. *Oncogene* **2006**, *25*, 4633–4646. [CrossRef]
2. Gu, L.; Yi, Z.; Zhang, Y.; Ma, Z.; Zhu, Y.; Gao, J. Low dose of 2-deoxy-D-glucose kills acute lymphoblastic leukemia cells and reverses glucocorticoid resistance via N-linked glycosylation inhibition under normoxia. *Oncotarget* **2017**, *8*, 30978–30991. [CrossRef]
3. Pui, C.-H.; Evans, W.E. Treatment of acute lymphoblastic leukemia. *N. Engl. J. Med.* **2006**, *354*, 166–178. [CrossRef]
4. Lomelino, C.L.; Andring, J.T.; McKenna, R.; Kilberg, M.S. Asparagine synthetase: Function, structure, and role in disease. *J. Biol. Chem.* **2017**, *292*, 19952–19958. [CrossRef]
5. Ueno, T.; Ohtawa, K.; Mitsui, K.; Kodera, Y.; Hiroto, M.; Matsushima, A.; Inada, Y.; Nishimura, H. Cell cycle arrest and apoptosis of leukemia cells induced by L-asparaginase. *Leukemia* **1997**, *11*, 1858–1861. [CrossRef]
6. Sugimoto, K.; Suzuki, H.I.; Fujimura, T.; Ono, A.; Kaga, N.; Isobe, Y.; Sasaki, M.; Taka, H.; Miyazono, K.; Komatsu, N. A clinically attainable dose of L-asparaginase targets glutamine addiction in lymphoid cell lines. *Cancer Sci.* **2015**, *106*, 1534–1543. [CrossRef]
7. Zhang, L.; Marrano, P.; Wu, B.; Kumar, S.; Thorner, P.; Baruchel, S. Combined Antitumor Therapy with Metronomic Topotecan and Hypoxia-Activated Prodrug, Evofosfamide, in Neuroblastoma and Rhabdomyosarcoma Preclinical Models. *Clin. Cancer Res.* **2016**, *22*, 2697–2708. [CrossRef]
8. Murai, J.; Huang, S.N.; Das, B.B.; Renaud, A.; Zhang, Y.; Doroshow, J.H.; Ji, J.; Takeda, S.; Pommier, Y. Trapping of PARP1 and PARP2 by Clinical PARP Inhibitors. *Cancer Res.* **2012**, *72*, 5588–5599. [CrossRef]
9. Murai, J.; Huang, S.-Y.N.; Renaud, A.; Zhang, Y.; Ji, J.; Takeda, S.; Morris, J.; Teicher, B.; Doroshow, J.H.; Pommier, Y. Stereospecific PARP trapping by BMN 673 and comparison with olaparib and rucaparib. *Mol. Cancer Ther.* **2014**, *13*, 433–443. [CrossRef]
10. Horton, J.K.; Wilson, S.H. Predicting enhanced cell killing through PARP inhibition. *Mol. Cancer Res.* **2013**, *11*, 13–18. [CrossRef]
11. Smith, M.A.; Reynolds, C.P.; Kang, M.H.; Kolb, E.A.; Gorlick, R.; Carol, H.; Lock, R.B.; Keir, S.T.; Maris, J.M.; Billups, C.A.; et al. Synergistic activity of PARP inhibition by talazoparib (BMN 673) with temozolomide in pediatric cancer models in the pediatric preclinical testing program. *Clin. Cancer Res. Off. J. Am. Assoc. Cancer Res.* **2015**, *21*, 819–832. [CrossRef]
12. Pawlik, C.A.; Houghton, P.J.; Stewart, C.F.; Cheshire, P.J.; Richmond, L.B.; Danks, M.K. Effective schedules of exposure of medulloblastoma and rhabdomyosarcoma xenografts to topotecan correlate with in vitro assays. *Clin. Cancer Res. Off. J. Am. Assoc. Cancer Res.* **1998**, *4*, 1995–2002.
13. Zhou, Q.; Guo, P.; Wang, X.; Nuthalapati, S.; Gallo, J.M. Preclinical pharmacokinetic and pharmacodynamic evaluation of metronomic and conventional temozolomide dosing regimens. *J. Pharmacol. Exp. Ther.* **2007**, *321*, 265–275. [CrossRef]
14. van Geel, R.M.J.M.; Beijnen, J.H.; Schellens, J.H.M. Concise drug review: Pazopanib and axitinib. *Oncologist* **2012**, *17*, 1081–1089. [CrossRef]
15. Hartmann, J.T.; Lipp, H.-P. Camptothecin and podophyllotoxin derivatives: Inhibitors of topoisomerase I and II—mechanisms of action, pharmacokinetics and toxicity profile. *Drug Saf.* **2006**, *29*, 209–230. [CrossRef]
16. Roux, C.; Revon-Rivière, G.; Gentet, J.C.; Verschuur, A.; Scavarda, D.; Saultier, P.; Appay, R.; Padovani, L.; André, N. Metronomic Maintenance with Weekly Vinblastine after Induction with Bevacizumab-Irinotecan in Children with Low-grade Glioma Prevents Early Relapse. *J. Pediatr. Hematol. Oncol.* **2021**, *43*, E630–E634. [CrossRef]
17. Zapletalova, D.; Andr, N.; Deak, L.; Kyr, M.; Bajciova, V.; Mudry, P.; Dubska, L.; Demlova, R.; Pavelka, Z.; Zitterbart, K.; et al. Metronomic chemotherapy with the COMBAT regimen in advanced pediatric malignancies: A multicenter experience. *Oncology* **2012**, *82*, 249–260. [CrossRef]
18. Carcamo, B.; Francia, G. Cyclic Metronomic Chemotherapy for Pediatric Tumors: Six Case Reports and a Review of the Literature. *J. Clin. Med.* **2022**, *11*, 2849. [CrossRef]
19. Štěrba, J.; Pavelka, Z.; Šlampa, P. Concomitant radiotherapy and metronomic temozolomide in pediatric high-risk brain tumors. *Neoplasma* **2002**, *49*, 117–120.
20. Fousseyni, T.; Diawara, M.; Pasquier, E.; André, N. Children treated with metronomic chemotherapy in a low-income country: METRO-MALI-01. *J. Pediatr. Hematol. Oncol.* **2011**, *33*, 31–34. [CrossRef]
21. Stempak, D.; Gammon, J.; Halton, J.; Moghrabi, A.; Koren, G.; Baruchel, S. A pilot pharmacokinetic and antiangiogenic biomarker study of celecoxib and low-dose metronomic vinblastine or cyclophosphamide in pediatric recurrent solid tumors. *J. Pediatr. Hematol. Oncol.* **2006**, *28*, 720–728. [CrossRef]
22. Traore, F.; Togo, B.; Pasquier, E.; Dembélé, A.; André, N. Preliminary evaluation of children treated with metronomic chemotherapy and valproic acid in a low-income country: Metro-Mali-02. *Indian J. Cancer* **2013**, *50*, 250–253. [CrossRef]
23. Kieran, M.W.; Turner, C.D.; Rubin, J.B.; Chi, S.N.; Zimmerman, M.A.; Chordas, C.; Klement, G.; Laforme, A.; Gordon, A.; Thomas, A.; et al. A feasibility trial of antiangiogenic (metronomic) chemotherapy in pediatric patients with recurrent or progressive cancer. *J. Pediatr. Hematol. Oncol.* **2005**, *27*, 573–581. [CrossRef]
24. Manji, A.; Samson, Y.; Deyell, R.J.; Johnston, D.L.; Lewis, V.A.; Zorzi, A.P.; Berman, J.N.; Brodeur-Robb, K.; Morrison, E.; Kee, L.; et al. Low-Dose Metronomic Topotecan and Pazopanib (TOPAZ) in Children with Relapsed or Refractory Solid Tumors: A C17 Canadian Phase I Clinical Trial. *Cancers* **2022**, *14*, 2985. [CrossRef]
25. Ali, A.M.; El-Sayed, M.I. Metronomic chemotherapy and radiotherapy as salvage treatment in refractory or relapsed pediatric solid tumours. *Curr. Oncol.* **2016**, *23*, e253–e259. [CrossRef]

86. Pasqualini, C.; Rubino, J.; Brard, C.; Cassard, L.; André, N.; Rondof, W.; Scoazec, J.Y.; Marchais, A.; Nebchi, S.; Boselli, L.; et al. Phase II and biomarker study of programmed cell death protein 1 inhibitor nivolumab and metronomic cyclophosphamide in paediatric relapsed/refractory solid tumours: Arm G of AcSé-ESMART, a trial of the European Innovative Therapies for Children With Cance. *Eur. J. Cancer* **2021**, *150*, 53–62. [CrossRef]
87. Robison, N.J.; Campigotto, F.; Chi, S.N.; Manley, P.E.; Turner, C.D.; Zimmerman, M.A.; Chordas, C.A.; Werger, A.M.; Allen, J.C.; Goldman, S.; et al. A phase II trial of a multi-agent oral antiangiogenic (metronomic) regimen in children with recurrent or progressive cancer. *Pediatr. Blood Cancer* **2014**, *61*, 636–642. [CrossRef]
88. Verschuur, A.; Heng-Maillard, M.-A.; Dory-Lautrec, P.; Truillet, R.; Jouve, E.; Chastagner, P.; Leblond, P.; Aerts, I.; Honoré, S.; Entz-Werle, N.; et al. Metronomic Four-Drug Regimen Has Anti-tumor Activity in Pediatric Low-Grade Glioma; The Results of a Phase II Clinical Trial. *Front. Pharmacol.* **2018**, *9*, 00950. [CrossRef]
89. André, N.; Abed, S.; Orbach, D.; Alla, C.A.; Padovani, L.; Pasquier, E.; Gentet, J.C.; Verschuur, A. Pilot study of a pediatric metronomic 4-drug regimen. *Oncotarget* **2011**, *2*, 960–965. [CrossRef]
90. Heng-Maillard, M.A.; Verschuur, A.; Aschero, A.; Dabadie, A.; Jouve, E.; Chastagner, P.; Leblond, P.; Aerts, I.; De Luca, B.; André, N. SFCE METRO-01 four-drug metronomic regimen phase II trial for pediatric extracranial tumor. *Pediatr. Blood Cancer* **2019**, *66*, e27693. [CrossRef]
91. El kababri, M.; Benmiloud, S.; Cherkaoui, S.; El houdzi, J.; Maani, K.; Ansari, N.; Khoubila, N.; Kili, A.; El khorassani, M.; Madani, A.; et al. Metro-SMHOP 01: Metronomics combination with cyclophosphamide-etoposide and valproic acid for refractory and relapsing pediatric malignancies. *Pediatr. Blood Cancer* **2020**, *67*, 1–6. [CrossRef]
92. Bisogno, G.; De Salvo, G.L.; Bergeron, C.; Gallego Melcón, S.; Merks, J.H.; Kelsey, A.; Martelli, H.; Minard-Colin, V.; Orbach, D.; Glosli, H.; et al. Vinorelbine and continuous low-dose cyclophosphamide as maintenance chemotherapy in patients with high-risk rhabdomyosarcoma (RMS 2005): A multicentre, open-label, randomised, phase 3 trial. *Lancet Oncol.* **2019**, *20*, 1566–1575 [CrossRef]
93. Pramanik, R.; Agarwala, S.; Gupta, Y.K.; Thulkar, S.; Vishnubhatla, S.; Batra, A.; Dhawan, D.; Bakhshi, S. Metronomic chemotherapy vs best supportive care in progressive pediatric solid malignant tumors: A randomized clinical trial. *JAMA Oncol.* **2017**, *3*, 1222–1227. [CrossRef]
94. Pramanik, R.; Agarwala, S.; Sreenivas, V.; Dhawan, D.; Bakhshi, S. Quality of life in paediatric solid tumours: A randomised study of metronomic chemotherapy versus placebo. *BMJ Support. Palliat. Care* **2021**. [CrossRef]
95. Andre, N.; Cointe, S.; Barlogis, V.; Arnaud, L.; Lacroix, R.; Pasquier, E.; Dignat-George, F.; Michel, G.; Sabatier, F. Maintenance chemotherapy in children with ALL exerts metronomic-like thrombospondin-1 associated anti-endothelial effect. *Oncotarget* **2015**, *6*, 23008–23014. [CrossRef]
96. Vo, K.T.; Karski, E.E.; Nasholm, N.M.; Allen, S.; Hollinger, F.; Gustafson, W.C.; Long-Boyle, J.R.; Shiboski, S.; Matthay, K.K.; DuBois, S.G. Phase 1 study of sirolimus in combination with oral cyclophosphamide and topotecan in children and young adults with relapsed and refractory solid tumors. *Oncotarget* **2017**, *8*, 23851–23861. [CrossRef]
97. Pramanik, R.; Tyagi, A.; Agarwala, S.; Vishnubhatla, S.; Dhawan, D.; Bakhshi, S. Evaluation of Vascular Endothelial Growth Factor (VEGF) and Thrombospondin-1 as Biomarkers of Metronomic Chemotherapy in Progressive Pediatric Solid Malignancies. *Indian Pediatr.* **2020**, *57*, 508–511. [CrossRef]
98. Toh, Y.-M.; Li, T.-K. Mitoxantrone inhibits HIF-1α expression in a topoisomerase II-independent pathway. *Clin. Cancer Res. Off. J. Am. Assoc. Cancer Res.* **2011**, *17*, 5026–5037. [CrossRef]
99. André, N.; Carré, M.; Pasquier, E. Metronomics: Towards personalized chemotherapy? *Nat. Rev. Clin. Oncol.* **2014**, *11*, 413–431. [CrossRef]
100. Mariotto, A.B.; Enewold, L.; Zhao, J.; Zeruto, C.A.; Yabroff, K.R. Medical Care Costs Associated with Cancer Survivorship in the United States. *Cancer Epidemiol. Biomark. Prev.* **2020**, *29*, 1304–1312. [CrossRef] [PubMed]
101. André, N.; Orbach, D.; Pasquier, E. Metronomic Maintenance for High-Risk Pediatric Malignancies: One Size Will Not Fit All. *Trends Cancer* **2020**, *6*, 819–828. [CrossRef]
102. Choi, D.K.; Helenowski, I.; Hijiya, N. Secondary malignancies in pediatric cancer survivors: Perspectives and review of the literature. *Int. J. Cancer* **2014**, *135*, 1764–1773. [CrossRef] [PubMed]

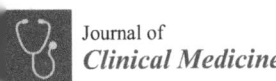

Review

Metronomic Chemotherapy for Metastatic Breast Cancer Treatment: Clinical and Preclinical Data between Lights and Shadows

Marina Elena Cazzaniga [1,2], Serena Capici [2], Nicoletta Cordani [1], Viola Cogliati [2], Francesca Fulvia Pepe [2], Francesca Riva [3] and Maria Grazia Cerrito [1,*]

1. School of Medicine and Surgery, Milano-Bicocca University, 20900 Monza, Italy
2. Phase 1 Research Centre, ASST Monza, 20900 Monza, Italy
3. Oncology Unit, ASST Monza, 20900 Monza, Italy
* Correspondence: mariagrazia.cerrito@unimib.it; Tel.: +39-039-2339037

Abstract: Metronomic chemotherapy (mCHT), defined as continuous administration of low-dose chemotherapeutic agents with no or short regular treatment-free intervals, was first introduced to the clinic in international guidelines in 2017, and, since then, has become one of the available strategies for the treatment of advanced breast cancer (ABC). Despite recent successes, many unsolved practical and theoretical issues remain to be addressed. The present review aims to identify the "lights and shadows" of mCHT in preclinical and clinical settings. In the preclinical setting, several findings indicate that one of the most noticeable effects of mCHT is on the tumor microenvironment, which, over the last twenty years, has been demonstrated to be pivotal in supporting tumor cell survival and proliferation. On the other hand, the direct effects on tumor cells have been less well-defined. In addition, critical items to be addressed are the lack of definition of an optimal biological dose (OBD), the method of administration of metronomic schedules, and the recognition and validation of predictive biomarkers. In the clinical context—where mCHT has mainly been used in a metastatic setting—low toxicity is the most well-recognised light of mCHT, whereas the type of study design, the absence of randomised trials and uncertainty in terms of doses and drugs remain among the shadows. In conclusion, growing evidence indicates that mCHT is a suitable treatment option for selected metastatic breast cancer (MBC) patients. Moreover, given its multimodal mechanisms of action, its addition to immunological and targeted therapies might represent a promising new approach to the treatment of MBC. More preclinical data are needed in this regard, which can only be obtained through support for translational research as the key link between basic science and patient care.

Keywords: metronomic chemotherapy; breast cancer; safety

1. Introduction

Metronomic chemotherapy (mCHT) refers to the minimum biologically effective dose of a chemotherapeutic agent able to induce antitumor activity when given as a continuous dosing regimen with no prolonged drug-free breaks. Standard-of-care chemotherapy, instead, is based on administration of the maximum tolerated dose (MTD) of a drug(s) given for several cycles, with prolonged drug-free breaks between administrations. Since its inception, mCHT was perceived as a therapy to be used in very advanced or palliative settings, especially in those cancers, such as breast cancer, for which more complex and modern therapies are available and mistakenly considered more effective [1]. Despite the difficult circumstances in which mCHT took its first steps, it soon became evident that it had some peculiar properties, mainly related to its various mechanisms of action, and that these properties could be exploited to optimise the sequencing of treatment.

For clinical application, mCHT was first introduced in international guidelines in 2017. The International Consensus Guidelines for advanced breast cancer (ABC) stated that "*Metronomic ChT is a reasonable treatment option for patients not requiring rapid tumour response. The better studied regimen is CM (low-dose oral cyclophosphamide and methotrexate); other regimens are being evaluated (including capecitabine and vinorelbine). Randomised trials are needed to accurately compare metronomic ChT with standard dosing regimens*". Clinical evidence gathered at that time, despite this being in early stages of development, supported a strong recommendation that the benefits outweighed the risks and harms even in the absence of randomised studies. A consensus on the published statement was reached by 88% of the panelists.

Since that point, mCHT became one of the strategies available for the treatment of ABC, even though the story of the treatment remained bedecked with lights and shadows. A significant concern is a lack of connection between laboratory data and the clinic: trial design has mainly been based on clinical outcomes without corresponding translational research aims or has been constrained by the very small number of patients enrolled. Improved linkage between preclinical and clinical research could reduce the gap between a correct diagnosis and the most favorable clinical outcome for the patient.

The purpose of the present review is to consider the lights and shadows of mCHT in preclinical and clinical settings, with the aim of highlighting both the positives and the missing aspects of this treatment approach.

With respect to preclinical research, we report data relating to the different mechanisms of action and the validation of some biomarkers, seeking to distinguish between established findings and work in progress, even though it is not always feasible to clearly demarcate these.

Regarding clinical research, among the lights, given the generally reported low incidence of severe side-effects related to mCHT, we decided to focus on these, together with quality-of-life (QoL) data, when available. Among the shadows, we reviewed study designs and end-points, and the presence of correlative biomarker studies, as these are areas requiring further exploration.

Considering the significant number of publications which relate to metronomic strategies in ABC patients, this review necessarily reports only key findings of research obtained in preclinical and clinical settings.

2. Materials and Methods

For the purposes of this review, we considered crucial studies with fully published results, which reported data concerning side-effects, QoL, symptom control or all of these. To better describe the toxicity of mCHT regimens, we included only studies that investigated pure metronomic regimens, in which drugs were administered at low dose, continuously, according to the definition of mCHT provided above [2]. We scanned databases using PubMed for keywords (e.g., *metronomic, breast cancer*), and, by using filters for the years *2010 to the present*), retrieved 247 results. We subsequently narrowed the field to clinical trials and randomized clinical trials, producing 64 results. The choice of selecting only papers published after 2010 was made due to the presence of different, and sometimes exhaustive, reviews published around that time, including one from our group. Amongst the clinical studies, we separately reported metronomic schedules with single or combination chemotherapy agents and metronomic schedules with chemotherapy agents combined with different targeted therapies, focusing on ABC. Our choice was informed by the lack of clinical trials in the early period, except for two which had enrolled a small number of patients.

For preclinical data, we conducted a literature search on PubMed and Web of Science using the terms "preclinical model of breast cancer and metronomic chemotherapy" and "mechanisms of action and biomarkers and metronomic chemotherapy" and selected the most relevant studies from 2000 to 2022. From the entire literature search, we retrieved 110 results, 67 of which were regarded as potentially relevant, 45 of which, in turn, were retained and fully reviewed.

3. Results
3.1. Preclinical Setting Lights

During the last twenty years, significant advances have been made in the understanding of the biology of cancer, including the interaction of tumour cells with their microenvironment. Several points of intervention for its treatment have emerged. For example, the importance and the mechanism of action of specific drugs have been highlighted, and it has also been understood that the way these molecules are administered—the dose and schedule—is very important [3], leading to the recognition of the importance of mCHT. Several mechanisms of action of mCHT have been identified, which include: (i) the prevention of tumour angiogenesis; (ii) direct effects on cancer cells; (iii) the induction of cellular senescence; and (iv) modulation of the immune system—with which the tumour cells interact directly—and of adjacent stromal cells. However, several challenges remain, particularly in terms of determining the mechanisms of action and identifying predictive biomarkers to identify those patients who will most benefit from mCHT.

We report what, in our opinion, can be considered "lights"—mechanisms and biomarkers that are well-documented for mCHT—and "shadows", i.e., areas that require further research.

3.1.1. Mechanisms of Action

Tumour-associated angiogenesis is defined as the sprouting of new micro-vessels from pre-existing ones; these new blood vessels can support tumour growth. However, neo-angiogenesis can also arise from cells recruited from the bone marrow, or that differentiate from cancer stem cells, in a process called "vascular mimicry" [4].

In recent years, research in this field has focused on understanding how different therapies act to prevent or block angiogenesis, mainly by inhibiting VEGF, which is the signal gradient towards which the growing vascular sprouts move. The anti-angiogenic effect of anticancer drugs at the MTD preferentially impacts proliferating endothelial cells (ECs), some of which participate in the germination of new tumour micro-vessels. Unfortunately, these effects are reversed during the two to three week pauses between subsequent treatments, as occurs with standard chemotherapy schedules. The anti-angiogenic stimulus of chemotherapy appeared to be improved when drugs were administered metronomically, in small doses, on a frequent schedule (daily, several times a week, or weekly), and continuously for prolonged periods, as shown in xenotransplant models, including for drug-resistant tumours [2]. Klement et al. established that orthotopic xenografts of human breast cancer responded significantly to continuous low-dose chemotherapy regimens when used in combination with a second anti-angiogenic drug, i.e., anti-VEGFR-2 antibodies, which led to inhibition of tumour angiogenesis and reduced tumour size [5].

To determine the sensitivity to angiogenic therapy of primary orthotopic breast cancer xenografts compared to distant metastases, Bridgeman and colleagues evaluated histological data, in which primary tumours exhibited intense angiogenesis while lung metastases did not. In the lungs, there was evidence of "vessel co-optation", which is the capturing of existing vessels by tumour cells—particularly in a vascular-rich organ like the lung—migrating along the vessels of the host organ, thus supporting the metastatic process. These data confirmed the previous findings of Pezzella in 1996, who was the first to demonstrate the ability of cancer cells to enlist existing vessels to feed the growing tumour. Pezzella also suggested that the co-optation of the vessel constituted a mechanism of intrinsic resistance or a means of lowering the response to anti-angiogenic drugs.

Cancer cells, particularly those from highly metastatic tumours, are also capable of vasculogenic mimicry to escape anti-angiogenic therapy. Cancer cells can differentiate and enhance EC-like characteristics by expressing VE-cadherin and ephrin A2. This process is associated with increased tumour invasiveness and relapses [6].

Various preclinical studies have indicated that proliferating microvascular ECs represent the primary targets when tumours are treated with mCHT. Low-dose chemotherapy directly affects the tumour vessel through growth arrest and apoptosis of activated ECs. mCHT inhibits the expression of pro-angiogenic factors, such as VEGF, VEGFR2, bFGF, and

SDF1, and induces the production of angiogenesis inhibitors, such as thrombospondin-1, in both stromal and cancer cells, platelet factor-4, and endostatin. Moreover, mCHT induces apoptosis in circulating ECs and inhibits endothelial progenitor cell (EPC) mobilisation [7,8]. In addition, combined treatment of anti-angiogenic and cytotoxic drugs synergistically hampered tumour progression and prolonged survival in tumour-bearing animal models [9,10]. An interesting study evaluated the molecular mechanisms of topotecan administered in mCHT mode, alone or in combination with pazopanib (an antiangiogenic tyrosine kinase inhibitor), in primary and metastatic orthotopic models of triple-negative breast cancer (TNBC); the impact of hypoxic conditions was also examined. The combination of metronomic topotecan and pazopanib significantly improved antitumor activity compared to monotherapy with both drugs, and prolonged survival, even in the context of advanced metastatic cancer, with important changes in tumor angiogenesis, tumor cell proliferation, apoptosis, HIF1α levels, and HIF-1 target gene expression [11].

Together, these data suggest that mCHT impacts on the altered blood flow of tumour vessels through their functional normalisation, rendering the delivery of anticancer drugs to the tumour more effective. Tumour vessel normalisation represents an emerging concept for mCHT-based tumour treatment.

The modulation of the immune system directly affects tumour cells and adjacent stromal cells [12] and the effect of chemotherapy on these components has been studied in different experimental settings. For example, the Kerbel group performed a preclinical study using an orthotopic model of syngeneic murine TNBC (EMT6/P) treated with the immune checkpoint inhibitor anti-CTLA4. The use of the monoclonal antibody partially inhibited tumour growth and this inhibitory effect was increased when the anti-CTLA4 antibody was combined with a low-dose cyclophosphamide (CTX) regimen, but not when the anti-CTLA4 antibody was combined with high-dose injection of CTX plus a low oral dose of CTX [13]. These results were further corroborated and expanded when the authors compared three different CTX protocols for anti-cancer efficacy in three murine breast cancer models. In an EMT6/P model, three different CTX regimens were studied: the MTD protocol, a low dose daily/continuous oral metronomic CTX, and medium dose intermittent CTX (CTX140 1q6d regimen) where the drug was injected in a medium dose, every six days. The latter protocol was more effective in inhibiting primary tumour growth than the MTD or continuous oral low daily dose CTX. In addition, CTX140 1q6d also produced anti-cancer results by stimulating the innate and adaptive immune systems. In fact, CTX140 1q6d upregulated PD-L1 expression on CD45+ and CD45− cells within the tumour microenvironment. Consistent with these preclinical data, a clinical study reported that therapy with an mCHT schedule in TNBC-patients expressing higher levels of PD-L1 in the tumour microenvironment resulted in better responses [14]. Orecchioni et al. investigated the effects of mCHT VNR, CTX and 5-FU, alone or in combination with checkpoint inhibitors, on the circulating immune cells of mice injected in the mammary fat pad with 4T1 TNBC cells. They found a synergistic effect in reducing circulating T, B, and NK cells when chemotherapy was given with anti-PD-L1. Notably, they observed that the reduction in the different immune cells triggered by mCHT in peripheral blood was not mirrored by a similar decrease in the intratumoral immune cell infiltrate [15].

Figure 1 describes the main mechanisms of action of mCHT.

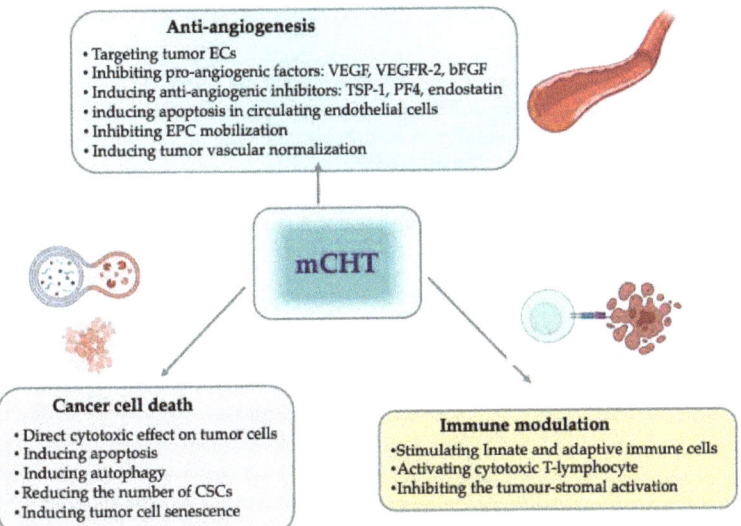

Figure 1. Mechanisms of action of metronomic chemotherapy (mCHT). The beneficial effects of mCHT are mediated by the inhibition of angiogenesis, the direct inhibition of tumour cell proliferation, and the stimulation of the immune system. Inhibition of angiogenesis plays a fundamental role in mCHT. The anti-angiogenic effects include direct inhibition of endothelial cells (ECs) proliferation via inhibition of pro-angiogenic factors, such as vascular-endothelial growth factor (VEGF), vascular endothelial growth factor receptor 2 (VEGF-R2), basic fibroblast growth factor (bFGF), and upregulation of endogenous angiogenic inhibitors, such as Thrombospondin 1 (TSP-1) endostatin, and platelet factor 4 (PF4), and inhibition of endogenous endothelial progenitor cells (EPCs) mobilization. Direct cytotoxic effects on tumor cells and decreased cancer stem cells (CSCs) population are also observed. mCHT also stimulates anticancer immunity by increasing cytotoxic activity of immune cell effectors and by inhibiting tumour-stromal activation. Figure created with BioRender.com.

3.1.2. Biomarkers

In the last decade, considerable efforts have been made in the preclinical setting to identify valuable biomarkers that could be used to stratify breast cancer patients and monitor the effectiveness of the mCHT regimen [16,17]. Potential biomarkers have been studied to demonstrate, for example, its anti-angiogenic action. They include circulating blood biomarkers, such as VEGF, angiopoietin, thrombospondin $\frac{1}{2}$(TSP-1/2) and circulating ECs [7,18], polymorphisms of a single nucleotide (e.g., VEGF, IL6, IL8) [19], and immunohistochemistry (e.g., VEGF and TSP-2). Techniques applied have also included functional imaging (e.g., dynamic contrast-enhanced magnetic resonance imaging or dynamic contrast-enhanced computed tomography) [20] and laser speckle flowmetry to evaluate the efficacy of mCHT CTX treatment in tumor shrinkage and tumor vasculature response [21]. More recently, it has been shown, in a preclinical study of patient-derived xenografts (PDXs) from CDK12HIGH and CDK12LOW human breast cancers, that CDK12 overexpression can predict response to metronomic methotrexate-based therapy. In addition, a retrospective analysis of lymph-node-positive breast cancer patients, randomized to receive metronomic cyclophosphamide plus methotrexate (CM) chemotherapy or no chemotherapy after completion of standard adjuvant treatments, confirmed CDK12 expression as a valuable biomarker in breast cancer patients [22].

3.2. Preclinical Setting—Shadows

3.2.1. Mechanisms of Action

Preclinical and clinical evidence suggests a direct effect of mCHT on cancer cells [1]. For instance, it has been shown that protracted exposure to paclitaxel (PTX)—a taxane usually administered to treat breast cancer—induced a stronger cytotoxic effect than a short exposure, indicating that dose and duration are essential factors in the anticancer activity of PTX in human cancers, and prolonged exposure might increase this effect [12]. Recently, Roy et al. documented the efficacy of methylglyoxal, a highly reactive glycolytic metabolite, on breast cancer stem cells, and that its combination in an mCHT schedule with doxorubicin or cisplatin enhanced cytotoxicity towards MCF-7 and MDA-MB-231 cell lines [23].

Salem et al., demonstrated that low doses of the muscarinic agonist carbachol, combined with PTX, reduced MCF-7 cell growth in vitro, likely via down-regulation of the cancer stem cell population [24]. Recently, we confirmed that the mechanism of action of anticancer agents, such as 5-fluorouracil (5-FU) and vinorelbine (VNR), can be significantly different when given metronomically compared to administration following an MTD schedule [25]. We showed that, in TNBC cells, metronomic combinations of VNR and 5-FU could inhibit cell growth by inducing apoptosis and autophagy, and by significantly increasing cellular senescence [25]. Many studies have demonstrated effects of senescence, which may be involved in cancer prevention but also in its aggressiveness. There is both light and shadow with respect to the role of senescence in cancer. Additional studies are necessary to better understand the role of senescence in cancer and assess whether it is beneficial or detrimental for patients.

Considering the different effects of the combinatorial regimens of mCHT, it is reasonable to assume that further mechanisms remain to be discovered.

3.2.2. Biomarkers

Several biomarkers have been studied in TNBC to identify new actionable targets [26]. Among them FGFR1 amplification (the most frequent aberrancy implicated in tumorigenesis) was found in 18–33% of samples. Notably, antibodies against the different FGFR isoforms are already being tested in different preclinical settings with good efficacy. Therefore, the combination of anti-FGFR antibodies with mCHT might also be envisioned for the future. Remarkably, it has already been shown in preclinical studies on TNBC cells that when PD-1 mAbs are combined with metronomic-PTX treatment, the efficacy of anti-PD-1 is improved. These studies attempted to respond to a clinical need, i.e., the unsatisfactory effect of PD-1/PD-L1 monoclonal antibodies used alone [27]. In another study, the authors analyzed the immunomodulatory effects of EphA2-ILs-DTXp, a targeted nanoliposomal taxane, in combination with checkpoint inhibitors. They found, in an EMT-6 breast cancer model, that metronomic dosing of docetaxel improved tumour growth suppression by increasing the activity of CD8+ T cells [28]. Earlier, Francia et al. showed, in Her-2-positive human metastatic breast cancer xenografts, that the efficacy of trastuzumab was enhanced when combined with metronomic low-dose CTX [29]. Recent preclinical studies have used CTX combined with other drugs to treat breast cancer with varying success [30].

Significant attention has also been paid to the identification of non-invasive imaging markers of response to chemotherapy treatment [31]; for example, therapy-induced responses, including apoptosis and proliferation, have been traced in preclinical cancer models using label-free optical imaging techniques, such as spatial frequency domain imaging [32].

Another important aspect that deserves attention concerns the optimal biological dose (OBD) of drugs, defined as the smallest effective dose that causes the highest tumour volume shrinkage with no or minimal toxicity. Several preclinical models have been used to evaluate the toxicological and biological effects of treatments, although none is considered perfect for determining drug OBD. For this reason, to obtain accurate results, it is important to select the most suitable preclinical model to study. In a pioneering paper, Shaked and colleagues [33] identified the OBD of various mCHT regimens in four different preclinical cancer models, including breast cancer. Each OBD obtained by the authors was associated with the highest reduction in circulating VEGFR2-positives

Critical issues remain to be addressed regarding the administration of metronomic schedules and the recognition and validation of predictive biomarkers. These aspects were underlined in a recent study [34] in which the authors highlighted the importance of the pharmacokinetic effects of mCHT, which are often overlooked, even though they are of fundamental significance, considering the implications of this understanding for both preclinical research and the design of clinical trials.

Overall, solid and reliable biomarkers (i.e., diagnostic, predictive) are still needed to predict which patients are more likely to benefit from mCHT.

A summary of the mechanisms of action and biomarkers that have been established (lights) and those that need further investigation (shadows) related to mCHT are outlined in Figure 2.

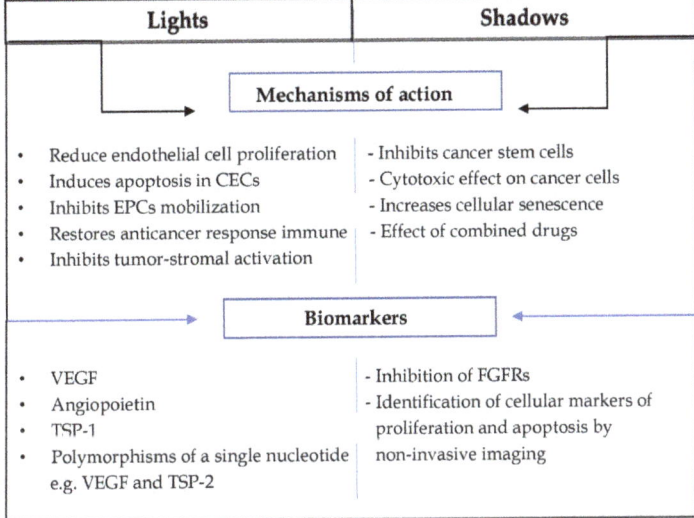

Figure 2. The scheme summarises the mechanisms of action and biomarkers that have been determined (highlights) and those that need further investigation (shadows) related to mCHT. Circulating endothelial cells (CECs); endothelial progenitor cells (EPCs); vascular endothelial growth factor (VEGF); thrombospondin-1 and -2 (TSP-1, and TSP-2); fibroblast growth factor receptors (FGFRs).

3.3. Clinical Setting—Lights

Breast cancer was the first type of tumour investigated for application of mCHT. In patients with ABC, the main goals remain QoL improvement and disease symptom reduction, rather than tumour response. In this context, mCHT provides an excellent alternative to conventional chemotherapy, especially considering the low incidence of side-effects. The most studied drugs are CTX, methotrexate (MTX), VNR and capecitabine (CAPE), alone, or combined with other chemotherapy agents or targeted therapies.

3.3.1. mCHT Alone

As highlighted in different reviews, CTX was the first and is the most studied drug, usually administered at a continuous dose of 50 mg/day. The metronomic dose used in several clinical trials was set, on an empirical basis, to be 50 mg p.o. daily [35]; subsequent steps included, first, the addition of MTX [24] and, subsequently, of biological agents.

Different trials [36–38] have studied metronomic CTX in ABC patients, mostly in those heavily pre-treated using several lines of treatment. Overall, Grade 3 leukopenia and neutropenia, ranged between 3–10% of patients, whereas Grade 4 was reported in approximately 4% of patients.

A retrospective analysis [36] of 61 patients with endocrine-resistant ABC who already received two lines of chemotherapy treated with oral CTX at the dose of 50 mg/day (Cohort 1, N = 22) or CTX at the same dose, together with MTX 2.5 mg orally twice a week (Cohort 2, N = 39), reported Grade 3 leukopenia in 5% of the cases treated with CTX alone and 3% of cases in those treated with CTX + MTX. All other toxicities, such as nausea/vomiting, mucositis and diarrhoea were Grade 1 or Grade 2. Symptom control was achieved in 54% of the cases.

Similar results were described by Lu et al. [39], who retrospectively reviewed data regarding the efficacy and safety of CTX+MTX in 186 ABC patients. The authors reported a very good safety profile for this combination; the incidence of any grade of leukopenia and neutropenia was 0.6%. Other toxicities, specifically, nausea and AST/ALT elevation, which were mostly related to MTX, were below 10% (7.1% and 3%, respectively).

The combination of CTX with etoposide was explored by Mutlu et al. [38] in a retrospective analysis of 77 heavily pre-treated ABC patients. The patients received continuous oral CTX at a dose of 50 mg/day and oral etoposide given as 50 mg twice a day for two days per week. The toxicities related to mCHT were low and mainly haematologic: G3 and G4 leukopenia were reported in 10.4% and 3.9% of the cases, respectively, and G3 and G4 thrombocytopenia in 2.6 and 0% of cases, respectively. No Grade 4 emesis was observed. In this study, the addition of etoposide, a drug with well-known haematologic toxicity, slightly increased the incidence of haematologic events, which was usually very low, as described above.

Another much-studied drug is VNR, alone, or, most commonly, in combination with CAPE, CTX, or both. Despite the availability of Phase 1 trial data [40], which, for VNR, suggested a recommended dose of 50 mg thrice a week when used as a single agent, some trials tested alternative schedules, such as 30 mg/day, without interruptions. This schedule was studied in a multicentre, open-label, single-arm study which enrolled nine patients and was closed early due to one Grade 5 toxicity (febrile neutropenia) [41].

Many more studies have explored the combination of VNR with CAPE, CTX, or both [42]. One of the most extensive studies conducted considering combinations of different metronomic drugs was that undertaken by Montagna et al. [42]; a total of 43 patients in a naïve group and 65 in a pre-treated group received 40 mg VNR thrice a week plus 500 mg CAPE thrice a day, together with CTX at a dose of 50 mg/day (VEX), administered continuously. Among the considerable strengths of this study was the prospective design, enabling corroboration of evidence that the incidence of side-effects with mCHT is very low; the most frequent G3 treatment-related adverse events were neutropenia (5%), increase in transaminases (5%) and hand and foot syndrome (7%).

Similarly, the XeNa trial [43] reported a lower incidence of some severe adverse events in the metronomic group compared with the standard regimen (fatigue: 9.7% vs. 17.2%). This was a large, randomised Phase 2 study that enrolled 120 Her2- ABC patients; the patients were randomised to receive either the standard schedule of VNR (60 mg/m^2 day 1 + day 8 in the first cycle, followed by 80 mg/m^2 day 1 + day 8 in the following cycles) or metronomic VNR 50 mg three times a week. Capecitabine 1000 mg/m^2 twice a day for days 1–14 was administered in both groups.

Finally, Krajnak et al. [44] retrospectively analysed 35 MBC patients treated with a combination of CTX 50 mg daily and MTX 2.5 mg every second day; discontinuation due to adverse events occurred in 9% of the patients, whereas only 11% of the patients stopped MTX, mainly due to gastro-intestinal toxicity.

Our own research on mCHT has comprised different studies over the years, starting with the VICTOR-1 study [45], which established the maximum tolerated dose (MTD) of VNR as 40 mg thrice a week in combination with fixed doses of CAPE (500 mg thrice a day); these results were subsequently confirmed in the multicentre VICTOR-2 study [46], and reinforced in the VICTOR-6 real-world study [47]. In all these studies, we only observed mild (Grade 1–2) toxicities (Grade 1–2: nausea/vomiting 15.4%; hematologic effects 14%, diarrhoea 12%), even in the large population analysed in the VICTOR-6 trial (600 patients), or subgroups of patients, such as those aged over 75 years.

Keeping in mind that the main aim in the treatment of ABC patients is the improvement of OS, the duration of the clinical benefit produced by a defined regimen is a crucial element: Montagna et al. [48] recently analysed data for their cohort of ABC patients enrolled in a clinical trial of mCHT (VNR + CTX + CAPE), reporting a PFS rate at three years of 25.4%. The main Grade 3–4 adverse event observed was hand-foot syndrome (7%), with no evidence of specific or more important, cumulative or delayed toxicities with mCHT, which was confirmed as a very well-tolerated strategy.

3.3.2. mCHT in Combination with Targeted Agents

Many other authors have investigated the combination of CTX + MTX with other anti-cancer agents, such as the VEGFR inhibitor vandetanib (VAN) [49], and non-anticancer drugs, such as thalidomide [50], dalteparin and prednisone or idiotype vaccine; however, outcomes showed non-significant therapeutic improvements. Due to its safety profile and the ease of administration, mCHT has been studied in combination with different targeted agents, mainly anti-Her2, anti-VEGF or tyrosine-kinase inhibitors (TKIs). Although the combination with targeted agents has led to a renewed interest in mCHT, the side-effects related to biological drugs partially cancel the significant advantage in terms of toxicity provided by this modality of administration. Nevertheless, these combinations represent an alternative to CHT standard-dose regimens and are of especial value for frail or elderly patients.

mCHT in Combination with Anti-HER2 Agents

The largest and most well-conducted study regarding the combination of mCHT with anti-HER2 agents was carried out by Wildiers et al. [51] in frail ABC patients, defined by age (70 years or older and 60 years or older) but without the presence of comorbidities. Patients were randomized to receive metronomic oral CTX 50 mg per day plus trastuzumab and pertuzumab, or trastuzumab and pertuzumab alone at standard doses. The most frequent grade 3–4 adverse events in the mCHT arm were hypertension (12%), diarrhoea (12%), dyspnoea (10%), fatigue (5%), pain (5%), and a thromboembolic event occurred in 10% of the patients. CTX discontinuation was necessary for 22 patients (54%). Grade 3 adverse events were heart failure (5%), diarrhoea, fatigue, pain and anorexia (5% for each of the four adverse events). The incidence of these events was very similar to that reported in the control arm and were more likely to have been related to the anti-HER2 agents rather than mCHT. This study was one of the few that analysed patients' quality of life [52]. The authors assessed HRQoL using the EORTC QLQ-C30 and the EORTC Elderly specific module QLQ-ELD14 at baseline, and weeks 9, 27, and 52. The primary HRQoL domains were global health status/QoL scale (GHQs), fatigue and pain. No statistically significant differences in terms of HRQoL domain changes were detected over time between the two treatments.

Other authors [53] investigated the combination of mCHT (VNR 40 mg thrice a week), in combination with trastuzumab, reporting very few adverse events, the most important being neutropenia, which was observed in 10% of the patients.

mCHT in Combination with Anti-Angiogenic Drugs

The combination of mCHT with anti-angiogenic agents is probably one of the most promising associations, particularly when CTX is part of the regimens, given that its peculiar anti-angiogenic properties have been demonstrated in preclinical [13] and clinical settings [54–57]. As already illustrated above, mCHT inhibits circulating ECs and EPCs, and modulates pro- and anti-angiogenic molecules, such as VEGF, thrombospondin-1 and VEGFR2, amongst others [58].

Different drugs have been tested in combination with bevacizumab (the monoclonal antibody against VEGF-A), with CTX being the most used at a dose of 50 mg/day, in combination with either CAPE [54,56] or MTX [55]. Grade 3 or 4 adverse effects that occurred in the trials were hypertension, leukopenia, neutropenia and transaminitis. One study [54] explored, together with efficacy, the relationship among circulating ECs and circulating EPCs and the response and outcomes of the patients.

Similar toxicities were observed in a Phase III study which randomized ABC patients to receive bevacizumab with either PTX (arm A) or daily oral CAPE-CTX (arm B, CAPE 500 mg x 3/daily + CTX 50 mg/day) as a first-line treatment [56]. A major strength of this study was the direct comparison between mCHT and standard chemotherapy in terms of QoL evaluation, which considered physical well-being, measured by self-assessment questionnaire. The questionnaire included indicators of physical well-being, mood, coping effort, overall treatment burden, health perception, appetite, tiredness, hair loss, nausea/vomiting, and numbness/tingling in the hands/feet. The incidence of primary endpoint-defining adverse events was similar between the two arms (25% vs. 24%; $p = 0.96$); 17 patients stopped treatment because of unacceptable toxicities, 12 (17%) in the standard CHT arm and 5 (7%) in the mCHT arm. Although the study failed to meet its primary endpoint, it provided important information regarding the QoL of ABC patients treated with mCHT; these reported substantially less hair loss ($p < 0.0001$) and less numbness with increasing time ($p < 0.01$) than those treated with standard CHT, and a tendency toward a lower overall treatment burden ($p = 0.11$).

Considering that different mechanisms account for the anti-angiogenic effect of mCHT, such as the selective inhibition of proliferation and/or induction of apoptosis of activated endothelial cells, the selective inhibition of endothelial cell migration, increase in the expression level of TSP-1 and sustained decrease in the levels and viability of bone marrow-derived EPCs, other authors have tested mCHT in combination with celecoxib, sorafenib, and vandetanib.

Together these studies indicate that the combination of mCHT and anti-angiogenic agents is feasible, with a slight increase in toxicities, mainly related to the anti-angiogenic drug; in our opinion, what is missing in this area is a systematic, prospective collection and analysis of biomarkers, which could definitively validate the principal mechanisms of action of mCHT.

mCHT in Combination with other Targeted Agents

Different combinations of mCHT have been explored to date including with celecoxib [59,60]), sorafenib [61], veliparib [62,63] and some others.

Perroud et al. postulated that the high expression in BC of the prostaglandin synthase enzyme cyclooxygenase-2 (COX2) could be a reasonable basis to combine metronomic CTX with the anti-COX2 agent celecoxib. These authors also evaluated many different biomarkers of angiogenesis, such as VEGF, TSP-1 and others, as well as QoL. Together with an excellent safety profile, specifically, the absence of G3 adverse events, the authors, when investigating biomarkers of angiogenesis, observed a decrease in VEGF concentration, whereas TSP-1 did not change significantly over the period, nor did the percentage of circulating EPCs and ECs. The authors also evaluated quality of life using the FACT-B questionnaire, reporting a marginally significant increase in functional well-being and a significant increase in additional concerns.

The same authors [60] investigated the combination above in a larger set of ABC patients, confirming the toxicity profile.

Another interesting combination of letrozole 2.5 mg/day plus CTX 50 mg/day and sorafenib every fifth day at a dose of 400 mg bid was explored as neoadjuvant treatment in a cohort of 13 early BC patients [61]. These authors also evaluated the expression of some biomarkers, such as VEGF-A and CD31, reporting a significant reduction at Day 14 and at definitive surgery in comparison to baseline. In contrast, a reduction in VEGF-A expression was detected only when comparing levels at the time of surgery with baseline. The authors also demonstrated that the concentration of sorafenib was not affected by dosing in combination with CTX, whereas mean plasma concentrations of CTX were significantly lower following concomitant administration of sorafenib and letrozole compared with concomitant administration of letrozole alone. The toxicity of this combination was notable and would be incompatible with clinical practice. The advantages of this study included the comprehensive evaluation of different parameters, such as ^{18}FDG-PET changes over the time, which showed a significant reduction in SUV uptake at the surgery in comparison to baseline in all patients and for all biomarkers (i.e., CD31 significantly suppressed; VEGF-A expression significantly suppressed in response to treatment).

Finally, one of the most intriguing combinations tested is that of mCHT with poly [ADP-ribose] polymerase (PARP) inhibitors (PARPi). The rationale for this combination relies on the activity of PARPi in mutated BRCA patients, which can increase the DNA damage caused by chemotherapy; moreover, considering that these agents are administered orally, they could be paired with mCHT in an all-oral regimen.

Veliparib was investigated in combination with CTX in two different studies, one of which was a Phase 1 trial, [62,63], in different cohorts of heavily pre-treated TNBC patients. Overall, the combination did not improve the activity of CTX as a single-agent in the comparison study, though toxicity was acceptable and Grade 3–4 event percentages were below 10%.

Considering the high potential of combining low-dose, oral therapies with subcutaneous formulations of some anti-HER2 agents (e.g., trastuzumab, pertuzumab/trastuzumab), with novel and more potent oral TKIs, such as neratinib or tucatinib, or with novel therapies, further studies should be undertaken which aim to clarify: (1) the best mCHT backbone for targeted therapy; (2) the most appropriate drugs to enhance the biological activity of chosen interventions; and (3) which biomarkers best reflect the biological effects of drugs used in metronomic regimens. It would be beneficial for these future studies to include QoL evaluation, patient adherence, and biomarker evaluation. In our opinion, it is scientifically meaningless to continue to see published small, mostly retrospective, collections of cases, instead of joining forces to design a prospective, academic study with well-defined aims and end-points (including head-to-head comparisons, prospective QoL evaluation, biomarker assessment, etc).

Table 1 summarises the toxicities observed in the main studies.

Table 1. Summary of toxicities observed in the main studies.

Author (Year)	Regimen	Toxicity Grade 1–2 [1]	Toxicity Grade 3–4 [1]
Krajnak (2021) [41]	VNR 30 mg/day, continuously	Increased AST/ALT 22%	Febrile neutropenia (Grade 5)
Wang (2021) [53]	VNR 40 mg 3/week + trastuzumab 6 mg/kg (loading dose)	Nausea 15% Leukopenia 15% Increased ALT/AST 15% Diarrhoea 10% Peripheral neuropathy 10%	Neutropenia 10%
Brems-Eskildsen (2020) [43]	Arm A: VNR 60 mg/m^2 day 1 + day 8 in the first cycle followed by 80 mg/m^2 day 1 + day 8 + CAPE 1000 mg bid × 14 days, Q21 Arm B: VNR 50 mg 3/week + CAPE 1000 mg bid × 14 days, Q21	Arm A vs. Arm B Diarrhoea 53.2% vs. 46.5% Nausea 43.5% vs. 32.7% Mucositis 40.3% vs. 41.4% Fatigue 32.2% vs. 29.3% Hand-foot 48.4% vs. 44.8% Constipation 29% vs. 29.3% Neuropathy 29% vs. 25.9% Neutropenia 25.8% vs. 24.1% Dyspnea 24.2% vs. 18.9% Increased ALT/AST 20.9% vs. 17.2% Joint affection 19.4% vs. 17.2% Pain 19.3% Leucopenia 16.1% vs. 13.7% Fever 14.5% vs. 18.9% Abdominal pain 14.5% vs. 17.2% Back pain 11.3%	Fatigue 9.7% vs. 17.2%

Table 1. Cont.

Author (Year)	Regimen	Toxicity Grade 1–2 [1]	Toxicity Grade 3–4 [1]
Cazzaniga (2019) [64]	Different schedules	Nausea/vomiting 15.4% Hematologic 14.0% Diarrhoea 12% Fatigue 10.3%	<10%
Montagna (2022) [48]	VNR 40 mg 3/week + CTX 50 mg/day + CAPE 500 mg 3/day	Not reported	Hand-foot syndrome 7%
Perroud HA (2013) [59]	CTX 50 mg/daily + celecoxib 200 mg bid	Leucopenia G1 13.3% Neutropenia G1 6.7% Thrombocytopenia G1 6.7%	None
Bazzola (2015) [61]	Letrozole 2.5 mg/day + CTX 50 mg + sorafenib 400 mg bid every 5th day	Neutropenia G2 13.3% Anaemia G2 26.7% Alopecia 76.9% Neutropenia 38.5% Sensory neuropathy 38.5% Weight loss 38.5% Hand-foot syndrome 30.7% Fatigue 30.7% Rash 30.7% Dehydration 30.7% Anorexia 30.7% Arthralgias 23% Joint function 23% Hypertension 15.4% Mucositis 15.4% Acne 23%	Hand-foot syndrome 69.3% Rash 69.3% Diarrhoea 46.1% Dehydration 23%

[1] Reported if incidence > 10%.

As described in a recent review published by our group [1], this excellent toxicity profile is associated with well-documented clinical activity in various types of cancer and in ABC patients.

In a recently published systematic literature analysis [65], Lien et al. reviewed the status of knowledge regarding mCHT across different types of cancer. They reported that the main cancer types included in mCHT trials were breast (26.25%) and prostate tumours (11.25%) and the main agent was CTX (43%). Differences in terms of adverse event reporting were noted. Most of the studies used the NCI-CTCAE (any version) criteria, while seven used the WHO criteria. The authors emphasized that, despite the differences in reporting, mCHT was found to lead to low toxicity rates; in particular, no toxicity affected more than 6% of all pooled patients. The availability of such a systematic literature review compensates, to some extent, for the high heterogeneity observed in mCHT trials, at least with respect to toxicity.

Finally, it is our opinion that one of the most important lights of mCHT was its role during the COVID-19 pandemic. Even if the pandemic no longer represents an urgent emergency for public health services, we believe that it has provided an important lesson for the entire healthcare system, which should probably be reorganised in some areas to address future emergencies. In this context, the low toxicity profile of mCHT, together with its documented efficacy in some cancer types, above all ABC, should enable physicians to continue to treat patients in settings other than hospitals, such as the home, reducing admissions to hospital as much as possible.

3.4. Clinical Setting—Shadows

The prominent shadows regarding the use of mCHT in ABC patients include the different regimens and schedules applied, even when the same drugs are used, the small number of patients enrolled in the different trials, the retrospective design of most studies, and the almost complete absence of prospective randomized trials. The only randomized trial available to date has been the XeNa trial, which has some limitations, above all, the study design, which was not set up to provide a direct comparison between the two arms, and the use of a non-metronomic schedule for CAPE, which affected the toxicity results obtained. These are only some of the issues that require to be addressed to ensure that mCHT can be applied as a therapeutic strategy.

The need for an empirical basis for determining the optimal OBD and in monitoring the therapeutic activity of the drugs used in a metronomic schedule is a crucial point; for those drugs, such as CTX which is associated with a precise and known effect (angiogenesis), the OBD can be easily determined by assessing the maximum reduction in viable peripheral blood circulating VEGFR-2 or EPCs [66]. Monitoring of VEGFR-2 blood levels during treatment can also be easily achieved, as a useful dynamic biomarker to evaluate the response. Unfortunately, not all the drugs used in the different metronomic schedules are clearly associated with a precise mechanism of action, and not all the mechanisms are evaluable by a specific biomarker. For example, the well-known effect on T-reg down regulation observed with some metronomic schedules is only a partial and incomplete expression of the immune system stimulation.

In our opinion, the main limitation remains the absence of randomised studies for the vast majority of combinations and settings: fortunately, some trials [60] have filled this gap and some others are due, such as TEMPO BREAST (EudraCT number 2014-003860-19), which compared iv vs. a metronomic oral formulation of VNR as the first-line of treatment in 164 HR + /HER2-ABC patients randomly assigned to one of two treatment arms, and METEORA (NCT02954055), a multi-center, randomised phase II trial that randomised women with ER-positive, HER2-negative (human epidermal growth factor receptor 2-negative) metastatic or locally relapsed breast cancer in a ratio of 1:1, to receive a metronomic regimen of VNR plus CTX and CAPE, or the conventional paclitaxel monotherapy, the results for which are awaited soon.

Another important shadow is the almost total absence of QoL evaluation, even in trials that enrolled large populations of ABC patients; this has been performed sporadically but, unfortunately, was not planned for in most of the prospective studies.

4. Discussion

mCHT for the treatment of breast cancer treatment started slowly at the beginning of the 2000s; at that time, most physicians believed that it was nothing more than a palliative therapy, confining its use to very late stages in care.

With increasing evidence coming from scientists all around the world who tested mCHT in single arm, proof-of-concept studies in cancers different from breast (e.g., lung, prostate, paediatric, head and neck and ovarian cancers, glioblastoma), it became evident that mCHT could play a different role.

Even after many years of clinical use, especially as part of treatment of ABCs, the use of mCHT remains a matter of debate in the scientific community. Physicians are divided between those who have adopted it in their clinical practice, based mainly on its safety profile, and those who remain fierce opponents, citing many different reasons. Research is required to look deeper into developing strategies to improve the efficacy of drugs and significantly reduce toxicity.

In this paper, we have reviewed the available data regarding mCHT in ABC patients, seeking to highlight the lights and shadows of this strategy. Among the "lights" of mCHT, we considered the safety profile of the different drugs as options for treatment of ABC patients, alone or in combination with targeted agents, and the data regarding QoL. As well covered in the literature analysis by Lien et al. [65], despite differences in reporting, mCHT has been found to lead to low toxicity rates, in particular no toxicity affected more than 6% of pooled patients. This represents, in our opinion, the brightest light of mCHT.

In the preclinical setting, we evaluated as "lights," the well-described mechanisms that prevent or block angiogenesis, mainly by inhibiting VEGF and, to some extent, the effect of mCHT immunomodulation.

Among the "shadows", we discussed the absence of prospective randomised trials, the design and the end-points adopted in some studies, and the heterogeneity of existing schedules, even for the same drug. Recently, Mishra-Kalyani et al. considered the role of control arms in oncology [67]; they suggest that, even though randomised control trials allow for a comparison of treatment arms with minimal concern for confounding by known and unknown factors, in some situations, and for some strategies, a randomised study is not feasible. These authors suggest that, when such designs are not possible, the incorporation of external control data into the study design could get around the obstacle. In the absence of the possibility of conducting prospective randomised phase 3 studies in different settings of BC and for different populations (TNBC, Luminal, HER2 + ve), we hope that this suggested shortcut will allow a definitive comparison between standard and metronomic strategies.

From the preclinical point of view, the "shadows" are represented by all the aspects still to be clarified, including the different factors that might facilitate the use of combinatorial regimens of mCHT. These include understanding of the mechanisms of action of metronomic schedules and the recognition and validation of predictive biomarkers, which, if identified, would provide valuable support for clinical application.

Our aim is to encourage readers to extend the amount of available data collected on mCHT for the treatment of ABC patients and, perhaps, to push them to consider this strategy in their clinical practice for some patients, in some emergency situations, or in low- or middle-income countries, where a low-cost strategy, such as mCHT, might partially rebalance disparities.

5. Conclusions

The efficacy of other agents in mCHT treatment combined with antiangiogenic treatment should be investigated. An example of a promising approach is the use of Bruton's tyrosine kinase (BTK) inhibitors, such as ibrutinib, which was developed to treat several blood cancers, but has recently been shown to act effectively in solid tumours [68,69]. These drugs hit multiple targets and are associated with numerous expected outcomes. It has already been shown that ibrutinib has an antimetastatic effect on MCF-7 cells by activating the MAPK/NF-kB/AP-1 pathway and inhibiting MMP-9 expression [70]; reducing the viability of Erb2-positive (Erb2+) breast cancer cell lines by inhibiting the phosphorylation of receptor tyrosine kinases ErbB1, ErbB2, ErbB3 [71]; inhibits xenograft tumour growth by decreasing HER2, BTK, Akt, Erk, and increasing cleaved caspase-3 [72]; and affects anti-tumour immunity by reprogramming myeloid-derived suppressor cells (MDSCs) to mature DCs thus preventing tumour growth and metastasis, as demonstrated in a murine model of breast cancer [73].

Preclinical models of breast cancer could be developed to gain a more in-depth understanding of the basis of resistance, relapse, or progression of mCHT therapy, as well as to perform precise therapeutic tests of mCHT treatment by using mice with metastatic disease or mice carrying patient-derived breast cancer tissue, to characterize and improve the efficacy of antitumor combination therapies in vivo, as suggested by Kerbel [74].

From this extensive analysis focused on lights and shadows, we can conclude that mCHT *per se* is not associated with severe toxicities, especially haematological or gastrointestinal effects, as detailed in the studies reported in this review, and as described in other similar papers [75,76]. However, mCHT loses this advantage, which is peculiar to this method, when different agents, with their related toxicities, or other chemotherapy drugs administered at standard doses, are co-administered [43,59].

Considering that improvement in the QoL of ABC patients, by reducing treatment toxicity, is one of the main goals of the Global Alliance Against Cancer, we strongly believe that current strategies, such as immunotherapy, should be studied in association with mCHT.

Global efforts should be combined so as not to throw away such a precious amount of data. More modern study designs should be used to clearly demonstrate if mCHT should be incorporated into our current strategies for treatment.

Author Contributions: Conceptualization, M.E.C. and M.G.C.; methodology, M.E.C. and M.G.C.; writing—original draft preparation, M.E.C., N.C., S.C., V.C., F.F.P., F.R. and M.G.C.; writing—review and editing, M.E.C. and M.G.C.; supervision, M.E.C. All authors have read and agreed to the published version of the manuscript.

Funding: This research received no external funding.

Acknowledgments: We would like to acknowledge Maddalena Mongera for administrative and technical support and the Centro Studi Raffaella Trabattoni for donations in kind (APC).

Conflicts of Interest: The authors declare no conflict of interest.

References

1. Cazzaniga, M.E.; Cordani, N.; Capici, S.; Cogliati, V.; Riva, F.; Cerrito, M.G. Metronomic Chemotherapy. *Cancers* **2021**, *13*, 2236. [CrossRef] [PubMed]
2. Hanahan, D.; Bergers, G.; Bergsland, E. Less is more, regularly: Metronomic dosing of cytotoxic drugs can target tumor angiogenesis in mice. *J. Clin. Investig.* **2000**, *105*, 1045–1047. [CrossRef]
3. Browder, T.; Butterfield, C.E.; Kraling, B.M.; Shi, B.; Marshall, B.; O'Reilly, M.S.; Folkman, J. Antiangiogenic scheduling of chemotherapy improves efficacy against experimental drug-resistant cancer. *Cancer Res.* **2000**, *60*, 1878–1886.
4. Wechman, S.L.; Emdad, L.; Sarkar, D.; Das, S.K.; Fisher, P.B. Vascular mimicry: Triggers, molecular interactions and in vivo models. *Adv. Cancer Res.* **2020**, *148*, 27–67. [CrossRef] [PubMed]
5. Klement, G.; Huang, P.; Mayer, B.; Green, S.K.; Man, S.; Bohlen, P.; Hicklin, D.; Kerbel, R.S. Differences in therapeutic indexes of combination metronomic chemotherapy and an anti-VEGFR-2 antibody in multidrug-resistant human breast cancer xenografts. *Clin. Cancer Res.* **2002**, *8*, 221–232.
6. Fouladzadeh, A.; Dorraki, M.; Min, K.K.M.; Cockshell, M.P.; Thompson, E.J.; Verjans, J.W.; Allison, A.; Bonder, C.S.; Abbott, D. The development of tumour vascular networks. *Commun. Biol.* **2021**, *4*, 1111. [CrossRef]
7. Natale, G.; Bocci, G. Does metronomic chemotherapy induce tumor angiogenic dormancy? A review of available preclinical and clinical data. *Cancer Lett.* **2018**, *432*, 28–37. [CrossRef] [PubMed]
8. Kerbel, R.S.; Kamen, B.A. The anti-angiogenic basis of metronomic chemotherapy. *Nat. Rev. Cancer* **2004**, *4*, 423–436. [CrossRef] [PubMed]
9. Vasudev, N.S.; Reynolds, A.R. Anti angiogenic therapy for cancer: Current progress, unresolved questions and future directions. *Angiogenesis* **2014**, *17*, 471–494. [CrossRef] [PubMed]
10. Ghosh Dastidar, D.; Ghosh, D.; Chakrabarti, G. Tumour vasculature targeted anti-cancer therapy. *Vessel Plus* **2020**, *4*, 14. [CrossRef]
11. Di Desidero, T.; Xu, P.; Man, S.; Bocci, G.; Kerbel, R.S. Potent efficacy of metronomic topotecan and pazopanib combination therapy in preclinical models of primary or late stage metastatic triple-negative breast cancer. *Oncotarget* **2015**, *6*, 42396–42410. [CrossRef]
12. Andre, N.; Tsai, K.; Carre, M.; Pasquier, E. Metronomic Chemotherapy: Direct Targeting of Cancer Cells after all? *Trends Cancer* **2017**, *3*, 319–325. [CrossRef] [PubMed]
13. Parra, K.; Valenzuela, P.; Lerma, N.; Gallegos, A.; Reza, L.C.; Rodriguez, G.; Emmenegger, U.; Di Desidero, T.; Bocci, G.; Felder, M.S.; et al. Impact of CTLA-4 blockade in conjunction with metronomic chemotherapy on preclinical breast cancer growth. *Br. J. Cancer* **2017**, *116*, 324–334. [CrossRef]
14. Khan, K.A.; Ponce de Leon, J.L.; Benguigui, M.; Xu, P.; Chow, A.; Cruz-Munoz, W.; Man, S.; Shaked, Y.; Kerbel, R.S. Immunostimulatory and anti-tumor metronomic cyclophosphamide regimens assessed in primary orthotopic and metastatic murine breast cancer. *NPJ Breast Cancer* **2020**, *6*, 29. [CrossRef] [PubMed]
15. Orecchioni, S.; Talarico, G.; Labanca, V.; Calleri, A.; Mancuso, P.; Bertolini, F. Vinorelbine, cyclophosphamide and 5-FU effects on the circulating and intratumoural landscape of immune cells improve anti-PD-L1 efficacy in preclinical models of breast cancer and lymphoma. *Br. J. Cancer* **2018**, *118*, 1329–1336. [CrossRef]
16. Shaked, Y.; Emmenegger, U.; Francia, G.; Chen, L.; Lee, C.R.; Man, S.; Paraghamian, A.; Ben-David, Y.; Kerbel, R.S. Low-dose metronomic combined with intermittent bolus-dose cyclophosphamide is an effective long-term chemotherapy treatment strategy. *Cancer Res.* **2005**, *65*, 7045–7051. [CrossRef]
17. Daenen, L.G.; Shaked, Y.; Man, S.; Xu, P.; Voest, E.E.; Hoffman, R.M.; Chaplin, D.J.; Kerbel, R.S. Low-dose metronomic cyclophosphamide combined with vascular disrupting therapy induces potent antitumor activity in preclinical human tumor xenograft models. *Mol. Cancer Ther.* **2009**, *8*, 2872–2881. [CrossRef] [PubMed]
18. Fukumura, D.; Kloepper, J.; Amoozgar, Z.; Duda, D.G.; Jain, R.K. Enhancing cancer immunotherapy using antiangiogenics: Opportunities and challenges. *Nat. Rev. Clin. Oncol.* **2018**, *15*, 325–340. [CrossRef] [PubMed]

19. Cramarossa, G.; Lee, E.K.; Sivanathan, L.; Georgsdottir, S.; Lien, K.; Santos, K.D.; Chan, K.; Emmenegger, U. A systematic literature analysis of correlative studies in low-dose metronomic chemotherapy trials. *Biomark Med.* **2014**, *8*, 893–911. [CrossRef] [PubMed]
20. Rajasekaran, T.; Ng, Q.S.; Tan, D.S.; Lim, W.T.; Ang, M.K.; Toh, C.K.; Chowbay, B.; Kanesvaran, R.; Tan, E.H. Metronomic chemotherapy: A relook at its basis and rationale. *Cancer Lett.* **2017**, *388*, 328–333. [CrossRef]
21. Kim, H.; Lee, Y.; Lee, S.; Kim, J.G. Changes in Breast-tumor Blood Flow in Response to Hypercapnia during Chemotherapy with Laser Speckle Flowmetry. *Curr. Opt. Photonics* **2019**, *3*, 555–565. [CrossRef]
22. Filippone, M.G.; Gaglio, D.; Bonfanti, R.; Tucci, F.A.; Ceccacci, E.; Pennisi, R.; Bonanomi, M.; Jodice, G.; Tillhon, M.; Montani, F.; et al. CDK12 promotes tumorigenesis but induces vulnerability to therapies inhibiting folate one-carbon metabolism in breast cancer. *Nat. Commun.* **2022**, *13*, 2642. [CrossRef] [PubMed]
23. Roy, A.; Sarker, S.; Upadhyay, P.; Pal, A.; Adhikary, A.; Jana, K.; Ray, M. Methylglyoxal at metronomic doses sensitizes breast cancer cells to doxorubicin and cisplatin causing synergistic induction of programmed cell death and inhibition of stemness. *Biochem. Pharmacol.* **2018**, *156*, 322–339. [CrossRef]
24. Salem, A.R.; Martinez Pulido, P.; Sanchez, F.; Sanchez, Y.; Espanol, A.J.; Sales, M.E. Effect of low dose metronomic therapy on MCF-7 tumor cells growth and angiogenesis. Role of muscarinic acetylcholine receptors. *Int. Immunopharmacol.* **2020**, *84*, 106514. [CrossRef]
25. Cerrito, M.G.; De Giorgi, M.; Pelizzoni, D.; Bonomo, S.M.; Digiacomo, N.; Scagliotti, A.; Bugarin, C.; Gaipa, G.; Grassilli, E.; Lavitrano, M.; et al. Metronomic combination of Vinorelbine and 5Fluorouracil is able to inhibit triple-negative breast cancer cells. Results from the proof-of-concept VICTOR-0 study. *Oncotarget* **2018**, *9*, 27448–27459. [CrossRef]
26. Sukumar, J.; Gast, K.; Quiroga, D.; Lustberg, M.; Williams, N. Triple-negative breast cancer: Promising prognostic biomarkers currently in development. *Expert Rev. Anticancer Ther.* **2021**, *21*, 135–148. [CrossRef]
27. Chen, Q.; Xia, R.; Zheng, W.; Zhang, L.; Li, P.; Sun, X.; Shi, J. Metronomic paclitaxel improves the efficacy of PD-1 monoclonal antibodies in breast cancer by transforming the tumor immune microenvironment. *Am. J. Transl. Res.* **2020**, *12*, 519–530.
28. Kamoun, W.S.; Dugast, A.S.; Suchy, J.J.; Grabow, S.; Fulton, R.B.; Sampson, J.F.; Luus, L.; Santiago, M.; Koshkaryev, A.; Sun, G.; et al. Synergy between EphA2-ILs-DTXp, a Novel EphA2-Targeted Nanoliposomal Taxane, and PD-1 Inhibitors in Preclinical Tumor Models. *Mol. Cancer Ther.* **2020**, *19*, 270–281. [CrossRef]
29. Francia, G.; Man, S.; Lee, C.J.; Lee, C.R.; Xu, P.; Mossoba, M.E.; Emmenegger, U.; Medin, J.A.; Kerbel, R.S. Comparative impact of trastuzumab and cyclophosphamide on HER-2-positive human breast cancer xenografts. *Clin. Cancer Res.* **2009**, *15*, 6358–6366. [CrossRef]
30. Vergato, C.; Doshi, K.A.; Roblyer, D.; Waxman, D.J. Type-I Interferon Signaling Is Essential for Robust Metronomic Chemo-Immunogenic Tumor Regression in Murine Breast Cancer. *Cancer Res. Commun.* **2022**, *2*, 246–257. [CrossRef]
31. Fowler, A.M.; Mankoff, D.A.; Joe, B.N. Imaging Neoadjuvant Therapy Response in Breast Cancer. *Radiology* **2017**, *285*, 358–375. [CrossRef] [PubMed]
32. Tabassum, S.; Tank, A.; Wang, F.; Karrobi, K.; Vergato, C.; Bigio, I.J.; Waxman, D.J.; Roblyer, D. Optical scattering as an early marker of apoptosis during chemotherapy and antiangiogenic therapy in murine models of prostate and breast cancer. *Neoplasia* **2021**, *23*, 294–303. [CrossRef] [PubMed]
33. Shaked, Y.; Pham, E.; Hariharan, S.; Magidey, K.; Beyar-Katz, O.; Xu, P.; Man, S.; Wu, F.T.; Miller, V.; Andrews, D.; et al. Evidence Implicating Immunological Host Effects in the Efficacy of Metronomic Low-Dose Chemotherapy. *Cancer Res.* **2016**, *76*, 5983–5993. [CrossRef] [PubMed]
34. Bocci, G.; Kerbel, R.S. Pharmacokinetics of metronomic chemotherapy: A neglected but crucial aspect. *Nat. Rev. Clin. Oncol.* **2016**, *13*, 659–673. [CrossRef]
35. Colleoni, M.; Gray, K.P.; Gelber, S.; Lang, I.; Thurlimann, B.; Gianni, L.; Abdi, E.A.; Gomez, H.L.; Linderholm, B.K.; Puglisi, F.; et al. Low-Dose Oral Cyclophosphamide and Methotrexate Maintenance for Hormone Receptor-Negative Early Breast Cancer: International Breast Cancer Study Group Trial 22-00. *J. Clin. Oncol.* **2016**, *34*, 3400–3408. [CrossRef]
36. Gebbia, V.; Boussen, H.; Valerio, M.R. Oral metronomic cyclophosphamide with and without methotrexate as palliative treatment for patients with metastatic breast carcinoma. *Anticancer Res.* **2012**, *32*, 529–536.
37. Jung, L.; Miske, A.; Indorf, A.; Nelson, K.; Gadi, V.K.; Banda, K. A Retrospective Analysis of Metronomic Cyclophosphamide, Methotrexate, and Fluorouracil (CMF) Versus Docetaxel and Cyclophosphamide (TC) as Adjuvant Treatment in Early Stage, Hormone Receptor Positive, HER2 Negative Breast Cancer. *Clin. Breast Cancer* **2022**, *22*, e310–e318. [CrossRef]
38. Mutlu, H.; Musri, F.Y.; Artac, M.; Kargi, A.; Ozdogan, M.; Bozcuk, H. Metronomic oral chemotherapy with old agents in patients with heavily treated metastatic breast cancer. *J. Cancer Res. Ther.* **2015**, *11*, 287–290. [CrossRef]
39. Lu, Q.; Lee, K.; Xu, F.; Xia, W.; Zheng, Q.; Hong, R.; Jiang, K.; Zhai, Q.; Li, Y.; Shi, Y.; et al. Metronomic chemotherapy of cyclophosphamide plus methotrexate for advanced breast cancer: Real-world data analyses and experience of one center. *Cancer Commun.* **2020**, *40*, 222–233. [CrossRef]
40. Briasoulis, E.; Pappas, P.; Puozzo, C.; Tolis, C.; Fountzilas, G.; Dafni, U.; Marselos, M.; Pavlidis, N. Dose-ranging study of metronomic oral vinorelbine in patients with advanced refractory cancer. *Clin. Cancer Res.* **2009**, *15*, 6454–6461. [CrossRef]
41. Krajnak, S.; Decker, T.; Schollenberger, L.; Rose, C.; Ruckes, C.; Fehm, T.; Thomssen, C.; Harbeck, N.; Schmidt, M. Phase II study of metronomic treatment with daily oral vinorelbine as first-line chemotherapy in patients with advanced/metastatic HR+/HER2- breast cancer resistant to endocrine therapy: VinoMetro-AGO-B-046. *J. Cancer Res. Clin. Oncol.* **2021**, *147*, 3391–3400. [CrossRef]

42. Montagna, E.; Palazzo, A.; Maisonneuve, P.; Cancello, G.; Iorfida, M.; Sciandivasci, A.; Esposito, A.; Cardillo, A.; Mazza, M.; Munzone, E.; et al. Safety and efficacy study of metronomic vinorelbine, cyclophosphamide plus capecitabine in metastatic breast cancer: A phase II trial. *Cancer Lett.* **2017**, *400*, 276–281. [CrossRef] [PubMed]
43. Brems-Eskildsen, A.S.; Linnet, S.; Dano, H.; Luczak, A.; Vestlev, P.M.; Jakobsen, E.H.; Neimann, J.; Jensen, C.B.; Dongsgaard, T.; Langkjer, S.T. Metronomic treatment of vinorelbine with oral capecitabine is tolerable in the randomized Phase 2 study XeNa including patients with HER2 non-amplified metastatic breast cancer. *Acta Oncol.* **2021**, *60*, 157–164. [CrossRef] [PubMed]
44. Krajnak, S.; Battista, M.; Brenner, W.; Almstedt, K.; Elger, T.; Heimes, A.S.; Hasenburg, A.; Schmidt, M. Explorative Analysis of Low-Dose Metronomic Chemotherapy with Cyclophosphamide and Methotrexate in a Cohort of Metastatic Breast Cancer Patients. *Breast Care* **2018**, *13*, 272–276. [CrossRef] [PubMed]
45. Cazzaniga, M.E.; Torri, V.; Riva, F.; Porcu, L.; Cicchiello, F.; Capici, S.; Cortinovis, D.; Digiacomo, N.; Bidoli, P. Efficacy and safety of vinorelbine-capecitabine oral metronomic combination in elderly metastatic breast cancer patients: VICTOR-1 study. *Tumori* **2017**, *103*, e4–e8. [CrossRef]
46. Cazzaniga, M.E.; Cortesi, L.; Ferzi, A.; Scaltriti, L.; Cicchiello, F.; Ciccarese, M.; Della Torre, S.; Villa, F.; Giordano, M.; Verusio, C.; et al. Metronomic chemotherapy with oral vinorelbine (mVNR) and capecitabine (mCAPE) in advanced HER2-negative breast cancer patients: Is it a way to optimize disease control? Final results of the VICTOR-2 study. *Breast Cancer Res. Treat.* **2016**, *160*, 501–509. [CrossRef]
47. Cazzaniga, M.E.; Pinotti, G.; Montagna, E.; Amoroso, D.; Berardi, R.; Butera, A.; Cagossi, K.; Cavanna, L.; Ciccarese, M.; Cinieri, S.; et al. Metronomic chemotherapy for advanced breast cancer patients in the real world practice: Final results of the VICTOR-6 study. *Breast* **2019**, *48*, 7–16. [CrossRef] [PubMed]
48. Montagna, E.; Pagan, E.; Cancello, G.; Sangalli, C.; Bagnardi, V.; Munzone, E.; Sale, E.O.; Malengo, D.; Cazzaniga, M.E.; Negri, M.; et al. The prolonged clinical benefit with metronomic chemotherapy (VEX regimen) in metastatic breast cancer patients. *Anticancer Drugs* **2022**, *33*, e628–e634. [CrossRef] [PubMed]
49. Mayer, E.L.; Isakoff, S.J.; Klement, G.; Downing, S.R.; Chen, W.Y.; Hannagan, K.; Gelman, R.; Winer, E.P.; Burstein, H.J. Combination antiangiogenic therapy in advanced breast cancer: A phase 1 trial of vandetanib, a VEGFR inhibitor, and metronomic chemotherapy, with correlative platelet proteomics. *Breast Cancer Res. Treat.* **2012**, *136*, 169–178. [CrossRef]
50. Colleoni, M.; Orlando, L.; Sanna, G.; Rocca, A.; Maisonneuve, P.; Peruzzotti, G.; Ghisini, R.; Sandri, M.T.; Zorzino, L.; Nole, F.; et al. Metronomic low-dose oral cyclophosphamide and methotrexate plus or minus thalidomide in metastatic breast cancer: Antitumor activity and biological effects. *Ann. Oncol.* **2006**, *17*, 232–238. [CrossRef] [PubMed]
51. Wildiers, H.; Tryfonidis, K.; Dal Lago, L.; Vuylsteke, P.; Curigliano, G.; Waters, S.; Brouwers, B.; Altintas, S.; Touati, N.; Cardoso, F.; et al. Pertuzumab and trastuzumab with or without metronomic chemotherapy for older patients with HER2-positive metastatic breast cancer (EORTC 75111-10114): An open-label, randomised, phase 2 trial from the Elderly Task Force/Breast Cancer Group. *Lancet. Oncol.* **2018**, *19*, 323–336. [CrossRef]
52. Dal Lago, L.; Uwimana, A.L.; Coens, C.; Vuylsteke, P.; Curigliano, G.; Brouwers, B.; Jagiello-Gruszfeld, A.; Altintas, S.; Tryfonidis, K.; Poncet, C.; et al. Health-related quality of life in older patients with HER2+ metastatic breast cancer: Comparing pertuzumab plus trastuzumab with or without metronomic chemotherapy in a randomised open-label phase II clinical trial. *J. Geriatr. Oncol.* **2022**, *5*, 582–593. [CrossRef]
53. Wang, Z.; Liu, J.; Ma, F.; Wang, J.; Luo, Y.; Fan, Y.; Yuan, P.; Zhang, P.; Li, Q.; Li, Q.; et al. Safety and efficacy study of oral metronomic vinorelbine combined with trastuzumab (mNH) in HER2-positive metastatic breast cancer: A phase II trial. *Breast Cancer Res. Treat.* **2021**, *188*, 441–447. [CrossRef] [PubMed]
54. Dellapasqua, S.; Bertolini, F.; Bagnardi, V.; Campagnoli, E.; Scarano, E.; Torrisi, R.; Shaked, Y.; Mancuso, P.; Goldhirsch, A.; Rocca, A.; et al. Metronomic cyclophosphamide and capecitabine combined with bevacizumab in advanced breast cancer. *J. Clin. Oncol.* **2008**, *26*, 4899–4905. [CrossRef]
55. Garcia-Saenz, J.A.; Martin, M.; Calles, A.; Bueno, C.; Rodriguez, L.; Bobokova, J.; Custodio, A.; Casado, A.; Diaz-Rubio, E. Bevacizumab in combination with metronomic chemotherapy in patients with anthracycline- and taxane-refractory breast cancer. *J. Chemother.* **2008**, *20*, 632–639. [CrossRef]
56. Rochlitz, C.; Bigler, M.; von Moos, R.; Bernhard, J.; Matter-Walstra, K.; Wicki, A.; Zaman, K.; Anchisi, S.; Kung, M.; Na, K.J.; et al. SAKK 24/09: Safety and tolerability of bevacizumab plus paclitaxel vs. bevacizumab plus metronomic cyclophosphamide and capecitabine as first-line therapy in patients with HER2-negative advanced stage breast cancer—A multicenter, randomized phase III trial. *BMC Cancer* **2016**, *16*, 780. [CrossRef]
57. Palazzo, A.; Dellapasqua, S.; Munzone, E.; Bagnardi, V.; Mazza, M.; Cancello, G.; Ghisini, R.; Iorfida, M.; Montagna, E.; Goldhirsch, A.; et al. Phase II Trial of Bevacizumab Plus Weekly Paclitaxel, Carboplatin, and Metronomic Cyclophosphamide With or Without Trastuzumab and Endocrine Therapy as Preoperative Treatment of Inflammatory Breast Cancer. *Clin. Breast Cancer* **2018**, *18*, 328–335. [CrossRef] [PubMed]
58. Bertolini, F.; Paul, S.; Mancuso, P.; Monestiroli, S.; Gobbi, A.; Shaked, Y.; Kerbel, R.S. Maximum tolerable dose and low-dose metronomic chemotherapy have opposite effects on the mobilization and viability of circulating endothelial progenitor cells. *Cancer Res.* **2003**, *63*, 4342–4346.
59. Perroud, H.A.; Rico, M.J.; Alasino, C.M.; Queralt, F.; Mainetti, L.E.; Pezzotto, S.M.; Rozados, V.R.; Scharovsky, O.G. Safety and therapeutic effect of metronomic chemotherapy with cyclophosphamide and celecoxib in advanced breast cancer patients. *Future Oncol.* **2013**, *9*, 451–462. [CrossRef]

60. Perroud, H.A.; Alasino, C.M.; Rico, M.J.; Mainetti, L.E.; Queralt, F.; Pezzotto, S.M.; Rozados, V.R.; Scharovsky, O.G. Metastatic breast cancer patients treated with low-dose metronomic chemotherapy with cyclophosphamide and celecoxib: Clinical outcomes and biomarkers of response. *Cancer Chemother. Pharmacol.* **2016**, *77*, 365–374. [CrossRef]
61. Bazzola, L.; Foroni, C.; Andreis, D.; Zanoni, V.; Cappelletti, M.R.; Allevi, G.; Aguggini, S.; Strina, C.; Milani, M.; Venturini, S.; et al. Combination of letrozole, metronomic cyclophosphamide and sorafenib is well-tolerated and shows activity in patients with primary breast cancer. *Br. J. Cancer* **2015**, *112*, 52–60. [CrossRef] [PubMed]
62. Kummar, S.; Wade, J.L.; Oza, A.M.; Sullivan, D.; Chen, A.P.; Gandara, D.R.; Ji, J.; Kinders, R.J.; Wang, L.; Allen, D.; et al. Randomized phase II trial of cyclophosphamide and the oral poly (ADP-ribose) polymerase inhibitor veliparib in patients with recurrent, advanced triple-negative breast cancer. *Investig. New Drugs* **2016**, *34*, 355–363. [CrossRef]
63. Anampa, J.; Chen, A.; Wright, J.; Patel, M.; Pellegrino, C.; Fehn, K.; Sparano, J.A.; Andreopoulou, E. Phase I Trial of Veliparib, a Poly ADP Ribose Polymerase Inhibitor, Plus Metronomic Cyclophosphamide in Metastatic HER2-negative Breast Cancer. *Clin. Breast Cancer* **2018**, *18*, e135–e142. [CrossRef]
64. Cazzaniga, M.E.; Munzone, E.; Bocci, G.; Afonso, N.; Gomez, P.; Langkjer, S.; Petru, E.; Pivot, X.; Sanchez Rovira, P.; Wysocki, P.; et al. Pan-European Expert Meeting on the Use of Metronomic Chemotherapy in Advanced Breast Cancer Patients: The PENELOPE Project. *Adv. Ther.* **2019**, *36*, 381–406. [CrossRef]
65. Lien, K.; Georgsdottir, S.; Sivanathan, L.; Chan, K.; Emmenegger, U. Low-dose metronomic chemotherapy: A systematic literature analysis. *Eur. J. Cancer* **2013**, *49*, 3387–3395. [CrossRef]
66. Shaked, Y.; Emmenegger, U.; Man, S.; Cervi, D.; Bertolini, F.; Ben-David, Y.; Kerbel, R.S. Optimal biologic dose of metronomic chemotherapy regimens is associated with maximum antiangiogenic activity. *Blood* **2005**, *106*, 3058–3061. [CrossRef] [PubMed]
67. Mishra-Kalyani, P.S.; Amiri Kordestani, L.; Rivera, D.R.; Singh, H.; Ibrahim, A.; DeClaro, R.A.; Shen, Y.; Tang, S.; Sridhara, R.; Kluetz, P.G.; et al. External control arms in oncology: Current use and future directions. *Ann. Oncol.* **2022**, *33*, 376–383. [CrossRef] [PubMed]
68. Grassilli, E.; Cerrito, M.G.; Lavitrano, M. BTK, the new kid on the (oncology) block? *Front. Oncol.* **2022**, *12*, 944538. [CrossRef]
69. Grassilli, E.; Cerrito, M.G.; Bonomo, S.; Giovannoni, R.; Conconi, D.; Lavitrano, M. p65BTK Is a Novel Biomarker and Therapeutic Target in Solid Tumors. *Front. Cell Dev. Biol.* **2021**, *9*, 690365. [CrossRef] [PubMed]
70. Kim, J.M.; Park, J.; Noh, E.M.; Song, H.K.; Kang, S.Y.; Jung, S.H.; Kim, J.S.; Park, B.H.; Lee, Y.R.; Youn, H.J. Bruton's agammaglobulinemia tyrosine kinase (Btk) regulates TPAinduced breast cancer cell invasion via PLCgamma2/PKCbeta/NFkappaB/AP1dependent matrix metalloproteinase9 activation. *Oncol. Rep.* **2021**, *45*, 56. [CrossRef] [PubMed]
71. Grabinski, N.; Ewald, F. Ibrutinib (ImbruvicaTM) potently inhibits ErbB receptor phosphorylation and cell viability of ErbB2-positive breast cancer cells. *Investig. New Drugs* **2014**, *32*, 1096–1104. [CrossRef] [PubMed]
72. Wang, X.; Wong, J.; Sevinsky, C.J.; Kokabee, L.; Khan, F.; Sun, Y.; Conklin, D.S. Bruton's Tyrosine Kinase Inhibitors Prevent Therapeutic Escape in Breast Cancer Cells. *Mol. Cancer Ther.* **2016**, *15*, 2198–2208. [CrossRef] [PubMed]
73. Varikuti, S.; Singh, B.; Volpedo, G.; Ahirwar, D.K.; Jha, B.K.; Saljoughian, N.; Viana, A.G.; Verma, C.; Hamza, O.; Halsey, G.; et al. Ibrutinib treatment inhibits breast cancer progression and metastasis by inducing conversion of myeloid-derived suppressor cells to dendritic cells. *Br. J. Cancer* **2020**, *122*, 1005–1013. [CrossRef] [PubMed]
74. Kerbel, R.S. A Decade of Experience in Developing Preclinical Models of Advanced- or Early-Stage Spontaneous Metastasis to Study Antiangiogenic Drugs, Metronomic Chemotherapy, and the Tumor Microenvironment. *Cancer J.* **2015**, *21*, 274–283. [CrossRef]
75. Scharovsky, O.G.; Rico, M.J.; Mainetti, L.E.; Perroud, H.A.; Rozados, V.R. Achievements and challenges in the use of metronomics for the treatment of breast cancer. *Biochem. Pharmacol.* **2020**, *175*, 113909. [CrossRef]
76. Krajnak, S.; Battista, M.J.; Hasenburg, A.; Schmidt, M. Metronomic Chemotherapy for Metastatic Breast Cancer. *Oncol. Res. Treat.* **2022**, *45*, 12–17. [CrossRef]

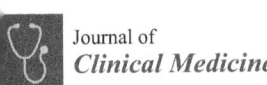

Review

Metronomic Chemotherapy in Prostate Cancer

Piotr J. Wysocki [1,2,*], Maciej T. Lubas [2] and Malgorzata L. Wysocka [3,*]

1. Department of Oncology, Medical College, Jagiellonian University, 30-252 Krakow, Poland
2. Department of Oncology, Krakow University Hospital, 30-688 Krakow, Poland; mlubas@su.krakow.pl
3. Oncoaid, ul. Sliska 7/2, 30-504 Krakow, Poland
* Correspondence: piotr.wysocki@uj.edu.pl (P.J.W.); mkw1606@gmail.com (M.L.W.); Tel.: +48-12-424-7180 (P.J.W.)

Abstract: Despite the significant expansion of the therapeutic armamentarium associated with the introduction of novel endocrine therapies, cytotoxic agents, radiopharmaceuticals, and PARP inhibitors, progression of metastatic castration-resistant prostate cancer (mCRPC) beyond treatment options remains the leading cause of death in advanced prostate cancer patients. Metronomic chemotherapy (MC) is an old concept of wise utilization of cytotoxic agents administered continuously and at low doses. The metronomic is unique due to its multidimensional mechanisms of action involving: (i) inhibition of cancer cell proliferation, (ii) inhibition of angiogenesis, (iii) mitigation of tumor-related immunosuppression, (iv) impairment of cancer stem cell functions, and (v) modulation of tumor and host microbiome. MC has been extensively studied in advanced prostate cancer before the advent of novel therapies, and its actual activity in contemporary, heavily pretreated mCRPC patients is unknown. We have conducted a prospective analysis of consecutive cases of mCRPC patients who failed all available standard therapies to find the optimal MC regimen for phase II studies. The metronomic combination of weekly paclitaxel 60 mg/m^2 i.v. with capecitabine 1500 mg/d p.o. and cyclophosphamide 50 mg/d p.o. was selected as the preferred regimen for a planned phase II study in heavily pretreated mCRPC patients.

Keywords: metronomic chemotherapy; prostate cancer; CRPC; castration; cyclophosphamide; capecitabine; paclitaxel; immunomodulation; angiogenesis; microbiome

1. Standard Systemic Treatment of Advanced Prostate Cancer

Endocrine therapy, basically androgen deprivation (ADT), is the standard treatment of prostate cancer (PC). This neoplasm arises from prostate gland epithelial cells located in lobules and ducts, whose growth and differentiation are tightly regulated by androgens, mainly testosterone. Therefore, well-differentiated prostate cancers are usually susceptible to androgen deprivation which allows for long-term inhibition of disease progression. However, many prostate cancers are poorly differentiated (Gleason ≥ 8 or grading ≥ 4), and therefore the sensitivity to endocrine treatment is low and short. Historically, surgical castration, and later, pharmacological castration, represented the only option of systemic treatment with proven activity in prostate cancer, and chemotherapy was generally assumed as not active in this disease [1]. The development of resistance to androgen deprivation (castration) is usually associated with increased expression and/or hypersensitivity of androgen receptors in PC cells and autocrine and paracrine production of androgens beyond the control hypothalamus–pituitary–gonadal axis [2,3]. Therefore, since, at the initial stage of castration resistance, PC cells demonstrate increased instead of decreased endocrine sensitivity, novel generations of hormonal agents like abiraterone acetate or irreversible androgen receptor (AR) blockers (enzalutamide, daralutamide, and apalutamide) could show high anticancer activity leading to prolonged disease control and improved patients' outcomes [4–8]. However, prostate cancer cells will ultimately become resistant to endocrine treatment by activating various hormone-unrelated molecular mechanisms, leading to increased aggressiveness and proliferation. However, these features of castration resistant prostate cancer reflect increased sensitivity of PC cells to antiproliferative cytotoxic agents such as microtubule inhibitors. Docetaxel was the first chemotherapy drug shown in 2004, to improve the overall survival of metastatic castration-resistant prostate cancer (mCRPC) patients [9]. Additionally, due to its inhibitory impact on AR transcriptional activity, docetaxel's antitumor potential was also confirmed in metastatic castration-sensitive PC (mCSPC), where it was combined in first-line of treatment with androgen deprivation [10,11]. The increased chemotherapy sensitivity of CRPC cells, which results from AR-independency and increased proliferation rate, is not restricted to a single class of cytotoxic drugs (microtubule depolymerization inhibitors—taxanes). In hormone-refractory PC various cytotoxic agents have demonstrated clinical activity, but only large phase III clinical studies on taxanes had sufficient power to prove a significant improvement of outcomes with the use of chemotherapy.

With the widespread of novel, highly active endocrine agents, the incidence of a previously rare phenomenon of neuroendocrine differentiation increased significantly [12]. Cells with neuroendocrine features occur in approx. 1% of primary prostate tumors, but neuroendocrine differentiation is present in 25% of end-stage metastatic castration-resistant disease cases [13]. The loss of adenocarcinoma phenotype and transformation into small cells with neuroendocrine features is one of the ways the androgen-deprived PC utilizes to get rid of androgen dependency. Characteristic features of small-cell neuroendocrine tumors are high aggressiveness, rapid proliferation, and sensitivity to chemotherapy platinum-based regimens usually used to treat neuroendocrine cancers such as small-cell lung cancer [14] However, the sensitivity of prostate cancer to platinum compounds, which is atypical for this tumor besides neuroendocrine differentiation, can also result from prostate cancer genetic background. Inherited mutations of genes responsible for homologous recombination (homologous recombination deficiency—HRD) are relatively rare, with germinal mutations of the two most important cancer predisposition genes—*BRCA1* or *BRCA2* found in 0.4% and 1–2% of PC patients, respectively [15,16]. On the other hand, somatic or germinal mutations in genes responsible for double-strand DNA repair can be detected in 11.8% of tumor tissues from mCRPC patients [17]. Moreover, in a screening phase of a phase III study evaluating olaparib in mCRPC patients, at least one mutation/deletion (germline or somatic) within 15 genes responsible for homologous recombination was detected in 28% of patients (778 of 2792 tumors with HRD) [18]. Deleterious mutations in *BRCA1* and *BRCA2* genes in prostate cancer cells are predictive of the olaparib activity, which has been shown to significantly improve the overall survival of advanced mCRPC patients. However, recent data suggest the presence of HRD is also predictive of the activity of DNA-damaging cytotoxic agents. Therefore, in heavily pretreated mCRPC patients alkylating agents such as platinum compounds or cyclophosphamide can be more effective than previously, based on data from clinical studies conducted 2–3 decades ago, considered.

2. Challenges Associated with the Use of Standard Chemotherapy in Prostate Cancer

Prostate cancer is relatively resistant to chemotherapy. Before the introduction of docetaxel, the only available cytotoxic drug with any activity against prostate cancer was mitoxantrone [19]. However, when combined with prednisone, the benefit of this topoisomerase II inhibitor was superior to prednisone alone only in terms of pain control and quality of life, but not in terms of overall survival. In 2004, docetaxel was approved for the treatment of mCRPC patients based on two landmark studies—TAX327 and SWOG 9916, which demonstrated significant improvement in OS with docetaxel-based regimens compared to mitoxantrone [9,20]. Particularly, in TAX327 study, which compared 3-weekly docetaxel (75 mg/m^2 q3w) with weekly docetaxel (30 mg/m^2 q1w) and with mitoxantrone (all drugs combined with prednisone 10 mg/daily), the 3-weekly regimen significantly improved median OS compared to mitoxantrone (HR = HR = 0.79, 95%CI 0.67–0.93) [9]. The median OS was 19.2, 17.8, and 16.3 months, in docetaxel q3w, docetaxel q2w, and mitoxantrone arms, respectively. Additionally, both docetaxel-based regimens significantly improved patients' quality of life (QOL) compared to mitoxantrone [21]. However, the significant improvement of outcomes with docetaxel administered at 3-week intervals came at the cost of increased toxicity. Grade ≥ 3 adverse events such as neutropenia, fatigue, diarrhea, neuropathy, stomatitis, dyspnea, and peripheral edema were significantly more frequent in docetaxel q3w than mitoxantrone arm.

The toxicity of standard docetaxel dose can be reduced by administering the drug in shorter intervals at a reduced dose. The TAX327 study has not confirmed the clinical utility of weekly docetaxel at 30 mg/m^2, but a phase III study of a Scandinavian PROSTY group demonstrated at least similar activity of biweekly docetaxel 50 mg/m^2 compared to the standard dosing. The biweekly administration of docetaxel was associated with significant improvement of the primary endpoint, which was time-to-treatment failure (TTF), compared to the 3-weekly regimen [22]. The median TTF was 5.6 months vs 4.9 months, for 2-weekly and 3-weekly regimens, respectively. Typical adverse events occurred less frequently with the lower, biweekly dose of docetaxel. Unexpectedly, secondary endpoints such as OS and PFS were significantly improved with biweekly docetaxel. There were statistically significant differences in overall QOL values and pain values favoring the biweekly treatment arm regarding patient-reported outcomes [23].

Over time, despite numerous attempts to improve the activity of docetaxel-based chemotherapy regimens by combining them with targeted agents, 3- or 2-weekly monotherapy with docetaxel remained the chemotherapy of choice for mCRPC patients [24–28].

Another taxane, cabazitaxel, is the second and the last cytotoxic agent with proven, significant activity in patients with advanced, castration-resistant prostate adenocarcinoma. A phase III TROPIC study comparing cabazitaxel 25 mg/m^2 q3w (+prednisone) with mitoxantrone (+prednisone) in mCRPC patients following failure of docetaxel-based chemotherapy demonstrated significant superiority of cabazitaxel [29]. The median OS and PFS were 15.1 months vs. 12.7 months and 2.8 months vs 1.4 months in cabazitaxel and mitoxantrone arms, respectively. The hazard ratio for death of men treated with cabazitaxel compared with those taking mitoxantrone was 0.70 (95% CI 0.59–0.83). However, again the improvement in outcomes came at the cost of increased toxicity; 5% of patients treated with cabazitaxel and 2% treated with mitoxantrone died within 30 days of the last infusion. Still, none of the deaths in the cabazitaxel arm was associated with disease progression. The most frequent adverse events were associated with hematological toxicity (neutropenia, leukopenia, and anemia), and neutropenic fever occurred in 8% of patients. Subsequently, a non-inferiority phase III PROSELICA study aimed to compare a lower dose of cabazitaxel (20 mg/m^2 q3w) with the standard dose [30]. The non-inferiority endpoint of at least 50% of OS benefit with low-dose cabazitaxel compared to the standard dose was achieved. Grade ≥ 3 adverse events were 39.7% for the low-dose cabazitaxel and 54.5% for the standard dose. Health-related quality of life did not differ between cohorts. However, significant differences were observed in favor of standard-dose cabazitaxel for PSA response and time to PSA progression (HR = 1.195; 95% CI 1.025 to 1.393).

There is no doubt that improvement in outcomes of prostate cancer patients achieved with taxane-based chemotherapy regimens came at the cost of toxicity, which, especially in elderly and fragile patients, may represent a significant drawback. However, attempts to optimize chemotherapy with dose reduction or decreased intensity may lead to inferior outcomes in at least a fraction of mCRPC patients in a real-world setting. Moreover, most mCRPC patients treated in clinical practice are old and present with a deteriorating performance status due to advanced disease and long-term systemic treatment. Therefore, after docetaxel treatment failure, many of them are no more candidates for further, intensive anticancer treatment, including but not restricted to cabazitaxel-based therapy. Since there is no further treatment option for many of such patients but hospice care, novel, low-toxic therapeutic approaches that would give a chance to improve survival and maintain quality of life, such as metronomic chemotherapy, are urgently needed.

3. Metronomic Chemotherapy—Mechanisms of Action

Metronomic chemotherapy (MC) is a concept of continuous administration of cytotoxic drugs at low doses. Unlike standard chemotherapy regimens, which usually use maximal-tolerated doses (MTD) of chemotherapeutics and require long (usually >2 weeks) recovery periods, the metronomic chemotherapy safety profile allows for continuous, very frequent drug administration [31,32]. Metronomic chemotherapy is mainly based on oral drugs, which patients can take even several times a day. Standard chemotherapy regimens based on MTD are very useful for treating aggressive cancers with a high proliferation rate [33,34]. Highly proliferating tumors, in which 90–100% of cells are actively dividing, can wholly and rapidly respond to aggressive chemotherapy. However, the usual proliferation rate of most solid tumors in adults is lower, and Ki67 scores are far below 50% (often below 15% [35,36]), which means that far beyond 50% of tumor cells (non-proliferating cells) can survive administration of chemotherapy at MTD at wide intervals. In order to control such slowly proliferating tumors, tumor cells must be exposed continuously to antiproliferative agents which will impede cellular division whenever it occurs. It is thus clear that such a long-term exposure of tumor cells to anticancer agents can only be achieved by continuous administration of cytotoxic drugs. However, the MC not only means continuous inhibition of tumor-cell proliferation but also activation of other, clinically essential mechanisms of action, which represent crucial hallmarks of metronomic chemotherapy.

3.1. Inhibition of Angiogenesis

Angiogenesis is a crucial step in tumor development since its overgrowth beyond 2–3 mm in diameter must be associated with the development of tumor-associated vasculature [37]. The angiogenic switch is related to releasing proangiogenic factors by hypoxic cancer cells, which stimulate endothelial cells in nearby blood vessels to proliferate and migrate towards the tumor center. Some initial observations suggested that many cytotoxic drugs could inhibit the activation of endothelial cells, but the effect subsided during the withdrawal of medications in treatment-free intervals [38]. Therefore, the antiangiogenic potential of standard MTD-based chemotherapies is, at best, weak and intermittent. In contrast, metronomic chemotherapy administered continuously exerts continuous antiproliferative activity on endothelial cells, thus inhibiting their potential to create pathological vasculature. Numerous studies showed that metronomic chemotherapy inhibited the proliferation and circulation of endothelial cells and endothelial progenitor cells (CEPs) and reduced the differentiation of immature endothelial cells [39–41]. Moreover, MC can inhibit the secretion of proangiogenic factors by directly inhibiting hypoxia-inducible factor 1α (HIF1α) activity in tumor cells while simultaneously increasing the production of antiangiogenic molecules. It has been recently demonstrated that MTD-based chemotherapy can promote metastatic dissemination via activation of a transcriptional program dependent on HIF-1α and HIF-2α, and that this effect could be mitigated by switching from MTD to metronomic chemotherapy [42]. Bocci et al. demonstrated that metronomically administered cyclophosphamide inhibits the synthesis of thrombospondin-1 (TSP-1) and directly mediates growth arrest and apoptosis of endothelial cells.

Additionally, they showed the inhibition of angiogenesis in human tumor-bearing immunodeficient mice treated with low daily doses of CTX [43]. Later, it was demonstrated by several groups that the antiangiogenic effect is not restricted to cyclophosphamide but can be observed with many chemotherapy drugs administered in a metronomic manner [44,45]. Over the years, it turned out that metronomic chemotherapy stimulates the production of numerous antiangiogenic factors such as: endostatin, angiostatin, soluble VEGF receptors (sVEGFRs), and pigment epithelium-derived factor (PEDF) [46].

3.2. Immunomodulation

The immunological effects of chemotherapeutic drugs are extremely diverse and complex [47,48]. The classical assumption was that standard MTD-based chemotherapy is highly immunosuppressive, owning to its myelosuppressive activity. However, many studies suggested that chemotherapy-induced myelosuppression correlates with improved outcomes [49]. In a retrospective analysis of the TROPIC trial, severe neutropenia in mCRPC patients with initially high NLR (neutrophil-to-lymphocyte ratio) treated with cabazitaxel was associated with significantly improved OS and PFS [50]. It is, however, unknown whether these improved outcomes resulted from depletion of immunosuppressive mononuclear cells or whether the neutropenia only reflected the high cytotoxic activity of cabazitaxel in particular patients. On the other hand, a significant amount of data supports the beneficial impact of metronomic chemotherapy on anticancer immune responses. The immunostimulatory effects of metronomic chemotherapy include (i) induction of immunogenic cancer cell death [51], (ii) preferential depletion of regulatory T (Treg) cells [52–55], (iii) enhancement of antigen-presentation through stimulation of dendritic cells activity (DC) [56] and increased immunogenicity of cancer cells [57], (iv) inhibition of myeloid-derived suppressor cells (MDSC) [58], and (v) activation of immune effector cells, such as tumor-specific T cells [59,60] and γδT cells [61].

3.3. Targeting Cancer Stem Cells

Cancer stem cells (CSC) represent a population of cancer-initiating cells characterized by a slow proliferation rate, self-renewal capability, and resistance to chemotherapy and irradiation. In various in vitro models, metronomic chemotherapy impeded the survival and proliferation of CSCs. In a pancreatic tumor xenograft model, metronomic administration of cyclophosphamide reduced the number of CD133+ precursor cells and CD133+/CD44+/CD24+ cancer stem cells [62]. Similarly, metronomic, but not MTD-based, cyclophosphamide inhibited the function of C6 rat glioma CSCs [63]. In a preclinical model of luminal breast cancer, metronomic paclitaxel reduced the population of CD44+/CD24- stem cells [64]. Expansion of stem-like tumor-initiating cells correlates with the development of chemoresistance and metastatic potential of cancer cells. In animal models, MTD chemotherapy, regardless of cytotoxic agents used, induced persistent STAT-1 and NF-κB activity in carcinoma-associated fibroblasts leading to secretion of CXCR2-activating chemokines [65]. Stimulation of CXCR2 on cancer cells converts them into tumor-initiating CSC responsible for invasive behaviors and paradoxically enhanced tumor aggression after therapy. In contrast, the same overall dose of cytotoxic agents administered as an MC regimen prevented therapy-induced CXCR2 paracrine signaling, thus enhancing treatment response and extending the survival of tumor-bearing mice [65].

3.4. Modulation of Gut and Tumor Microbiome

Over the last few years, increasing attention has been paid to the host gut microbiome defined as the collection of genomes from all microorganisms in the gastrointestinal tract, especially within the intestines. However, it has been demonstrated that the microbiome in general (not only the gut, but also local or even intratumoral microbiome) is associated with the pathogenesis of various cancers such as colorectal, breast, ovarian, lung, and prostate cancers [66–70]. For example, compared to a healthy population, the fecal gut microbiome in CRC patients is enriched with *Prevotella*, *Collinsella*, and *Peptostreptococcus* and contained significantly lower concentrations of Escherichia-Shigella [70]. The gut microbiota of patients diagnosed with PC on transrectal biopsy was significantly enriched with *Bacteroides* spp. compared to patients with negative biopsy results [71]. In prostate cancer, the microbiota of tumor and peri-tumoral regions had higher relative abundance of *Staphylococcus* spp. than normal areas. Still, the normal areas had a higher abundance of *Streptococcus* spp. than the tumor and the peri-tumoral regions [72].

With the advent of novel immunotherapies, the role of the microbiome has become even more important in the context of its significant role in shaping responses to checkpoint inhibitors. The gut microbiota plays an important role in regulating systemic immune responses [73–75], and the role of intestinal microbiota in mediating immune activation in response to chemotherapeutic agents has been clearly demonstrated [76,77]. In an animal melanoma model, the presence of *Bifidobacterium* correlated with the activation of antitumor immune mechanisms by anti-PD1 checkpoint inhibitors, and oral administration of *Bifidobacterium* alone improved tumor control to the same degree as PD-L blockade [78]. Moreover, a combination of anti-PD-L1 antibody with oral administration of *Bifidobacterium* completely blocked the growth of melanoma tumors in mice. Many studies showed that administration of wide-spectrum antibiotics before initiation of treatment with checkpoint inhibitors could completely abolish the efficacy of immunotherapy in patients with various tumors [79–82]. Similar observations on the lack of activity of checkpoint inhibitors come from studies in germ-free animals that resemble the effect of gut microbiome eradication with the use of antibiotics. Transplantation of fecal microbiota from immune-responding melanoma patients into germ-free mice leads to improved tumor control, augmented T cell responses, and greater efficacy of anti-PD-L1 therapy [83]. Similarly, fecal transplantation from responding melanoma patients into germ-free or antibiotic-pretreated mice could restore antitumor immune responses and induce rejection of implanted tumors, which was not observed when such animals were transplanted with fecal microbiota from non-responding patients [84]. The observation in animal models has been recently replicated in humans. In a phase II clinical trial, 15 melanoma patients refractory to anti PD-1 therapy received responder-derived fecal microbiota transplantation combined with pembrolizumab Of the 15 treated patients, 6 achieved clinical benefit (one partial response and five disease stabilization) and durable changes in microbiome composition. Responding patients demonstrated an increased abundance of taxa known to be associated with response to anti-PD-1, increased CD8+ T cell activation, and decreased frequency of interleukin-8-expressing myeloid cells [85].

Escherichia coli, a common species found in benign prostate hyperplasia (BPH) tissue, induces inflammation and tissue damage leading to neoplastic transformation in prostate epithelial cells. Ma et al. demonstrated that specific microbes, such as *Listeria monocytogenes*, *Lactobacillus crispatus*, and *Thermus thermophilus*, prevented tumor formation and growth, while other microbes, such as *Nevskia ramosa* and *S. aureus*, displayed cancer-promoting properties by inducing inflammation, immunosuppression, and promoting prostate cancer stem cells (PCSC) responsible for the development of metastases [86]. Ma et al. have demonstrated that particular bacterial species—Listeria monocytogenes, Methylobacterium radiotolerans JCM 2831, Xanthomonas albilineans GPE PC73, and Bradyrhizobium japonicum—correlated respectively with well-differentiated phenotype, earlier disease stage, lower PSA level, and lower AR expression. A particular species of *Bacteroides*, which is a genus of Gram-negative, anaerobic bacteria, may contribute to the development of high-risk prostate cancer.

The impact of metronomic chemotherapy and its difference from MTD-based microchemotherapy on the gut and intratumoral microbiome is not well recognized yet. An observational study by Zhu et al. suggested that gut microbiota diversity is higher in breast cancer patients than in healthy controls [87], but additional studies demonstrated that the diversity could be decreased with the use of metronomic capecitabine, but not MTD-dosed chemotherapy [88]. Since the impact of MC on tumors and host microbiomes can represent a novel mechanism action of MC, we have initiated a prospective analysis of the impact of various metronomic chemotherapy regimens in breast, ovarian, and prostate cancer patients, and the preliminary results shall be posted soon.

4. Metronomic Chemotherapy in Prostate Cancer

Various metronomic chemotherapy-based regimens have been evaluated in advanced PC patients over the last three decades. However, most studies were conducted before the introduction of novel hormonal or cytotoxic agents such as abiraterone acetate, enzalutamide, apalutamide, darolutamide, or cabazitaxel. All the above agents have been approved for the treatment of CRPC patients based on large, well-conducted phase III clinical trials. In comparison, the benefit of MC has been usually evaluated in small, non-randomized trials or retrospective analyses. Accordingly, metronomic chemotherapy should not be considered as a standard option at the early stages of mCRPC, if highly active, well-tolerated novel hormonal agents are freely available. Therefore, MC represents a therapeutic option in mCRPC who failed all available therapies, are unfit for standard chemotherapies, or have no access to standard mCRPC treatments, e.g., in low- or middle-income countries [89]. Nevertheless, many studies demonstrated the activity of MC in advanced mCRPC patients before the advent of novel, active therapies dedicated for this population. Selected studies are summarized in Table 1. In addition to showing the antitumor activity of MC, which was reflected by biochemical responses (PSA decline) in 30–50% of patients, all of the summarized studies demonstrated a very favorable safety profile of MC. This observation underscores the clinical utility of MC, especially in elderly and frail patients, who represent the majority of mCRPC patients. In a recent study, Calvani et al. demonstrated that metronomic cyclophosphamide (50 mg/d p.o.) combined with corticosteroids (dexamethasone 1 mg/d p.o. or prednisone 10 mg/d p.o.) induced biochemical responses (at least 50% PSA reduction) in half of the studied population. However, only two analyzed patients could be considered standard contemporary candidates (pretreatment with docetaxel and novel hormonal agents) for metronomic chemotherapy. Therefore, it is still challenging to draw any conclusions regarding the actual utility of MC in heavily pretreated mCRPC patients since many of the old studies included mCRPC patients for whom, nowadays, at least 1–2 standard treatment options are routinely available. Additionally, most of the listed studies combined MC with steroids (especially dexamethasone), which further complicates the validation of the plain MC activity in mCRPC patients. Several studies have recently demonstrated that a simple switch from prednisone to dexamethasone in mCRPC patients treated with an abiraterone + prednisone combination can lead to profound biochemical responses [90–92]. This observation underscores the risk of overestimating the benefit of MC, especially when patients are simultaneously receiving dexamethasone as a part of an antitumor treatment strategy for the first time. There is only a single study evaluating the activity of metronomic chemotherapy in pretreated (docetaxel and ≥1 novel endocrine agent) mCRPC patients. In such mCRPC patients, single-agent cyclophosphamide led to a relatively low rate of PSA responses (16%), with PSF and OS of 4 and 8.1 months, respectively. This study demonstrates that the promising activity of MC observed before the era of novel therapies may not be easily reproducible in contemporary, standardly pretreated mCRPC patients.

Table 1. Studies evaluating metronomic chemotherapy in prostate cancer.

Regmien	Number of Patients	Biochemical Response (>50% PSA Reduction)	PFS/OS (Months)	Ref
CTX 50 mg p.o. + DEX 1 mg p.o.	34	39%	NR/NR	[93]
CTX 50 mg p.o.	58	34.5% [1]	NR/NR	[94]
CTX 500 mg/m^2 i.v. induction (day 1.) → CTX 50 mg/d p.o. + CXB 200 mg p.o. bid + DEX 1 mg/d p.o.	28	32%	3.0/21.0	[95]
CTX 50 mg p.o. + DEX 1 mg p.o.	17	24%	NR/24.0	[96]
CTX 50–100 mg p.o. + prednisone 10 mg/d p.o.	18	44% [1]	4.7/NR	[97]
CTX 50 mg p.o. + prednisone 10 mg/d p.o.	23	26%	6.0/11.0	[98]
VRB 25 mg/m^2 iv 12× qw → q2w + prednisone 10 mg/d p.o.	14	36%	4.5/17	[99]
CTX 50 mg/d + MTX 2.4 mg po twice a week	58	25%	5.2/11.5	[100]
CTX 100 mg/d p.o. UFT 400 mg/d p.o. DEX 1 mg/d p.o.	57	63%	7.2/NR	[101]
CAP 1000 mg bid p.o. d 1–14 q21 + CTX 50 mg/d p.o. + thalidomide 100 mg/d p.o. + prednisone 5 mg bid p.o.	28	35.7%	4.7/19.5	[102]
DXL 35 mg/m^2 i.v. qw + CAP 625 mg/m^2 bid d 5–18 q4w (4 cycles)	44	68%	NR/17.7	[103]
CTX 50 mg/d p.o. + DEX 1 mg/d p.o.	24	33%	5.0/19.0	[104,105]
CTX 50 mg/d p.o. + DEX 1 mg/d p.o.	37	51%	11.0/28.0	[105,106]
CTX 50 mg/d p.o. [2]	74	16%	3.0/7.5	[106]

CTX—cyclophosphamide, VRB—vinorelbine, MTX—methotrexate, UFT—Tegafur/uracil, DXL—docetaxel, CAP—capecitabine, DEX—dexamethasone, PFS—progression-free survival, OS—overall survival, NR—not reported, [1]—any PSA decrease, p.o.—oral administration, i.v.—intravenous administration, bid-twice daily, [2]—typical, contemporary mCRPC patients (pretreated with DXL and novel endocrine agents).

5. Our Hunt for an Optimal MC Regimen in mCRPC Patients

We have conducted a prospective analysis of consecutive cases of patients treated with various MC regimens to find the most optimal MC combination for a subsequent phase II study. In order to define the real benefit of MC, none of the mCRPC patients was allowed to receive corticosteroids but all continued on pharmacological castration with LHRH analogs. The analysis included nine heavily pretreated patients (median two lines of systemic treatment for mCRPC) and the majority of patients were initially diagnosed with aggressive PC (median Gleason score of 9). Patients received the following combinations—(i) cyclophosphamide 50 mg/d p.o. + vinorelbine 30 mg q2d p.o. (two patients), (ii) cisplatin 25 mg/m^2 i.v. qw + cyclophosphamide 50 mg/d p.o. (two patients), (iii) paclitaxel 60 mg/m^2 qw + capecitabine 1500–2000 mg/d (depending on patient weight) p.o. (two patients), (iv) paclitaxel 60 mg/m^2 qw + capecitabine 1500 mg/d p.o + cyclophosphamide 50 mg/d (three patients). The biochemical responses (PSA decline by $\geq$50%) were observed in 0%, 50%, 100%, and 100% of patients, respectively. The patients tolerated all analyzed regimens very well, with G1–2 myelotoxicity being the most common adverse event. Based on the prospective analysis of consecutive cases of mCRPC patients treated with MC, the paclitaxel + capecitabine + cyclophosphamide combination has been chosen for further evaluation in a planned phase II clinical trial.

The choice of paclitaxel as a compound for our MC regimen requires explanation. Although cabazitaxel (the new-generation taxoid) is an active and approved agent for the treatment of docetaxel-pretreated mCRPC [50,107,108] patients and studies on standard-dose of paclitaxel failed to demonstrate its activity in prostate cancer [109]; some recent intriguing data justify the choice of paclitaxel as an element of our MC regimen. It is well known that paclitaxel, administered weekly, exerts robust antiangiogenic activity [110–112]. Our choice of paclitaxel in mCRPC is also justified by a recent study comparing weekly paclitaxel with cabazitaxel in advanced breast cancer. The study aimed to demonstrate the superiority of cabazitaxel 25 mg/m^2 q3w over weekly paclitaxel as a first-line treatment in 158 patients with metastatic breast cancer, many of whom have previously received docetaxel in the neoadjuvant or adjuvant setting. Surprisingly, both drugs demonstrated similar OS, PFS, and ORR [113], thus suggesting the need for reevaluation of weekly paclitaxel in docetaxel-pretreated mCRPC patients.

6. Conclusions

Metronomic chemotherapy represents a unique treatment option for many advanced cancer patients, including those diagnosed with mCRPC. However, it should be not considered as a first-line option in chemotherapy-fit mCRPC patients due to the lack of robust, prospective data suggesting its equality to standard treatment options, including novel antiandrogen agents (abiraterone, enzalutamide, darolutamide, and apalutamide) [4,6–8,114], chemotherapeutic agents (docetaxel and cabazitaxel) [21,22,115], or novel targeted therapies (olaparib in HRD mCRPC or Lutetium-177–PSMA-617) [18,116]. The use of MC based on the current state of knowledge should be restricted, in a typical population of mCRPC patients, to later lines of treatment, where no standard treatment options nor dedicated clinical trials are available. Moreover, recent disappointing data on the lack of activity of novel immunotherapies in mCRPC when administered as single agents [117] represent an intriguing hint to combining checkpoint inhibitors with immunomodulating MC regimens. However, the MC remains an option for earlier lines of therapy in fragile, elderly patients in whom standard treatment options (especially bi- or three-weekly chemotherapy regimens) may be intolerable. There is also no doubt that MC, with its multidirectional mechanism of action, represents a treatment option for mCRPC patients in low- and middle-income patients who do not have access to still relatively novel and expensive anticancer agents. Therefore, studies on metronomic chemotherapy in various clinical settings are critical from a global perspective.

Author Contributions: Conceptualization, P.J.W. and M.L.W.; methodology, P.J.W. and M.T.L.; formal analysis, P.J.W.; investigation, P.J.W. and M.T.L.; data curation, M.T.L.; writing—original draft preparation, P.J.W. and M.L.W.; writing—review and editing, P.J.W. All authors have read and agreed to the published version of the manuscript.

Funding: The research was funded by Jagiielonian University—Medical College grant No N41/DBS/000706.

Informed Consent Statement: Informed consent was obtained from all subjects receiving metronomic treatment analyzed in the study.

Conflicts of Interest: The authors declare no conflict of interest. ONCOAID is a diagnostic company privately owned by Wysocka, which provides microbiome and laboratory diagnostics for cancer patients.

References

1. Potocki, P.M.; Wysocki, P.J. Evolution of prostate cancer therapy. Part 1. *Oncol. Clin. Pract.* **2022**. [CrossRef]
2. Karantanos, T.; Corn, P.G.; Thompson, T.C. Prostate cancer progression after androgen deprivation therapy: Mechanisms of castrate resistance and novel therapeutic approaches. *Oncogene* **2013**, *32*, 5501–5511. [CrossRef]
3. Stanbrough, M.; Bubley, G.J.; Ross, K.; Golub, T.R.; Rubin, M.A.; Penning, T.M.; Febbo, P.G.; Balk, S.P. Increased expression of genes converting adrenal androgens to testosterone in androgen-independent prostate cancer. *Cancer Res.* **2006**, *66*, 2815–2825. [CrossRef] [PubMed]
4. Beer, T.M.; Armstrong, A.J.; Rathkopf, D.E.; Loriot, Y.; Sternberg, C.N.; Higano, C.S.; Iversen, P.; Bhattacharya, S.; Carles, J.; Chowdhury, S.; et al. Enzalutamide in metastatic prostate cancer before chemotherapy. *N. Engl. J. Med.* **2014**, *371*, 424–433. [CrossRef]
5. Scher, H.I.; Fizazi, K.; Saad, F.; Taplin, M.-E.; Sternberg, C.N.; Miller, K.; de Wit, R.; Mulders, P.; Chi, K.N.; Shore, N.D.; et al. Increased survival with enzalutamide in prostate cancer after chemotherapy. *N. Engl. J. Med.* **2012**, *367*, 1187–1197. [CrossRef] [PubMed]
6. de Bono, J.S.; Logothetis, C.J.; Molina, A.; Fizazi, K.; North, S.; Chu, L.; Chi, K.N.; Jones, R.J.; Goodman, O.B.; Saad, F.; et al. Abiraterone and increased survival in metastatic prostate cancer. *N. Engl. J. Med.* **2011**, *364*, 1995–2005. [CrossRef] [PubMed]
7. Ryan, C.J.; Smith, M.R.; de Bono, J.S.; Molina, A.; Logothetis, C.J.; de Souza, P.; Fizazi, K.; Mainwaring, P.; Piulats, J.M.; Ng, S.; et al. Abiraterone in metastatic prostate cancer without previous chemotherapy. *N. Engl. J. Med.* **2013**, *368*, 138–148. [CrossRef] [PubMed]
8. Saad, F.; Efstathiou, E.; Attard, G.; Flaig, T.W.; Franke, F.; Goodman, O.B.; Oudard, S.; Steuber, T.; Suzuki, H.; Wu, D.; et al. Apalutamide plus abiraterone acetate and prednisone versus placebo plus abiraterone and prednisone in metastatic, castration-resistant prostate cancer (ACIS): A randomised, placebo-controlled, double-blind, multinational, phase 3 study. *Lancet Oncol.* **2021**, *22*, 1541–1559. [CrossRef]
9. Berthold, D.R.; Pond, G.R.; Soban, F.; de Wit, R.; Eisenberger, M.; Tannock, I.F. Docetaxel plus prednisone or mitoxantrone plus prednisone for advanced prostate cancer: Updated survival in the TAX 327 study. *J. Clin. Oncol.* **2008**, *26*, 242–245. [CrossRef]
10. James, N.D.; Sydes, M.R.; Clarke, N.W.; Mason, M.D.; Dearnaley, D.P.; Spears, M.R.; Ritchie, A.W.S.; Parker, C.C.; Russell, M.; Attard, G.; et al. Addition of docetaxel, zoledronic acid, or both to Fi Rst-line long-term hormone therapy in prostate cancer (STAMPEDE): Survival results from an adaptive, multiarm, multistage, platform randomised controlled trial. *Lancet* **2016**, *387*, 1163–1177. [CrossRef]
11. Sweeney, C.J.; Chen, Y.-H.; Carducci, M.; Liu, G.; Jarrard, D.F.; Eisenberger, M.; Wong, Y.-N.; Hahn, N.; Kohli, M.; Cooney, M.M.; et al. Chemohormonal therapy in metastatic hormone-sensitive prostate cancer. *N. Engl. J. Med.* **2015**, *373*, 737–746. [CrossRef] [PubMed]
12. Aggarwal, R.; Huang, J.; Alumkal, J.J.; Zhang, L.; Feng, F.Y.; Thomas, G.V.; Weinstein, A.S.; Friedl, V.; Zhang, C.; Witte, O.N.; et al. Clinical and genomic characterization of treatment-emergent small-cell neuroendocrine prostate cancer: A multi-institutional prospective study. *J. Clin. Oncol.* **2018**, *36*, 2492–2503. [CrossRef] [PubMed]
13. Epstein, J.I.; Amin, M.B.; Beltran, H.; Lotan, T.L.; Mosquera, J.M.; Reuter, V.E.; Robinson, B.D.; Troncoso, P.; Rubin, M.A. Proposed morphologic classification of prostate cancer with neuroendocrine differentiation. *Am. J. Surg. Pathol.* **2014**, *38*, 756–767. [CrossRef] [PubMed]
14. Humeniuk, M.S.; Gupta, R.T.; Healy, P.; McNamara, M.; Ramalingam, S.; Harrison, M.; George, D.; Zhang, T.; Wu, Y.; Armstrong, A.J. Platinum sensitivity in metastatic prostate cancer: Does histology matter? *Prostate Cancer Prostatic Dis.* **2018**, *21*, 92–99. [CrossRef]
15. Kote-Jarai, Z.; Leongamornlert, D.; Saunders, E.; Tymrakiewicz, M.; Castro, E.; Mahmud, N.; Guy, M.; Edwards, S.; O'Brien, L.; Sawyer, E.; et al. BRCA2 is a moderate penetrance gene contributing to young-onset prostate cancer: Implications for genetic testing in prostate cancer patients. *Br. J. Cancer* **2011**, *105*, 1230–1234. [CrossRef]
16. Leongamornlert, D.; Mahmud, N.; Tymrakiewicz, M.; Saunders, E.; Dadaev, T.; Castro, E.; Goh, C.; Govindasami, K.; Guy, M.; O'Brien, L.; et al. Germline BRCA1 mutations increase prostate cancer risk. *Br. J. Cancer* **2012**, *106*, 1697–1701. [CrossRef]

17. Pritchard, C.C.; Mateo, J.; Walsh, M.F.; de Sarkar, N.; Abida, W.; Beltran, H.; Garofalo, A.; Gulati, R.; Carreira, S.; Eeles, R.; et al. Inherited DNA-repair gene mutations in men with metastatic prostate cancer. *N. Engl. J. Med.* **2016**, *375*, 443–453. [CrossRef]
18. de Bono, J.; Mateo, J.; Fizazi, K.; Saad, F.; Shore, N.; Sandhu, S.; Chi, K.N.; Sartor, O.; Agarwal, N.; Olmos, D.; et al. Olaparib for metastatic castration-resistant prostate cancer. *N. Engl. J. Med.* **2020**, *382*, 2091–2102. [CrossRef]
19. Tannock, I.F.; Osoba, D.; Stockler, M.R.; Ernst, D.S.; Neville, A.J.; Moore, M.J.; Armitage, G.R.; Wilson, J.J.; Venner, P.M.; Coppin, C.M.; et al. Chemotherapy with mitoxantrone plus prednisone or prednisone alone for symptomatic hormone-resistant prostate cancer: A canadian randomized trial with palliative end points. *J. Clin. Oncol.* **1996**, *14*, 1756–1764. [CrossRef]
20. Petrylak, D.P.; Tangen, C.M.; Hussain, M.H.A.; Lara, P.N., Jr.; Jones, J.A.; Taplin, M.E.; Burch, P.A.; Berry, D.; Moinpour, C.; Kohli, M.; et al. Docetaxel and estramustine compared with mitoxantrone and prednisone for advanced refractory prostate cancer. *N. Engl. J. Med.* **2009**, *351*, 1513–1520. [CrossRef]
21. Berthold, D.R.; Pond, G.R.; Roessner, M.; de Wit, R.; Eisenberger, M.; Tannock, I.F. Treatment of hormone-refractory prostate cancer with docetaxel or mitoxantrone: Relationships between prostate-specific antigen, pain, and quality of life response and survival in the TAX-327 study. *Clin. Cancer Res.* **2008**, *14*, 2763–2767. [CrossRef] [PubMed]
22. Kellokumpu-Lehtinen, P.L.; Harmenberg, U.; Joensuu, T.; McDermott, R.; Hervonen, P.; Ginman, C.; Luukkaa, M.; Nyandoto, P.; Hemminki, A.; Nilsson, S.; et al. 2-weekly versus 3-weekly docetaxel to treat castration-resistant advanced prostate cancer: A randomised, phase 3 trial. *Lancet Oncol.* **2013**, *14*, 117–124. [CrossRef]
23. Kellokumpu-Lehtinen, P.-L.I.; Harmenberg, U.; Hervonen, P.; Joensuu, T.K.; McDermott, R.S.; Ginman, C.; Luukkaa, M.; Nyandoto, P.; Hemminki, A.; Nilsson, S.; et al. Triweekly docetaxel versus biweekly docetaxel as a treatment for advanced castration resistant prostate cancer: Quality of life analysis. *J. Clin. Oncol.* **2014**, *32*, 23. [CrossRef]
24. Garcia, J.A.; Hutson, T.E.; Shepard, D.; Elson, P.; Dreicer, R. Gemcitabine and docetaxel in metastatic, castrate-resistant prostate cancer. *Cancer* **2011**, *117*, 752–757. [CrossRef] [PubMed]
25. Madan, R.A.; Karzai, F.H.; Ning, Y.M.; Adesunloye, B.A.; Huang, X.; Harold, N.; Couvillon, A.; Chun, G.; Cordes, L.; Sissung, T.; et al. Phase II trial of docetaxel, bevacizumab, lenalidomide and prednisone in patients with metastatic castration-resistant prostate cancer. *BJU Int.* **2016**, *118*, 590–597. [CrossRef] [PubMed]
26. Picus, J.; Halabi, S.; Kelly, W.K.; Vogelzang, N.J.; Whang, Y.E.; Kaplan, E.B.; Stadler, W.M.; Small, E.J. A phase 2 study of Estramustine, docetaxel, and bevacizumab in men with castrate-resistant prostate cancer. *Cancer* **2011**, *117*, 526–533. [CrossRef]
27. Gross, M.E.; Dorff, T.B.; Quinn, D.I.; Diaz, P.M.; Castellanos, O.O.; Agus, D.B. Safety and efficacy of docetaxel, bevacizumab, and everolimus for castration-resistant prostate cancer (CRPC). *Clin. Genitourin. Cancer* **2017**, *16*, e11–e21. [CrossRef]
28. Tannock, I.F.; Fizazi, K.; Ivanov, S.; Karlsson, C.T.; Fléchon, A.; Skoneczna, I.; Orlandi, F.; Gravis, G.; Matveev, V.; Bavbek, S.; et al. Aflibercept versus placebo in combination with docetaxel and prednisone for treatment of men with metastatic castration-resistant prostate cancer (VENICE): A phase 3, double-blind randomised trial. *Lancet Oncol.* **2013**, *14*, 760–768. [CrossRef]
29. de Bono, J.S.; Oudard, S.; Ozguroglu, M.; Hansen, S.; MacHiels, J.P.; Kocak, I.; Gravis, G.; Bodrogi, I.; MacKenzie, M.J.; Shen, L.; et al. Prednisone plus cabazitaxel or mitoxantrone for metastatic castration-resistant prostate cancer progressing after docetaxel treatment: A randomised open-label trial. *Lancet* **2010**, *376*, 1147–1154. [CrossRef]
30. Eisenberger, M.; Hardy-Bessard, A.C.; Kim, C.S.; Géczi, L.; Ford, D.; Mourey, L.; Carles, J.; Parente, P.; Font, A.; Kacso, G.; et al. Phase III study comparing a reduced dose of cabazitaxel (20 Mg/m^2) and the currently approved dose (25 Mg/m^2) in postdocetaxel patients with metastatic castration-resistant prostate cancer-PROSELICA. *J. Clin. Oncol.* **2017**, *35*, 3198–3206. [CrossRef]
31. Cazzaniga, M.; Cordani, N.; Capici, S.; Cogliati, V.; Riva, F.; Cerrito, M. Metronomic chemotherapy. *Cancers* **2021**, *13*, 2236. [CrossRef] [PubMed]
32. Cazzaniga, M.E.; Munzone, E.; Bocci, G.; Afonso, N.; Gomez, P.; Langkjer, S.; Petru, E.; Pivot, X.; Sánchez Rovira, P.; Wysocki, P.; et al. Pan-european expert meeting on the use of metronomic chemotherapy in advanced breast cancer patients: The PENELOPE project. *Adv. Ther.* **2019**, *36*, 381–406. [CrossRef] [PubMed]
33. Huuhtanen, R.L.; Wiklund, T.A.; Blomqvist, C.P.; Böhling, T.O.; Virolainen, M.J.; Tribukait, B.; Andersson, L.C. A high proliferation rate measured by cyclin a predicts a favourable chemotherapy response in soft tissue sarcoma patients. *Br. J. Cancer* **1999**, *81*, 1017–1021. [CrossRef] [PubMed]
34. Bonetti, A.; Zaninelli, M.; Rodella, S.; Molino, A.; Sperotto, L.; Piubello, Q.; Bonetti, F.; Nortilli, R.; Turazza, M.; Cetto, G.L. Tumor proliferative activity and response to first-line chemotherapy in advanced breast carcinoma. *Breast Cancer Res. Treat.* **1996**, *38*, 289–297. [CrossRef]
35. Richardsen, E.; Andersen, S.; Al-Saad, S.; Rakaee, M.; Nordby, Y.; Pedersen, M.I.; Ness, N.; Grindstad, T.; Movik, I.; Dønnem, T.; et al. Evaluation of the proliferation marker Ki-67 in a large prostatectomy cohort. *PLoS ONE* **2017**, *12*, e0186852. [CrossRef]
36. Fantony, J.J.; Howard, L.E.; Csizmadi, I.; Armstrong, A.J.; Lark, A.L.; Galet, C.; Aronson, W.J.; Freedland, S.J. Is Ki67 prognostic for aggressive prostate cancer? A multicenter real-world study. *Biomark. Med.* **2018**, *12*, 727–736. [CrossRef]
37. Folkman, J. Tumor angiogenesis: Therapeutic implications. *N. Engl. J. Med.* **2010**, *285*, 1182–1186. [CrossRef]
38. Hanahan, D.; Bergers, G.; Bergsland, E. Less is more, regularly: Metronomic dosing of cytotoxic drugs can target tumor angiogenesis in mice. *J. Clin. Investig.* **2000**, *105*, 1045–1047. [CrossRef]
39. Kerbel, R.S.; Kamen, B.A. The anti-angiogenic basis of metronomic chemotherapy. *Nat. Rev. Cancer* **2004**, *4*, 423–436. [CrossRef]

40. Park, M.; Kim, J.Y.; Kim, J.; Lee, J.H.; Kwon, Y.G.; Kim, Y.M. Low-dose metronomic doxorubicin inhibits mobilization and differentiation of endothelial progenitor cells through REDD1-mediated VEGFR-2 downregulation. *BMB Rep.* **2021**, *54*, 470–475. [CrossRef]
41. Kim, J.Y.; Kim, Y.M. Tumor endothelial cells as a potential target of metronomic chemotherapy. *Arch. Pharmacal Res.* **2019**, *42*, 1–13. [CrossRef] [PubMed]
42. Schito, L.; Rey, S.; Xu, P.; Man, S.; Cruz-Muñoz, W.; Kerbel, R.S. Metronomic chemotherapy offsets HIFα induction upon maximum-tolerated dose in metastatic cancers. *EMBO Mol. Med.* **2020**, *12*, e11416. [CrossRef] [PubMed]
43. Bocci, G.; Francia, G.; Man, S.; Lawler, J.; Kerbel, R.S. Thrombospondin 1, a mediator of the antiangiogenic effects of low-dose metronomic chemotherapy. *Proc. Natl. Acad. Sci. USA* **2003**, *100*, 12917–12922. [CrossRef]
44. Steinbild, S.; Arends, J.; Medinger, M.; Häring, B.; Frost, A.; Drevs, J.; Unger, C.; Strecker, R.; Hennig, J.; Mross, K. Metronomic antiangiogenic therapy with capecitabine and celecoxib in advanced tumor patients—Results of a phase II study. *Onkologie* **2007**, *30*, 629–635. [CrossRef] [PubMed]
45. Mpekris, F.; Baish, J.W.; Stylianopoulos, T.; Jain, R.K. Role of Vascular Normalization in Benefit from Metronomic Chemotherapy. *Proc. Natl. Acad. Sci. USA* **2017**, *114*, 1994–1999. [CrossRef]
46. Natale, G.; Bocci, G. Does metronomic chemotherapy induce tumor angiogenic dormancy? A review of available preclinical and clinical data. *Cancer Lett.* **2018**, *432*, 28–37. [CrossRef]
47. Galluzzi, L.; Senovilla, L.; Zitvogel, L.; Kroemer, G. The secret ally: Immunostimulation by anticancer drugs. *Nat. Rev. Drug. Discov.* **2012**, *11*, 215–233. [CrossRef]
48. Zitvogel, L.; Apetoh, L.; Ghiringhelli, F.; André, F.; Tesniere, A.; Kroemer, G. The anticancer immune response: Indispensable for therapeutic success? *J. Clin. Investig.* **2008**, *118*, 1991–2001. [CrossRef]
49. Konopka, K.; Micek, A.; Ochenduszko, S.; Streb, J.; Potocki, P.; Kwinta, Ł.; Wysocki, P.J. Combined neutrophil-to-lymphocyte and platelet-volume-to-platelet ratio (NLR and PVPR score) represents a novel prognostic factor in advanced gastric cancer patients. *J. Clin. Med.* **2021**, *10*, 3902. [CrossRef]
50. Meisel, A.; von Felten, S.; Vogt, D.R.; Liewen, H.; de Wit, R.; de Bono, J.; Sartor, O.; Stenner-Liewen, F. Severe neutropenia during cabazitaxel treatment is associated with survival benefit in men with metastatic castration-resistant prostate cancer (MCRPC): A post-hoc analysis of the tropic phase III trial. *Eur. J. Cancer* **2016**, *56*, 93–100. [CrossRef]
51. Tesniere, A.; Apetoh, L.; Ghiringhelli, F.; Joza, N.; Panaretakis, T.; Kepp, O.; Schlemmer, F.; Zitvogel, L.; Kroemer, G. Immunogenic cancer cell death: A key-lock paradigm. *Curr. Opin. Immunol.* **2008**, *20*, 504–511. [CrossRef] [PubMed]
52. Banissi, C.; Ghiringhelli, F.; Chen, L.; Carpentier, A.F. Treg depletion with a low-dose metronomic temozolomide regimen in a rat glioma model. *Cancer Immunol. Immunother.* **2009**, *58*, 1627–1634. [CrossRef] [PubMed]
53. Ghiringhelli, F.; Menard, C.; Puig, P.E.; Ladoire, S.; Roux, S.; Martin, F.; Solary, E.; le Cesne, A.; Zitvogel, L.; Chauffert, B. Metronomic cyclophosphamide regimen selectively depletes CD4$^+$CD25$^+$ regulatory T cells and restores T and NK effector functions in end stage cancer patients. *Cancer Immunol. Immunother.* **2007**, *56*, 641–648. [CrossRef] [PubMed]
54. Zhao, J.; Cao, Y.; Lei, Z.; Yang, Z.; Zhang, B.; Huang, B. Selective depletion of CD4$^+$CD25$^+$Foxp3$^+$ regulatory T cells by low-dose cyclophosphamide is explained by reduced intracellular ATP levels. *Cancer Res.* **2010**, *70*, 4850–4858. [CrossRef] [PubMed]
55. Kan, S.; Hazama, S.; Maeda, K.; Inoue, Y.; Homma, S.; Koido, S.; Okamoto, M.; Oka, M. Suppressive effects of cyclophosphamide and gemcitabine on regulatory T-cell induction in vitro. *Anticancer Res.* **2012**, *32*, 5363–5369. [PubMed]
56. Kaneno, R.; Shurin, G.V.; Tourkova, I.L.; Shurin, M.R. Chemomodulation of human dendritic cell function by antineoplastic agents in low noncytotoxic concentrations. *J. Transl. Med.* **2009**, *7*, 58. [CrossRef]
57. Kaneno, R.; Shurin, G.V.; Kaneno, F.M.; Naiditch, H.; Luo, J.; Shurin, M.R. Chemotherapeutic agents in low noncytotoxic concentrations increase immunogenicity of human colon cancer cells. *Cell Oncol.* **2011**, *34*, 97–106. [CrossRef]
58. Michels, T.; Shurin, G.V.; Naiditch, H.; Sevko, A.; Umansky, V.; Shurin, M.R. Paclitaxel promotes differentiation of myeloid-derived suppressor cells into dendritic cells in vitro in a TLR4-independent manner. *J. Immunotoxicol.* **2012**, *9*, 292–300. [CrossRef]
59. Sierro, S.R.; Donda, A.; Perret, R.; Guillaume, P.; Yagita, H.; Levy, F.; Romero, P. Combination of lentivector immunization and low-dose chemotherapy or PD-1/PD-L1 blocking primes self-reactive T cells and induces anti-tumor immunity. *Eur. J. Immunol.* **2011**, *41*, 2217–2228. [CrossRef]
60. Geary, S.M.; Lemke, C.D.; Lubaroff, D.M.; Salem, A.K. The combination of a low-dose chemotherapeutic agent, 5-fluorouracil, and an adenoviral tumor vaccine has a synergistic benefit on survival in a tumor model system. *PLoS ONE* **2013**, *8*, e67904. [CrossRef]
61. Todaro, M.; Meraviglia, S.; Caccamo, N.; Stassi, G.; Dieli, F. Combining conventional chemotherapy and γδ T cell-based immunotherapy to target cancer-initiating cells. *Oncoimmunology* **2013**, *2*, e25821. [CrossRef] [PubMed]
62. Vives, M.; Ginestà, M.M.; Gracova, K.; Graupera, M.; Casanovas, O.; Capellà, G.; Serrano, T.; Laquente, B.; Viñals, F. Metronomic chemotherapy following the maximum tolerated dose is an effective anti-tumour therapy affecting angiogenesis, tumour dissemination and cancer stem cells. *Int. J. Cancer* **2013**, *133*, 2464–2472. [CrossRef] [PubMed]
63. Kerbel, R.S.; Shaked, Y. The potential clinical promise of "multimodality" metronomic chemotherapy revealed by preclinical studies of metastatic disease. *Cancer Lett.* **2017**, *400*, 293–304. [CrossRef] [PubMed]
64. Salem, A.R.; Pulido, P.M.; Sanchez, F.; Sanchez, Y.; Español, A.J.; Sales, M.E. Effect of low dose metronomic therapy on MCF-7 tumor cells growth and angiogenesis. role of muscarinic acetylcholine receptors. *Int. Immunopharmacol.* **2020**, *84*, 106514. [CrossRef]

65. Chan, T.S.; Hsu, C.C.; Pai, V.C.; Liao, W.Y.; Huang, S.S.; Tan, K.T.; Yen, C.J.; Hsu, S.C.; Chen, W.Y.; Shan, Y.S.; et al. Metronomic chemotherapy prevents therapy-induced stromal activation and induction of tumor-initiating cells. *J. Exp. Med.* **2016**, *213*, 2967–2988. [CrossRef] [PubMed]
66. Che, B.; Zhang, W.; Xu, S.; Yin, J.; He, J.; Huang, T.; Li, W.; Yu, Y.; Tang, K. Prostate microbiota and prostate cancer: A new trend in treatment. *Front. Oncol.* **2021**, *11*, 805459. [CrossRef]
67. Katongole, P.; Sande, O.J.; Joloba, M.; Reynolds, S.J.; Niyonzima, N. The human microbiome and its link in prostate cancer risk and pathogenesis. *Infect. Agents Cancer* **2020**, *15*, 53. [CrossRef]
68. Sipos, A.; Ujlaki, G.; Mikó, E.; Maka, E.; Szabó, J.; Uray, K.; Krasznai, Z.; Bai, P. The role of the microbiome in ovarian cancer: Mechanistic insights into oncobiosis and to bacterial metabolite signaling. *Mol. Med.* **2021**, *27*, 33. [CrossRef]
69. Golombos, D.M.; Ayangbesan, A.; O'Malley, P.; Lewicki, P.; Barlow, L.M.; Barbieri, C.E.; Chan, C.; DuLong, C.; Abu-Ali, G.; Huttenhower, C.; et al. The role of gut microbiome in the pathogenesis of prostate cancer: A prospective, pilot study. *Urology* **2018**, *111*, 122–128. [CrossRef]
70. Sheng, Q.; Du, H.; Cheng, X.; Cheng, X.; Tang, Y.; Pan, L.; Wang, Q.; Lin, J. Characteristics of fecal gut microbiota in patients with colorectal cancer at different stages and different sites. *Oncol. Lett.* **2019**, *18*, 4834–4844. [CrossRef]
71. Alanee, S.; El-Zawahry, A.; Dynda, D.; Dabaja, A.; McVary, K.; Karr, M.; Braundmeier-Fleming, A. A prospective study to examine the association of the urinary and fecal microbiota with prostate cancer diagnosis after transrectal biopsy of the prostate using 16sRNA gene analysis. *Prostate* **2019**, *79*, 81–87. [CrossRef]
72. Cavarretta, I.; Ferrarese, R.; Cazzaniga, W.; Saita, D.; Lucianò, R.; Ceresola, E.R.; Locatelli, I.; Visconti, L.; Lavorgna, G.; Briganti, A.; et al. The microbiome of the prostate tumor microenvironment. *Eur. Urol.* **2017**, *72*, 625–631. [CrossRef] [PubMed]
73. Ivanov, I.I.; Honda, K. Intestinal commensal microbes as immune modulators. *Cell Host Microbe* **2012**, *12*, 496–508. [CrossRef] [PubMed]
74. Hooper, L.V.; Littman, D.R.; Macpherson, A.J. Interactions between the microbiota and the immune system. *Science* **2012**, *336*, 1268–1273. [CrossRef] [PubMed]
75. McAleer, J.P.; Kolls, J.K. Maintaining poise: Commensal microbiota calibrate interferon responses. *Immunity* **2012**, *37*, 10–12. [CrossRef]
76. Viaud, S.; Saccheri, F.; Mignot, G.; Yamazaki, T.; Daillère, R.; Hannani, D.; Enot, D.P.; Pfirschke, C.; Engblom, C.; Pittet, M.J.; et al. The intestinal microbiota modulates the anticancer immune effects of cyclophosphamide. *Science* **2013**, *342*, 971–976. [CrossRef]
77. Iida, N.; Dzutsev, A.; Stewart, C.A.; Smith, L.; Bouladoux, N.; Weingarten, R.A.; Molina, D.A.; Salcedo, R.; Back, T.; Cramer, S.; et al. Commensal bacteria control cancer response to therapy by modulating the tumor microenvironment. *Science* **2013**, *342*, 967–970. [CrossRef]
78. Sivan, A.; Corrales, L.; Hubert, N.; Williams, J.B.; Aquino-Michaels, K.; Earley, Z.M.; Benyamin, F.W.; Lei, Y.M.; Jabri, B.; Alegre, M.L.; et al. Commensal bifidobacterium promotes antitumor immunity and facilitates anti-PD-L1 efficacy. *Science* **2015**, *350*, 1084–1089. [CrossRef]
79. Elkrief, A.; Derosa, L.; Kroemer, G.; Zitvogel, L.; Routy, B. The negative impact of antibiotics on outcomes in cancer patients treated with immunotherapy: A new independent prognostic factor? *Ann. Oncol.* **2019**, *30*, 1572–1579. [CrossRef]
80. Schett, A.; Rothschild, S.I.; Curioni-Fontecedro, A.; Krähenbühl, S.; Früh, M.; Schmid, S.; Driessen, C.; Joerger, M. Predictive impact of antibiotics in patients with advanced non small-cell lung cancer receiving immune checkpoint inhibitors: Antibiotics immune checkpoint inhibitors in advanced NSCLC. *Cancer Chemother. Pharmacol.* **2020**, *85*, 121–131. [CrossRef]
81. Derosa, L.; Hellmann, M.D.; Spaziano, M.; Halpenny, D.; Fidelle, M.; Rizvi, H.; Long, N.; Plodkowski, A.J.; Arbour, K.C.; Chaft, J.E.; et al. Negative association of antibiotics on clinical activity of immune checkpoint inhibitors in patients with advanced renal cell and non-small-cell lung cancer. *Ann. Oncol.* **2018**, *29*, 1437–1444. [CrossRef] [PubMed]
82. Tinsley, N.; Zhou, C.; Tan, G.; Rack, S.; Lorigan, P.; Blackhall, F.; Krebs, M.; Carter, L.; Thistlethwaite, F.; Graham, D.; et al. Cumulative antibiotic use significantly decreases efficacy of checkpoint inhibitors in patients with advanced cancer. *Oncologist* **2020**, *25*, 55–63. [CrossRef] [PubMed]
83. Matson, V.; Fessler, J.; Bao, R.; Chongsuwat, T.; Zha, Y.; Alegre, M.L.; Luke, J.J.; Gajewski, T.F. The commensal microbiome is associated with anti-PD-1 efficacy in metastatic melanoma patients. *Science* **2018**, *359*, 104–108. [CrossRef] [PubMed]
84. Routy, B.; Chatelier, E.L.; Derosa, L.; Duong, C.P.M.; Alou, M.T.; Daillère, R.; Fluckiger, A.; Messaoudene, M.; Rauber, C.; Roberti, M.P.; et al. Gut microbiome influences efficacy of PD-1-based immunotherapy against epithelial tumors. *Science* **2018**, *359*, 91–97. [CrossRef] [PubMed]
85. Davar, D.; Dzutsev, A.K.; McCulloch, J.A.; Rodrigues, R.R.; Chauvin, J.M.; Morrison, R.M.; Deblasio, R.N.; Menna, C.; Ding, Q.; Pagliano, O.; et al. Fecal microbiota transplant overcomes resistance to anti-PD-1 therapy in melanoma patients. *Science* **2021**, *371*, 595–602. [CrossRef]
86. Ma, J.; Gnanasekar, A.; Lee, A.; Li, W.T.; Haas, M.; Wang-Rodriguez, J.; Chang, E.Y.; Rajasekaran, M.; Ongkeko, W.M. Influence of intratumor microbiome on clinical outcome and immune processes in prostate cancer. *Cancers* **2020**, *12*, 2524. [CrossRef]
87. Zhu, J.; Liao, M.; Yao, Z.; Liang, W.; Li, Q.; Liu, J.; Yang, H.; Ji, Y.; Wei, W.; Tan, A.; et al. Breast cancer in postmenopausal women is associated with an altered gut metagenome. *Microbiome* **2018**, *6*, 136. [CrossRef]
88. Guan, X.; Ma, F.; Sun, X.; Li, C.; Li, L.; Liang, F.; Li, S.; Yi, Z.; Liu, B.; Xu, B. Gut microbiota profiling in patients with HER2-negative metastatic breast cancer receiving metronomic chemotherapy of capecitabine compared to those under conventional dosage. *Front. Oncol.* **2020**, *10*, 902. [CrossRef]

99. André, N.; Banavali, S.; Snihur, Y.; Pasquier, E. Has the time come for metronomics in low-income and middle-income countries? *Lancet Oncol.* **2013**, *14*, e239–e248. [CrossRef]
90. Fenioux, C.; Louvet, C.; Charton, E.; Rozet, F.; Ropert, S.; Prapotnich, D.; Barret, E.; Sanchez-Salas, R.; Mombet, A.; Cathala, N.; et al. Switch from abiraterone plus prednisone to abiraterone plus dexamethasone at asymptomatic PSA progression in patients with metastatic castration-resistant prostate cancer. *BJU Int.* **2019**, *123*, 300–306. [CrossRef]
91. Yang, Z.; Ni, Y.; Zhao, D.; Zhang, Y.; Wang, J.; Jiang, L.; Chen, D.; Wu, Z.; Wang, Y.; He, L.; et al. Corticosteroid switch from prednisone to dexamethasone in metastatic castration-resistant prostate cancer patients with biochemical progression on abiraterone acetate plus prednisone. *BMC Cancer* **2021**, *21*, 919. [CrossRef] [PubMed]
92. Romero-Laorden, N.; Lozano, R.; Jayaram, A.; López-Campos, F.; Saez, M.I.; Montesa, A.; Gutierrez-Pecharoman, A.; Villatoro, R.; Herrera, B.; Correa, R.; et al. Phase II pilot study of the prednisone to dexamethasone switch in metastatic castration-resistant prostate cancer (MCRPC) patients with limited progression on abiraterone plus prednisone (SWITCH study). *Br. J. Cancer* **2018**, *119*, 1052–1059. [CrossRef] [PubMed]
93. Glode, L.M.; Barqawi, A.; Crighton, F.; Crawford, E.D.; Kerbel, R. Metronomic therapy with cyclophosphamide and dexamethasone for prostate carcinoma. *Cancer* **2003**, *98*, 1643–1648. [CrossRef]
94. Lord, R.; Nair, S.; Schache, A.; Spicer, J.; Somaihah, N.; Khoo, V.; Pandha, H. Low dose metronomic oral cyclophosphamide for hormone resistant prostate cancer: A phase II study. *J. Urol.* **2007**, *177*, 2136–2140. [CrossRef]
95. Fontana, A.; Galli, L.; Fioravanti, A.; Orlandi, P.; Galli, C.; Landi, L.; Bursi, S.; Allegrini, G.; Fontana, E.; di Marsico, R.; et al. Clinical and pharmacodynamic evaluation of metronomic cyclophosphamide, celecoxib, and dexamethasone in advanced hormone-refractory prostate cancer. *Clin. Cancer Res.* **2009**, *15*, 4954–4962. [CrossRef] [PubMed]
96. Nelius, T.; Klatte, T.; de Riese, W.; Haynes, A.; Filleur, S. Clinical outcome of patients with docetaxel-resistant hormone-refractory prostate cancer treated with second-line cyclophosphamide-based metronomic chemotherapy. *Med. Oncol.* **2010**, *27*, 363–367. [CrossRef]
97. Dabkara, D.; Ganguly, S.; Biswas, B.; Ghosh, J. Metronomic therapy in metastatic castrate-resistant prostate cancer: Experience from a tertiary cancer care center. *Indian J. Cancer* **2018**, *55*, 94–97. [CrossRef]
98. Ladoire, S.; Eymard, J.C.; Zanetta, S.; Mignot, G.; Martin, E.; Kermarrec, I.; Mourey, E.; Michel, F.; Cormier, L.U.C.; Ghiringhelli, F. Metronomic oral cyclophosphamide prednisolone chemotherapy is an effective treatment for metastatic hormone-refractory prostate cancer after docetaxel failure. *Anticancer Res.* **2010**, *30*, 4317–4323.
99. Robles, C.; Furst, A.J.; Sriratana, P.; Lai, S.; Chua, L.; Donnelly, E.; Solomon, J.; Sundaram, M.; Feun, L.; Savaraj, N. Phase II study of vinorelbine with low dose prednisone in the treatment of hormone-refractory metastatic prostate cancer. *Oncol. Rep.* **2003**, *10*, 885–889. [CrossRef]
100. Gebbia, V.; Boussen, H.; Valerio, M.R. Oral metronomic cyclophosphamide with and without methotrexate as palliative treatment for patients with metastatic breast carcinoma. *Anticancer Res.* **2012**, *32*, 529–536.
101. Hatano, K.; Nonomura, N.; Nishimura, K.; Kawashima, A.; Mukai, M.; Nagahara, A.; Nakai, Y.; Nakayama, M.; Takayama, H.; Tsujimura, A.; et al. Retrospective analysis of an oral combination of dexamethasone, uracil plus tegafur and cyclophosphamide for hormone-refractory prostate cancer. *Jpn. J. Clin. Oncol.* **2011**, *41*, 253–259. [CrossRef] [PubMed]
102. Meng, L.J.; Wang, J.; Fan, W.F.; Pu, X.L.; Liu, F.Y.; Yang, M. Evaluation of oral chemotherapy with capecitabine and cyclophosphamide plus thalidomide and prednisone in prostate cancer patients. *J. Cancer Res. Clin. Oncol.* **2011**, *138*, 333–339. [CrossRef] [PubMed]
103. Ferrero, J.M.; Chamorey, E.; Oudard, S.; Dides, S.; Lesbats, G.; Cavaglione, G.; Nouyrigat, P.; Foa, C.; Kaphan, R. Phase II trial evaluating a docetaxel-capecitabine combination as treatment for hormone-refractory prostate cancer. *Cancer* **2006**, *107*, 738–745. [CrossRef] [PubMed]
104. Yashi, M.; Nishihara, D.; Mizuno, T.; Yuki, H.; Masuda, A.; Kambara, T.; Betsunoh, H.; Abe, H.; Fukabori, Y.; Muraishi, O.; et al. Metronomic oral cyclophosphamide chemotherapy possibly contributes to stabilization of disease in patients with metastatic castration-resistant prostate cancer: A prospective analysis of consecutive cases. *Clin. Genitourin. Cancer* **2014**, *12*, E197–E203. [CrossRef]
105. Calvani, N.; Morelli, F.; Naglieri, E.; Gnoni, A.; Chiuri, V.E.; Orlando, L.; Fedele, P.; Cinieri, S. Metronomic chemotherapy with cyclophosphamide plus low dose of corticosteroids in advanced castration-resistant prostate cancer across the era of taxanes and new hormonal drugs. *Med. Oncol.* **2019**, *36*, 80. [CrossRef]
106. Caffo, O.; Facchini, G.; Biasco, E.; Ferraù, F.; Morelli, F.; Donini, M.; Buttigliero, C.; Calvani, N.; Guida, A.; Chiuri, V.E.; et al. Activity and safety of metronomic cyclophosphamide in the modern era of metastatic castration-resistant prostate cancer. *Future Oncol.* **2019**, *15*, 1115–1123. [CrossRef]
107. Angelergues, A.; Efstathiou, E.; Gyftaki, R.; Wysocki, P.J.; Lainez, N.; Gonzalez, I.; Castellano, D.E.; Ozguroglu, M.; Carbonero, I.G.; Flechon, A.; et al. Results of the FLAC european database of metastatic castration-resistant prostate cancer patients treated with docetaxel, cabazitaxel, and androgen receptor–targeted agents. *Clin. Genitourin. Cancer* **2018**, *16*, e777–e784. [CrossRef]
108. Żołnierek, J.; Poborski, W.; Rogowski, W.; Arłukowicz-Czartoryska, B.; Skalska, K.; Gola, M.; Kucharz, J.; Wysocki, P.J. Retrospective analysis of the efficacy and safety of cabazitaxel treatment in castration-resistant prostate cancer after docetaxel failure. *Oncol. Clin. Pract.* **2019**, *15*, 281–288. [CrossRef]
109. Obasaju, C.; Hudes, G.R. Paclitaxel and docetaxel in prostate cancer. *Hematol. Oncol. Clin. N. Am.* **2001**, *15*, 525–545. [CrossRef]

110. Ai, B.; Bie, Z.; Zhang, S.; Li, A. Paclitaxel targets VEGF-mediated angiogenesis in ovarian cancer treatment. *Am. J. Cancer Res.* **2016**, *6*, 1624–1635.
111. Madariaga, A.; Garg, S.; Bruce, J.P.; Thiryayi, S.; Mandilaras, V.; Rath, P.; Oza, A.M.; Dhani, N.C.; Cescon, D.W.; Lee, Y.C.; et al. Biomarkers of outcome to weekly paclitaxel in epithelial ovarian cancer. *Gynecol. Oncol.* **2020**, *159*, 539–545. [CrossRef] [PubMed]
112. Thomas, H.; Rosenberg, P. Role of weekly paclitaxel in the treatment of advanced ovarian cancer. *Crit. Rev. Oncol. Hematol.* **2002**, *44*, 43–51. [CrossRef]
113. Bahl, A.; Braybrooke, J.; Bravo, A.; Foulstone, E.; Ball, J.; Churn, M.; Dubey, S.; Spensley, S.; Bowen, R.; Waters, S.; et al. Randomized multicenter trial of 3 weekly cabazitaxel versus weekly paclitaxel chemotherapy in the first-line treatment of HER2 negative metastatic breast cancer (MBC). *J. Clin. Oncol.* **2021**, *39*, 1008. [CrossRef]
114. Sternberg, C.N.; Fizazi, K.; Saad, F.; Shore, N.D.; De Giorgi, U.; Penson, D.F.; Ferreira, U.; Efstathiou, E.; Madziarska, K.; Kolinsky, M.P.; et al. Enzalutamide and Survival in Nonmetastatic, Castration-Resistant Prostate Cancer. *N. Engl. J. Med.* **2020**, *382*, 2197–2206. [CrossRef] [PubMed]
115. Thiery-Vuillemin, A.; Fizazi, K.; Sartor, O.; Oudard, S.; Bury, D.; Thangavelu, K.; Ozatilgan, A.; Poole, E.M.; Eisenberger, M.; de Bono, J. An Analysis of Health-Related Quality of Life in the Phase III PROSELICA and FIRSTANA Studies Assessing Cabazitaxel in Patients with Metastatic Castration-Resistant Prostate Cancer. *ESMO Open* **2021**, *6*, 100089. [CrossRef] [PubMed]
116. Sartor, O.; de Bono, J.; Chi, K.N.; Fizazi, K.; Herrmann, K.; Rahbar, K.; Tagawa, S.T.; Nordquist, L.T.; Vaishampayan, N.; El-Haddad, G.; et al. Lutetium-177–PSMA-617 for metastatic castration-resistant prostate cancer. *N. Engl. J. Med.* **2021**, *385*, 1091–1103. [CrossRef] [PubMed]
117. Powles, T.; Yuen, K.C.; Gillessen, S.; Kadel, E.E.; Rathkopf, D.; Matsubara, N.; Drake, C.G.; Fizazi, K.; Piulats, J.M.; Wysocki, P.J.; et al. Atezolizumab with enzalutamide versus enzalutamide alone in metastatic castration-resistant prostate cancer: A randomized phase 3 trial. *Nat. Med.* **2022**, *28*, 144–153. [CrossRef]

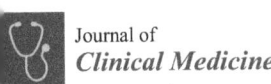

Review

Cyclic Metronomic Chemotherapy for Pediatric Tumors: Six Case Reports and a Review of the Literature

Benjamin Carcamo [1,2,*] and Giulio Francia [3,*]

1 Department of Pediatric Hematology Oncology, El Paso Children's Hospital, El Paso, TX 79905, USA
2 Department of Pediatrics, Texas Tech University Health Science Center, El Paso, TX 79430, USA
3 Border Biomedical Research Center, University of Texas at El Paso (UTEP), El Paso, TX 79968, USA
* Correspondence: benjamin.carcamo@ttuhsc.edu (B.C.); gfrancia@utep.edu (G.F.); Tel.: +1-915-479-8970 (B.C.); +1-915-747-8025 (G.F.); Fax: +1-915-242-8437 (B.C.); +1-915-747-5808 (G.F.)

Abstract: We report a retrospective case series of six Hispanic children with tumors treated with metronomic chemotherapy. The six cases comprised one rhabdoid tumor of the kidney, one ependymoma, two medulloblastomas, one neuroblastoma, and a type II neurocytoma of the spine. Treatment included oral cyclophosphamide daily for 21 days alternating with oral etoposide daily for 21 days in a backbone of daily valproic acid and celecoxib. In one case, celecoxib was substituted with sulindac. Of the six patients, three showed complete responses, and all patients showed some response to metronomic therapy with only minor hematologic toxicity. One patient had hemorrhagic gastritis likely associated with NSAIDs while off prophylactic antacids. These data add to a growing body of evidence suggesting that continuous doses of valproic acid and celecoxib coupled with alternating metronomic chemotherapy of agents such as etoposide and cyclophosphamide can produce responses in pediatric tumors relapsing to conventional dose chemotherapy.

Keywords: metronomic chemotherapy; pediatric tumors; cyclophosphamide; etoposide; valproic acid

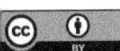

1. Introduction

Metronomic chemotherapy involves the continuous low-dose administration of chemotherapeutic drugs, and it is currently undergoing clinical evaluation for the treatment of various pediatric and adult malignancies [1–6]. For example, for adult tumors, a phase III clinical trial of metastatic colorectal cancer with maintenance metronomic capecitabine plus bevacizumab was reported, as were results of a phase III trial in early-stage breast cancer treated with bevacizumab plus metronomic cyclophosphamide and capecitabine [7,8]. For pediatric tumors, a number of phase II clinical trials have reported promising anti-tumor activity of metronomic chemotherapy, and these studies include those of Kieran and colleagues [9,10], of Andre and colleagues [11–17], and of the Baruchel group [18]. For both adult patients and pediatric tumors, the low toxicity that is frequently observed with this treatment strategy coupled with its (often) relatively low costs [4] make it an attractive treatment option. Preclinical studies [2,19,20] have shown that metronomic chemotherapy acts via inhibition of tumor angiogenesis, although additional mechanisms such as activation of the immune system have been proposed for regimens such as low-dose cyclophosphamide [21].

Metronomic chemotherapy may involve monotherapies, e.g., daily oral cyclophosphamide (CTX), but it can also be used to describe metronomic drug cocktails [22,23], including protocols that administer up to five different drugs [10] or more [24,25]. There are also evaluations involving the cyclical use of different drugs, an example of which is the work by Kieran and colleagues [9,10] on pediatric tumors. Here, we describe six children with pediatric cancer treated with cyclic alternating metronomic chemotherapy between 2002 and 2017.

These children had failed standard first line and salvage therapy and had refused or had no access to phase I or II studies. They were the only patients treated with this regimen during this period of time. The intention of the treatment was to provide palliation to children with refractory cancer that had exhausted all the therapeutic options available at the time and when parents requested additional treatment to prolong their children's life. It was not done to prove the validity of a metronomic regimen. The parents where consented to use a palliative regimen without curative intent so that they would understand the expected side effects of the individual drugs. They understood that it was not known if this treatment would prolong their life or not, and that the palliation was not done in the context of a study.

Metronomic chemotherapy included alternating 21-day cycles of etoposide (VP16) and CTX, along with the continuous administration of celecoxib and valproic acid. Sometimes due to individual reasons only celecoxib or valproic acid was used and sometimes celecoxib was substituted with sulindac. Oral continuous CTX at 50 mg/m^2/day had previously been used in metronomic regimens with minimal toxicity [26]. Oral VP16 at 50 mg/m^2/day for 21 days was chosen on the basis of evidence that continuous low-dose etoposide could enhance tumor cytotoxicity while lowering the risk of acute myeloid leukemia [27], and that 21 days of this dose with a 1 week rest had achieved partial response with moderate toxicity in recurrent disseminated medulloblastoma [28]. Alternating cycles of these drugs were chosen to decrease hematologic toxicity from etoposide and the emergence of drug resistance to either drug alone. Dose reduction was allowed for hematologic toxicity. Celecoxib is a selective COX2 inhibitor that has been well tolerated without cardiac toxicity at a dose of 2–16 mg/kg/day for prevention of adenomatous polyps in children [29]. The COX2 pathway is known to be involved in angiogenesis [30], and inhibition of angiogenesis has been reported to produce enhance the antitumor effects of metronomic chemotherapy [31], for which celecoxib was chosen at a dose of 250 mg/m^2/dose twice a day (equivalent to 8 mg/kg/day). Valproic acid (VA) is a histone deacetylase (HDAC) inhibitor with a long safety record in children with seizures that has shown antitumor effects in preclinical models of medulloblastoma, for which it was chosen at the standard pediatric dose of 15 mg/kg/day in two divided doses [32,33]. Furthermore, a major reason for the choice of these drugs was also their low toxicity profile, low cost, and availability. Medications were administered as capsules (the exception was for patient 3, for whom the liquid preparation of etoposide was mixed with cranberry juice). Our results suggest that this approach showed promising antitumor activity in six pediatric cases, and we propose that a cyclical regimen of 21 day VP16 followed by 21 day oral CTX on a backbone of continuous celecoxib and VA be further evaluated in these settings.

1.1. Patient 1

Patient 1 was a Hispanic boy who presented with metastatic rhabdoid tumor of the kidney at 34 months of life (Figure 1). He had a 7 cm × 11 cm mass in the left kidney, retroperitoneum invasion, and extension into the renal vein and inferior vena cava. He had metastasis to retroperitoneal lymph nodes and lungs, as well as rare micro-aggregates of cohesive abnormal large mononuclear cells suggestive of metastatic malignant tumor in the bone marrow by morphology alone (INH1 was not done). Bone marrow karyotype was 46,XY with no abnormal clones. He received vincristine–irinotecan, followed by cyclophosphamide–doxorubicin, followed by high-dose methotrexate as per regimen UH1 of AREN0321. This was followed by radical left nephrectomy at week 15. Subsequent evaluation revealed a residual 2 mm lung nodule but otherwise complete response. He subsequently received radiation to lungs and abdomen, followed by cycles of cyclophosphamide–carboplatin–etoposide and vincristine–doxorubicin–cyclophosphamide. Evaluation at the end of this therapy revealed recurrent disease to the lungs (two nodules measuring 3 mm and 1.5 mm in diameter) and an abnormal bone marrow clone, t(5;17)(q13;p13) in 15% of the cells. This cytogenetic abnormality has been previously reported in treatment-related myeloid neoplasia [34], and its presence was worrisome for early development of this condition from conventional chemotherapy and radiation, but there was no morphologic evidence of this entity at that time. No additional analysis was carried out, such as evaluation of INI1 loss. He was subsequently started on a metronomic regimen of VP16–CTX–celecoxib, and this maintenance regimen was effective at controlling the disease with no recurrent rhabdoid tumor or changes in the pulmonary nodules. Metronomic doses were as follows: VP16 37.5 mg/m^2 PO daily days 1–21, followed CTX 50 mg/m^2 PO daily days 22–42. Celecoxib was administered at 250 mg/m^2 PO twice a day and VA 15 mg/kg/day divided into two doses (dose adjusted to achieve levels of 100–150 ug/mL). He subsequently developed expansion of the original bone marrow clone (5;17)(q11.2p11.2) to 80% of metaphase cells, for which metronomic therapy was changed to bevacizumab (5 mg/kg every 3 weeks), temozolomide (60 mg/m^2/day on days 1–21), CTX (25 mg/m^2/day on days 22–42), VA (15 mg/kg/day divided into two doses) and celecoxib (250 mg/m^2 PO twice a day) after 17 months of treatment. He subsequently developed myelodysplastic changes consistent with treatment-related myeloid neoplasia, for which temozolomide and CTX were stopped 12 months later. These bone marrow myelodysplastic changes eventually progressed, in the absence of evidence of rhabdoid tumor reappearance, for which celecoxib–VA–bevacizumab were stopped, and he had a related donor allogenic bone marrow transplant 4 months later. He subsequently died of transplant-related infectious complications. He did not have evidence of recurrent rhabdoid tumor according to imaging studies at the time of his death. Autopsy was offered and declined. The rhabdoid tumor of this patient effectively responded to the metronomic chemotherapy for a period of 3 years.

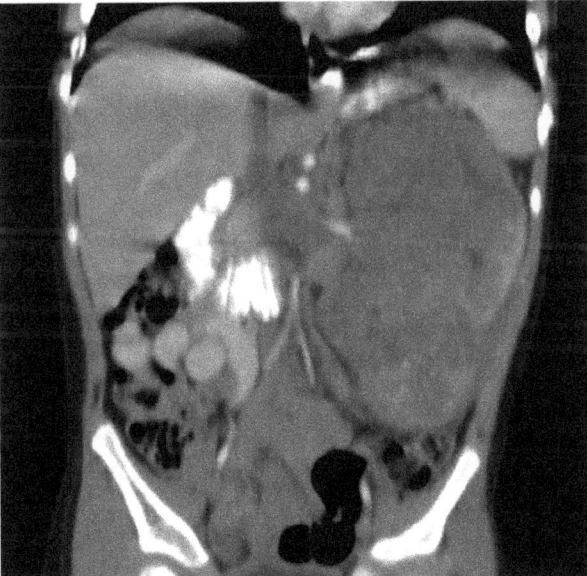

Figure 1. Patient 1: CT with contrast shows a large 11 × 7 cm left renal tumor with retroperitoneal infiltration, regional metastatic retroperitoneal adenopathy, and extension to renal vein and inferior vena cava. The patient also had innumerable solid circumscribed masses throughout the lung parenchyma bilaterally (not shown).

1.2. Patient 2

Patient 2 was diagnosed with anaplastic ependymoma when he presented with right hemianopsia, severe vision loss, and a 12 cm × 8 cm × 8 cm left temporo-occipital tumor at 6 years of life. He had two consecutive surgeries to remove the tumor, but a 1 cm unresectable lesion was left behind. He then received 5940 cGy field radiation to the tumor bed. Three months after radiation, he developed seizures, transient right arm paralysis, and recurrent disease to the left cerebral hemisphere, for which he received vincristine, carboplatin, and cyclophosphamide following the guidelines of ACNS0121 [35]. Three months later, he developed progressive disease with a large infiltrative enhancing mass (~5 cm) in the left temporal, occipital, and parietal lobes with involvement of the left thalamus, internal capsule, left external capsule, and insula, as well as leptomeningeal metastasis to the thoracic spine. He had no access to Phase I or II studies and was unable to travel for lack of insurance and migratory status, for which treatment was changed to palliation chemotherapy with oral VP16 (50 mg/m^2/day for 21 days) alternating with oral CTX (50 mg/m^2/day for 21 days) and continuous celecoxib (120 mg/m^2 PO bid) and VA. Celecoxib was subsequently changed to sulindac (8 mg/kg/day) due to drug access issues. He had an excellent response to palliation with resolution of all enhancing lesions and no evidence of residual disease after 2 years of therapy. (Figure 2). About this time VA was added to his seizure disorder management and continued until his last visit. He received 18 additional months of metronomic chemotherapy after complete response. He had no evidence of recurrent disease when he was lost to follow up 8 years from initial diagnosis and 4 years off metronomic chemotherapy. This patient showed complete response to the metronomic regimen.

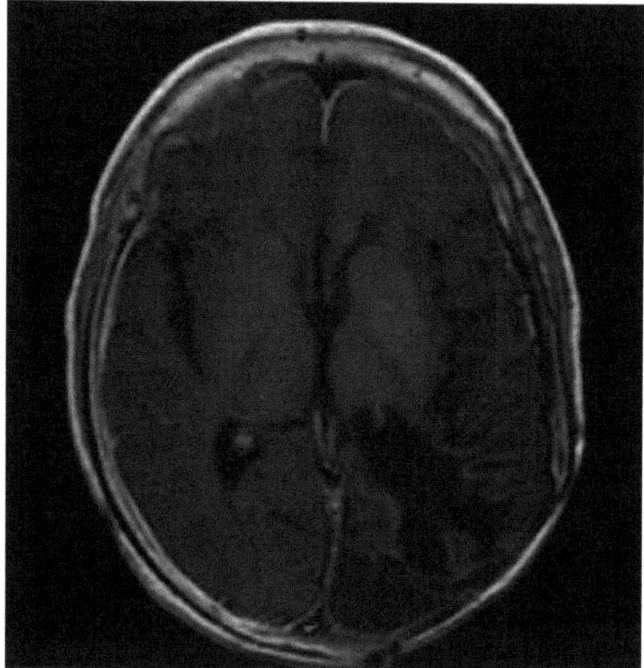

Figure 2. Patient 2: MRI shows confluent encephalomalacia gliosis in the left temporal and occipital lobes. There was no evidence of mass or pathologic enhancement 8 years from diagnosis and 4 years off therapy.

1.3. Patient 3

Patient 3 was a Hispanic girl diagnosed with medulloblastoma, when she presented with ataxia, dysmetria, increased head circumference and hydrocephalus at 10 months of age. She had gross total resection of a 5 × 5 × 4.5 cm posterior fossa tumor. Postoperative MRI revealed gross total resection and partial decompression of the fourth, third, and lateral ventricles. Following surgery, imaging studies showed no evidence residual disease or leptomeningeal involvement. However, ventricular fluid had evidence of microscopic disease with a five-cell cluster of malignant cells. Cerebrospinal fluid was negative. She received induction chemotherapy with cisplatin, cyclophosphamide, vincristine, and oral etoposide, followed 4 months later by radiotherapy to the posterior fossa, followed by another 8 months of chemotherapy as per POG 9631 [36]. Six months after therapy was completed, microscopic relapse was documented in cerebrospinal fluid with three clusters of malignant cells. Imaging studies failed to document gross leptomeningeal involvement. She started metronomic chemotherapy for relapsed medulloblastoma with 21 days of oral VP16 (35 mg/m^2/day) every 28 days. After 7 months of oral VP16, persistent microscopic disease was still present in the cerebrospinal fluid, and VA was added to the treatment. She achieved remission 5 months later, and serial cerebrospinal fluids remained consistently negative since then. She received a total of 39 months of metronomic chemotherapy including 21 months of etoposide and 31 months of VA. She was free of disease 5 years after metronomic chemotherapy was stopped.

1.4. Patient 4

Patient 4 was a Hispanic girl diagnosed with localized medulloblastoma without desmoplastic or anaplastic features when she presented with headaches, emesis, and blurred vision and a 4.9 × 4 × 4.5 cm heterogeneously enhancing tumor filling the fourth ventricle with associated moderate obstructive hydrocephalus at 5 years of age. Following gross total resection of the tumor, residual linear enhancement in the tumor bed was documented. She subsequently received 2340 cGy radiation to the craniospinal axis with a 3060 cGy boost to the posterior fossa (5400 cGy total) with concomitant vincristine after surgery. This was followed by 8 months of maintenance with vincristine, cisplatin, lomustine alternating with vincristine and cyclophosphamide as per ACNS0331 [37].

Three months off therapy, she developed a first relapse (Figure 3A) with recurrent tumors in the anterior horn of the left lateral ventricle (two), posterior horn of the left lateral ventricle (one), and anterior horn of the right lateral ventricle (one). CSF showed one abnormal cell. She was treated with 7 weeks of temozolomide followed by 1400 cGy of radiation to the ventricles and Gamma Knife surgery to a residual nodule, followed by autologous peripheral blood stem-cell transplantation (PBSCT), followed by 6 months of isotretinoin.

Three months later, she experienced a second relapse (Figure 3B) with a 1.7 × 1.4 × 0.5 cm enhancing tumor in the fourth ventricle, for which she was started on metronomic chemotherapy with alternating temozolomide (60 mg/m^2/day; days 1–21) and CTX (30.9 mg/m^2/day; days 22–42), daily celecoxib (250 mg/m^2) and VA (15 mg/kg), and bevacizumab (5 mg/kg) every 3 weeks. After 3 months on metronomic chemotherapy (Figure 3C), a partial response was documented with improved enhancing lesions in the dorsal brainstem and inferior vermis. At 4 months (Figure 3D), she developed multiple cranial nerve neuropathies and heterogeneous enhancement with mild increased volume at the left midbrain at the level of the left cerebellar peduncle, for which temozolomide was changed to VP16 (24.6 mg/m^2). This was complicated by hematologic toxicity requiring several treatment interruptions and VP16 dose reductions. After 8 months on treatment, MRI showed resolution of the enhancing tumor, an interval decrease in T2 changes, and diffusion restriction in the left cerebellar peduncle (Figure 3E). After 10 months on treatment (Figure 3F), she developed an extensive infiltrative tumor involving the dorsal mesencephalon, pons, and lower brainstem, and she died of her disease 2 months later. This heavily treated patient refractory to aggressive standard salvage therapy experienced 8 months of response and survived 12 months on metronomic chemotherapy.

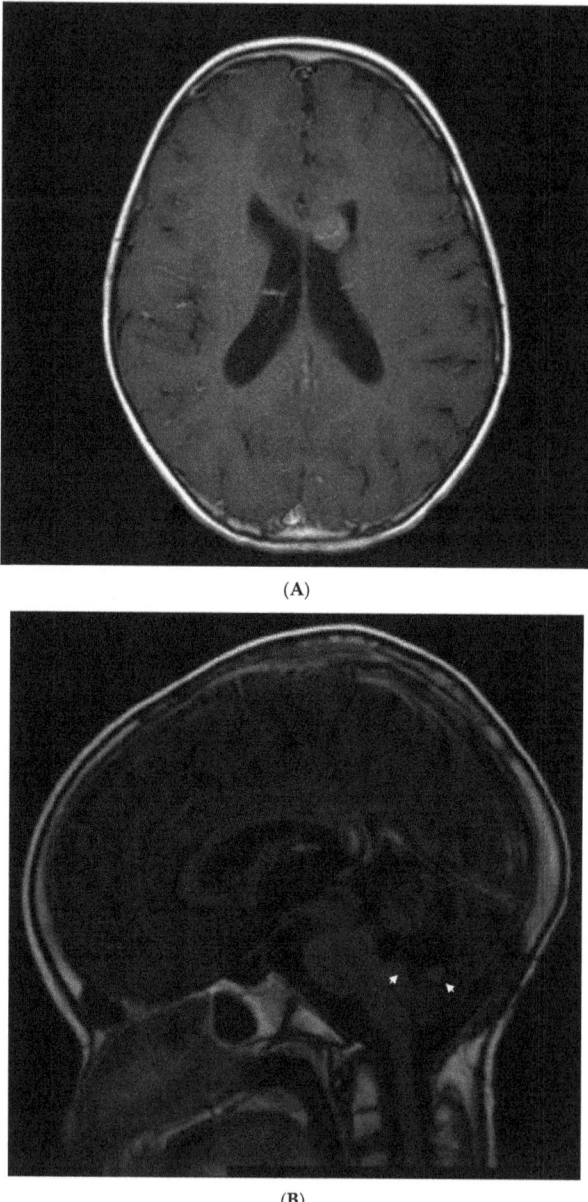

Figure 3. *Cont.*

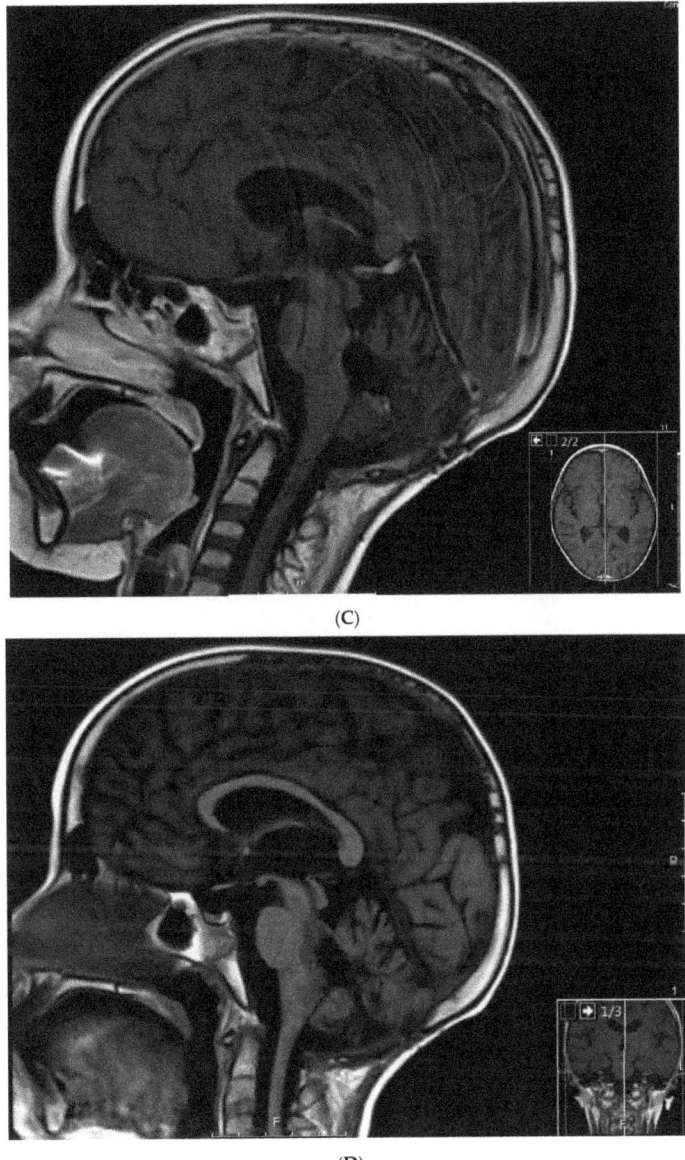

(C)

(D)

Figure 3. *Cont.*

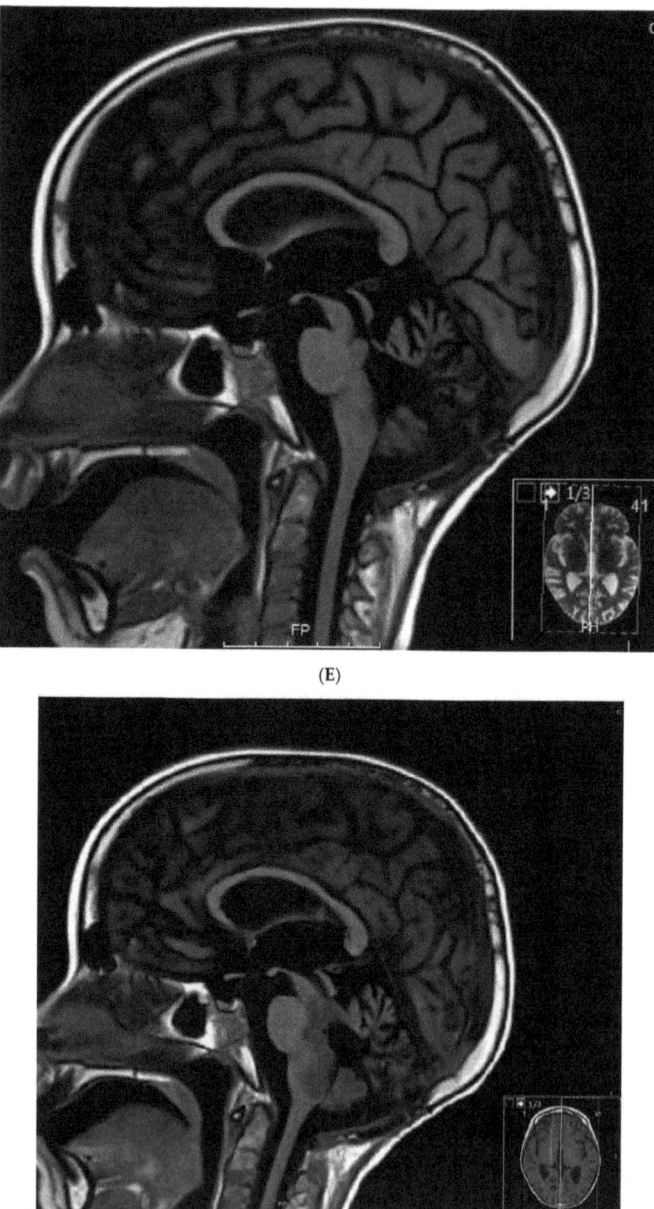

(E)

(F)

Figure 3. Patient 4: (**A**) image shows and enhancing tumor in the anterior horn of the left ventricle when she presented with first relapse of medulloblastoma. She achieved complete remission with salvage therapy; (**B**) image shows an enhancing tumor involving the anterior aspect and floor of the fourth ventricle (arrows) when she presented with second relapse; (**C**) image shows response to 3 months of metronomic therapy with decreased size and intensity of enhancing lesions; (**D**) image shows interval progression of the tumor seen in T2 FLAIR resulting in a change from temozolomide to etoposide at 4 months of treatment; (**E**) image shows resolution of the tumor mass and T2 FLAIR changes at 8 months of metronomic therapy; (**F**) image shows progressive disease at 10 months of treatment.

1.5. Patient 5

This patient was a Hispanic boy diagnosed with metastatic neuroblastoma when he presented with an 8 × 12 cm right suprarenal mass, extensive retroperitoneal and mesenteric lymphadenopathy, spinal cord compression, and metastatic bone disease to the right scapula and body of L1 at 9 years of age. He was treated with high-dose cisplatin and etoposide, cyclophosphamide, Adriamycin and vincristine, ifosfamide and etoposide, and carboplatin and etoposide, followed by subtotal resection of the retroperitoneal tumor and right kidney as per ANBL00P1 [38]. PBSCT was not available due to a lack of funds, for which he received two cycles of topotecan–cyclophosphamide, followed by 2160 cGy radiation to the tumor bed and spine, followed by 6 months of isotretinoin. He had no evidence of residual disease at the end of treatment. Seven months later, he developed recurrent neuroblastoma involving the right external iliac lymph nodes, for which he started palliative metronomic chemotherapy with oral VP16 (50 mg/m^2/day; days 1–21) alternating with oral CTX (75 mg/m^2/day; days 22–41) and continuous sulindac (4 mg/kg/day). He had hematologic toxicity requiring interruptions and dose reductions of both VP16 and CTX. Evaluation showed decreased tumor size at 5 and 8 months of therapy. He subsequently developed progressive disease after 11 months on therapy, for which sulindac was changed to celecoxib (500 mg/m^2/day). Two months later while off prophylactic antacids, the patient developed hemorrhagic gastritis, hematemesis, aspiration pneumonia, acute renal failure, and seizures, and died 13 months after starting metronomic chemotherapy.

1.6. Patient 6

This patient is a Hispanic girl found to have a large cervicomedullary tumor with a cervico-thoracic central syrinx with tumor seeding when she presented with right shoulder drop and right upper-extremity weakness at 3 years of age (Figure 4A). She had resection of the cervicomedullary portion of the tumor. Evaluation revealed a type 2 neurocytoma of the spine.

She subsequently received intensity-modulated radiotherapy to the tumor bed and residual cervico-thoracic tumor. Following radiation, a residual 11 mm expansile cervicomedullary nodule, centered at the C3–C4 level, was documented. Five months later, she developed progressive disease with increased size of the cervicomedullary nodule to 15 mm and development of a new second focus of enhancement on the ventral aspect of the spinal cord at C2. She was treated with topotecan, ifosfamide and carboplatin (TIP). She had significant hematologic toxicity and infectious complications during this treatment and no change in tumor size after nine cycles (Figure 4B), for which she was changed to metronomic chemotherapy with 21 days of temozolomide (60 mg/m^2 day) alternating with 21 days of CTX (50 mg/m^2), VA (15 mg/kg), celecoxib (250 mg/m^2/day) and bevacizumab (5 mg/kg IV every 3 weeks). Tumor response was noted 3 months after treatment with decreased tumor size to 9–10 mm (Figure 4C). Tumor size remained stable on subsequent studies, and temozolomide and CTX were stopped at 18 months, celecoxib and VA were stopped at 36 months, and bevacizumab was stopped at 48 months (Figure 4D). Metronomic chemotherapy was restarted after tumor progression was documented 10 months later (Table 1). She developed stable disease and treatment was stopped 15 months later. She remains with stable disease 4 years off therapy.

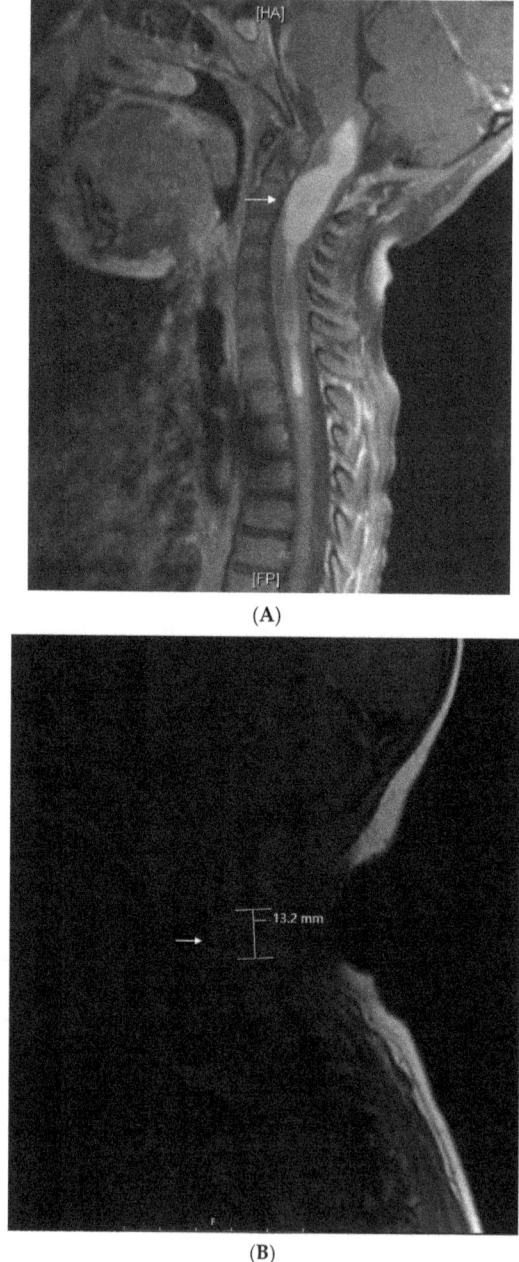

(A)

(B)

Figure 4. *Cont.*

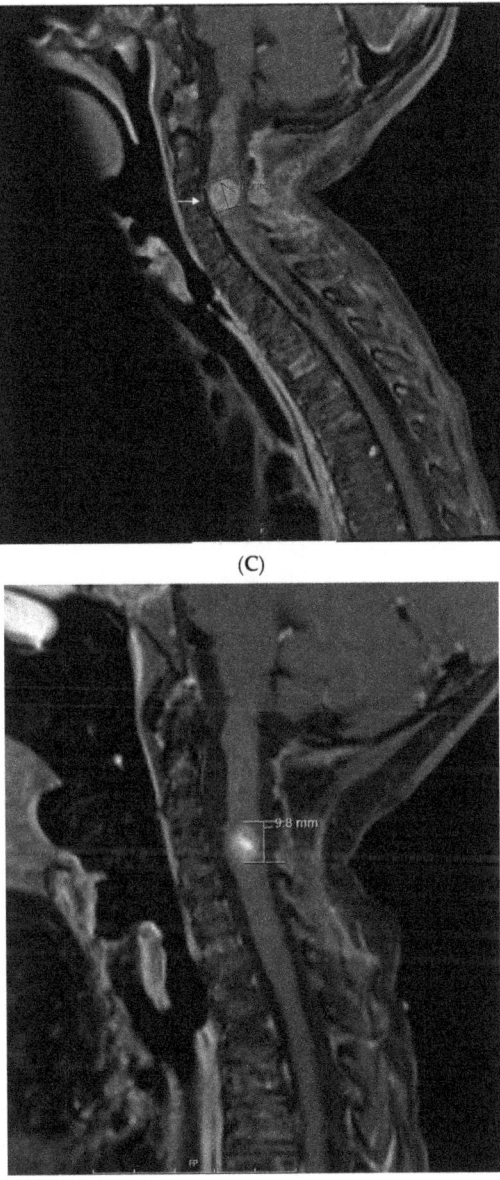

(C)

(D)

Figure 4. Patient 6: (**A**) MRI shows a 4.5 cm homogeneously enhancing expansile intramedullary tumor involving the medulla and upper cervical cord down to the level of C3–C4 (arrow) with an elongated syrinx extending inferiorly to the T3–T4 level; (**B**) the tumor was removed and treated with radiation but came back, for which it was treated with nine cycles of topotecan–ifosfamide–carboplatin with no significant change in tumor size (arrow) but significant toxicity, for which treatment was changed to metronomic chemotherapy; (**C**) after 3 months on metronomic chemotherapy, the patient recovered from toxicity and the tumor was slightly decreased; (**D**) the tumor was stable at the end of 4 years of metronomic chemotherapy.

Table 1. Summary of the 6 pediatric cases, treatment regimens, and clinical course.

Patient	Diagnosis	Regimen	Age at Initial Diagnosis	Best Response	Clinical Course
1	Rhabdoid tumor of the kidney (RTK) with lung and BM metastasis. Malignant myeloid clone at end of primary treatment. RTK relapse to bone marrow +/− lungs.	VP16-CTX, Celecoxib, VA	34 months	CR	Developed Treatment-related myeloid neoplasia and died from BMT complications in CR. CR 18 months at death. OS 3 years
2	Supratentorial Anaplastic Ependymoma. Local and distant relapse to spine.	VP16-CTX, Celecoxib, VA	6 years	CR	CR 5.5 years at last encounter Alive 8 years at last encounter
3	Medulloblastoma Infratentorial Microscopic leptomeningeal relapse	VP16 alone (VA added later)	10 months	CR	CR 5 years at last encounter Alive 7 years at last encounter
4	Medulloblastoma Infratentorial Second relapse	TMZ-CTX, VA, Celecoxib (TMZ changed to VP later)	5 years	PR	PR at 8 months lasted 2 months. Died of disease at 12 months
5	Metastatic neuroblastoma Retroperitoneal relapse	VP16-CTX, Sulindac (Sulindac changed to Celecoxib later)	9 years	PR	PR at 5 months lasted 6 months. Died of upper GI bleeding at 13 months.
6	Spinal cord neurocytoma Unresectable progressive tumor.	TMZ-CTX, VA, BV, Celecoxib	3 years	PR	PR at 3 months. Treatment stopped after 4 years of stable disease. PD 10 months later. She remains AWD on treatment

VP16 = etoposide, CTX = cyclophosphamide, VA = valproic acid, BV = bevacizumab, TMZ = temozolomide.

2. Discussion

Here, we report six cases of pediatric malignancies treated with metronomic chemotherapy that included alternating 21 days cycles of oral etoposide and cyclophosphamide in a backbone of celecoxib and/or valproic acid (Table 1). Because metronomic chemotherapy was used for palliation and not in the context of a study, some variation occurred due to medical and social issues such as individual choice, lack of insurance, and migration status. As noted, in some cases, bevacizumab and/or temozolomide were also administered. This treatment strategy produced significant tumor responses, including three complete responses. Three patients had hematologic toxicity with metronomic chemotherapy requiring interruptions and dose reductions. Two of these patients eventually progressed and died of their disease, and it is unclear whether the interruptions interfered with the metronomic effect. Patient 5 had hemorrhagic gastritis presumably from NSAIDs, for which this regimen should be used with prophylactic antacids as per current COG guidelines.

Three patients with brain tumors were treated. Unfortunately, they preceded easy access to molecular studies and, thus, are not reported according to the current WHO classification. The first patient (case 2) that used this regimen was treated in 2002. He had an anaplastic ependymoma that had failed surgery, radiation, and chemotherapy and had progressed with a large hemispheric tumor and spinal cord metastasis. He started treatment with alternating etoposide–cyclophosphamide on a backbone of celecoxib. Valproic acid was later added to the treatment for seizure control. He achieved a complete response at 2 years, stopped therapy 18 months later, and was still in remission 4 years off therapy when lost to follow-up 8 years later. Two patients with medulloblastoma were treated.

The first patient relapsed with clusters of malignant cells in CSF with normal imaging studies 6 months off therapy. The malignant cells persisted after 7 months of metronomic etoposide but resolved 5 months after adding valproic acid to the regimen. She remains free of disease 15 years off therapy. Since continuous celecoxib–valproic acid in the context of cyclic chemotherapy was well tolerated and the second patient may have responded to valproic acid, this medication was added to celecoxib in subsequent patients. The second medulloblastoma relapsed with brainstem involvement shortly after completing first- and second-line therapy. She was initially treated with alternating temozolomide–etoposide, bevacizumab, and continuous celecoxib–valproic acid but developed progressive disease 4 months later. She subsequently changed temozolomide to etoposide, achieved partial response 6 months later, and survived 12 months on metronomic chemotherapy. These three cases highlight the potential role of metronomic chemotherapy in refractory brain tumors. Recently, 29 children with refractory medulloblastoma were treated with a metronomic regimen that included alternating etoposide–cyclophosphamide, continuous thalidomide–celecoxib–fenofibrate, bevacizumab, and intraventricular liposomal cytarabine–etoposide (MEMMAT) [39]. EFS was 33% and 28% at 5 and 10 years, while OS was 44% and 39% at 5 and 10 years, respectively [39]. These results make MEMMAT the treatment of choice in refractory medulloblastoma. This regimen has some elements included in our regimen. For example, it contains alternating etoposide–cyclophosphamide and continuous celecoxib but lacks valproic acid. Since it is difficult to tell what elements in a complex metronomic regimen add to the activity, it is reasonable to explore our less complex regimen in patients that refuse invasive interventions or have poor access to care.

One patient with refractory metastatic neuroblastoma was treated after failing first-line therapy. He had no funds and was not able to travel to pursue second-line treatments including stem-cell transplant. He was treated with alternating etoposide–cyclophosphamide and sulindac. He had a partial response at 5 months but progressed at 11 months. Since then a regimen including cycles of 4 days of rapamycin–dasatinib followed by 5 days of irinotecan–temozolomide (RIST) showed impressive responses in refractory neuroblastoma with 90% response in 21 children including 12 CR and three PR, with 43% OS at 143 weeks [40]. While these results are impressive, rapamycin and dasatinib may not be readily available to patients with poor access to care. Most recently, 167 patients with high-risk stage 4 neuroblastoma without access to autologous stem-cell transplantation or anti-GD2 antibody therapy were treated with or without a metronomic regimen including continuous etoposide, cyclophosphamide, vinorelbine, topotecan, and celecoxib, including 106 patients in the metronomic arm and 61 in the non-metronomic arm. The 3 years of event-free survival (EFS) was 42.5% versus 29.4%, and overall survival (OS) was 71.1% versus 59.4%, respectively [41]. While the Corbacioglu et al. [40] report strongly supports RIST for refractory neuroblastoma, the report from Sun et al. [41] showing a benefit of oral metronomic chemotherapy comparable to autologous stem-cell transplant and anti-GD2 in high-risk Neuroblastoma suggests a possible role for metronomic chemotherapy in refractory neuroblastoma. Metronomic chemotherapy either with continuous drug delivery as reported by Sun et al. [41] or with alternating drugs as in this report needs to be further evaluated in these patients.

This report and previous reports by Kieran et al. [9,10], Andre et al. [11–13], Sharp et al. [18], Slavc et al. [39] and Sun [41], highlight possible metronomic regimen strategies for the treatment of refractory pediatric cancer. These metronomic strategies are summarized in Table 2.

Table 2. Summary of proposed metronomic regimens.

Study	Metronomic Regimen
Kieran 2005 [10]	Thalidomide 3 mg/kg oral daily days 1–42, Celecoxib 100–400 mg bid oral days 1–42 VP-16 50 mg/m^2/day oral days 1–21 CTX 2.5 mg/kg/day to a maximum of 100 mg oral days 22–42.
Kieran 2014 [9]	Celecoxib 100–400 mg bid oral days 1–42 Thalidomide 3 mg/kg oral daily days 1–42, Fenofibrate 90 mg/m^2 oral daily CTX 2.5 mg/kg/day to a max of 100 mg per day) days 1–21 VP16 50 mg/m^2/day days 22–42
Andre et al. 2008 [13]	VP-16 25 mg/m^2/day days 1–14 CTX 25 mg/m^2/day days 15–28 Celecoxib 100–400 mg/day days 1–28
MEMMAT Slavc et al. 2020 [39]	Etoposide 35–50 mg/m^2/day oral on days 1–21 of 42 day cycles CTX 2.5 mg/kg/day oral on days 22–42 of 42 day cycles Intrathecal Liposomal cytarabine 16–30 mg days 1, 4, 8, 11 of 28-day cycles Intrathecal VP16 0.5 mg days 18, 19, 20, 21, 21 of 28-day cycles. Bevacizumab 10 mg/kg IV every other week Thalidomide 3 mg/kg daily 1 year Celecoxib 50–400 mg oral daily 1 year Fenofibrate 90 mg/m^2 oral daily 1 year
Sun et al. 2021 [41]	VP16 25 mg/m^2 oral days 1–21 of 56–day cycles Topotecan 1.4 mg/m^2 oral daily on days 29–33 of 56-day cycles CTX 25–50 mg/m^2 oral daily days 1–56 of 56-day cycles. Vinorelbine 40 mg/m^2 oral weekly weeks 1–3 every 4 weeks Celecoxib 200 mg/m^2 oral twice a day 1 year
This manuscript	VP-16 50 mg/m^2/day days 1–21 CTX 2.5 mg/kg/day days 22–42 Celecoxib 250 mg/m^2/dose twice a day days 1–42 Valproic acid 7.5 mg/kg/dose twice a day days 1–42

We have previously used molecular genetics to identify a driving metabolic pathway within refractory Inflammatory Myofibroblastic Tumor that was specifically targeted with the TKI Lorlatinib with good response [42]. We also used proteomics in a refractory childhood embryonal tumor with multilayered rosettes of the brain to identify a driving metabolic pathway that was targeted with the TKI desatinib that and resulted in gross total resection of the tumor and prolong survival [43]. Unfortunately we have also found that these heavily pretreated tumors frequently become resistant to TKI after a few months of response [42]. One way to overcome this difficulty could be to add a backbone of metronomic chemotherapy that would target the micro environment, malignant angiogenesis and drug resistance, while the TKI would target aberrant metabolic pathways in the tumor, increase chemotherapy susceptibility and induce apoptosis.

While it has been noted that a VEGFR targeting TKI may blunt the ability of metronomic chemotherapy [44] to activate the immune system (suggesting antagonistic activity), we have previously shown that a metronomic chemotherapy plus a neutralizing anti-VEGFR antibody preclinically delays the growth of B16 melanoma lung metastases [45]. In addition, effective combination of the TKI sorafenib with metronomic chemotherapy has also been reported preclinically [46].

Collectively, these observations have led us to propose a study that incorporates tyrosine kinase inhibitors (TKI) to metronomic chemotherapy. Our backbone of choice to compare with TKI is celecoxib-valproic acid based on our experience and the growing interest in anti-histone drugs that have undergone trials with responses in difficult pediatric tumors [47]. All patients will receive alternating cyclophosphamide and etoposide as described in this report. This study depicted in Figure 5 will involve screening refractory patient's tumors for metabolic targets, and treating the patients with alternating etoposide-cyclophosphamide and either continuous celecoxib-valproic acid or continuous TKI if a targetable aberrant metabolic pathway is identified.

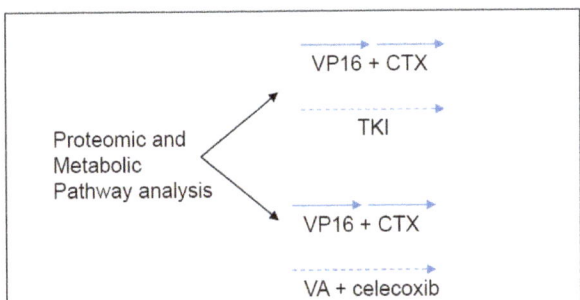

Figure 5. Schematic of future planned studies for pediatric cases eligible for metronomic chemotherapy. Proteomic and metabolic pathway analysis, where feasible, will be used to determine eligibility of patients to receive specific tyrosine kinase inhibitor (TKI) therapy coupled with metronomic chemotherapy, which involves alternating cycles of metronomic etoposide with metronomic cyclophosphamide. Patients not selected or not eligible for TKI-based therapies will receive valproic acid (VA) and celecoxib with metronomic chemotherapy as outlined in this manuscript.

The mechanisms via which metronomic chemotherapy produces antitumor effects are numerous [1] and are yet to be fully elucidated. Thus, in 2003, in collaboration with Bocci and colleagues [19], we reported that continuous low-dose CTX (as well as other drugs such as paclitaxel) can induce endothelial cells to overexpress the angiogenesis inhibitor protein thrombospondin-1. These data provide further evidence [48] for the antiangiogenic activity of metronomic chemotherapy. Other mechanisms include an alteration of intratumoral blood flow as observed following the administration of metronomic oral gemcitabine (LY2334737) as we previously observed in a preclinical model [20]. They also include the suppression of the homing of bone marrow-derived endothelial progenitor cells to the periphery of a tumor mass, as shown by Shaked and colleagues [49]. Additional mechanisms of action of metronomic chemotherapy, at least for drugs such as CTX, include immune activation, which likely occurs via suppression of regulatory T cells [21]. Furthermore, in collaboration with Emmenegger and colleagues [50], we reported that preclinical selection of tumors resistant to high-dose chemotherapy does not impair their response to subsequent metronomic regimens of the same drug [50]. These data suggest that mechanisms of tumor resistance to metronomic chemotherapy show little or no overlap with those for the same chemotherapeutics agent (e.g., CTX) given at pulsatile maximum tolerated doses. These results also suggest that a tumor relapsing to pulsatile high dose of a drug such as CTX may still show response to the same drug given on a metronomic schedule.

Metronomic chemotherapy has undergone a number of refinements since it was coined in 2000, to describe preclinical studies with drugs used in a continuous low-dose (as an antiangiogenic strategy or as a maintenance strategy), namely, CTX or vinblastine [48,51]. Since then, the concept of metronomic chemotherapy has evolved for the treatment of adult tumors, as well as in its application in pediatric oncology. Thus, for adult tumors, recent phase III clinical data in metastatic colorectal cancer showed improved progression-free survival in patients receiving maintenance low-dose capecitabine plus bevacizumab [7]. In addition, safety of administration was reported from a phase III clinical trial evaluating bevacizumab plus metronomic cyclophosphamide and capecitabine as first-line therapy in patients with HER2-negative advanced-stage breast cancer [8,52]. On the other hand, for pediatric tumors, reported protocols (as evident from a Pubmed search with the terms "metronomic" and "pediatric") include the long-term oral administration of daily low-dose mercaptopurine and weekly low-dose methotrexate for children with ALL [11]. They also include a metronomic vincristine/CTX/methotrexate/VA regimen given to children with refractory cancer of various tumor types [53]. Recently, there have been additional reports of metronomic chemotherapy improving survival in high-risk neuroblastoma patients [41], as well as other pediatric malignancies including Ewing sarcoma, osteosarcoma, and rhabdomyosarcoma [15], and studies have confirmed the low toxicity associated with this approach [54]. Alternating VP16 and cyclophosphamide metronomic regimens, with daily celecoxib, were combined with sirolimus in a phase I study of 18 pediatric relapsed or refractory solid and brain tumors, and the combination was found to be well tolerated [55]. It should be noted that among the first studies published on using chemotherapy metronomically for pediatric tumors were those of Kieran and colleagues [10] and of Andre and colleagues [13]. Thus, Kieran's group originally proposed continuous oral thalidomide and celecoxib with alternating oral etoposide and cyclophosphamide every 21 days. Recently, the same group reported a more complex strategy involving five drugs including metronomic CTX and etoposide, as shown in Table 2. Andre et al. proposed 2 weeks of metronomic etoposide followed by 2 weeks of metronomic CTX, plus celecoxib [13]. Because of the number of drugs involved in some regimens such as the one proposed by Kieran and colleagues (see Table 2), additional studies may be necessary to compare different permutations of the use of such drugs and the different orders in which such drugs are administered metronomically. Such studies may uncover whether specific combinations are important (e.g., CTX plus VA) or if the exact order of administration is critical (e.g., etoposide before CTX, or vice versa). In that respect, the six cases we report add data to a regimen of etoposide, CTX, and VA–celecoxib. Interestingly, with regard to VA–celecoxib as a backbone, we previously reported [20] that metronomic oral gemcitabine (LY2334737) has antitumor effects in preclinical mouse xenograft models. The LY2334737 oral gemcitabine prodrug is, once injected, metabolized into gemcitabine plus VA, suggesting that a metronomic oral gemcitabine schedule may unintentionally result in continuous administration of two drugs (gemcitabine and VA), although this possibility remains to be tested. Overall, these clinical and preclinical observations suggest that metronomic alternating regimens combined with continuous administration of celecoxib and VA have promising activity in tumors relapsing to pulsatile high-dose chemotherapy.

Author Contributions: Conceptualization, B.C.; writing—original draft preparation, B.C. and G.F.; writing—review and editing, B.C. and G.F. All authors have read and agreed to the published version of the manuscript.

Funding: G.F. was supported by NIH-NCI SC2CA211029 and SC1 GM136630-01 grants.

Institutional Review Board Statement: Not applicable.

Informed Consent Statement: Not applicable.

Data Availability Statement: Not applicable.

Acknowledgments: We thank Lidia Baiocchi, Guido Bocci, and Urban Emmenegger for their critical review of this manuscript. We also thank Karla Parra, Valerie Gallegos, and Paloma Valenzuela for assistance in assembling the documentation for this manuscript.

Conflicts of Interest: The authors declare no conflict of interest.

Abbreviations

cyclophosphamide (CTX), etoposide (VP16), valproic acid (VA).

References

1. Kerbel, R.S.; Kamen, B.A. The anti-angiogenic basis of metronomic chemotherapy. *Nat. Rev. Cancer* **2004**, *4*, 423–436. [CrossRef] [PubMed]
2. Derosa, L.; Galli, L.; Orlandi, P.; Fioravanti, A.; Di Desidero, T.; Fontana, A.; Antonuzzo, A.; Biasco, E.; Farnesi, A.; Marconcini, R.; et al. Docetaxel plus oral metronomic cyclophosphamide: A phase II study with pharmacodynamic and pharmacogenetic analyses in castration-resistant prostate cancer patients. *Cancer* **2014**, *120*, 3923–3931. [CrossRef] [PubMed]
3. Kerbel, R.S.; Grothey, A. Gastrointestinal cancer: Rationale for metronomic chemotherapy in phase III trials. *Nat. Rev. Clin. Oncol.* **2015**, *12*, 313–314. [CrossRef]
4. Bocci, G.; Kerbel, R.S. Pharmacokinetics of metronomic chemotherapy: A neglected but crucial aspect. *Nat. Rev. Clin. Oncol.* **2016**, *11*, 659–673. [CrossRef] [PubMed]
5. Munzone, E.; Colleoni, M. Clinical overview of metronomic chemotherapy in breast cancer. *Nat. Rev. Clin. Oncol.* **2015**, *12*, 631–644. [CrossRef]
6. Andre, N.; Banavali, S.; Pasquier, E. Paediatrics: Metronomics—Fulfilling unmet needs beyond level A evidence. *Nat. Rev. Clin. Oncol.* **2016**, *13*, 469–470. [CrossRef]
7. Simkens, L.H.; van Tinteren, H.; May, A.; ten Tije, A.J.; Creemers, G.J.; Loosveld, O.J.; de Jongh, F.E.; Erdkamp, F.L.; Erjavec, Z.; van der Torren, A.M.; et al. Maintenance treatment with capecitabine and bevacizumab in metastatic colorectal cancer (CAIRO3): A phase 3 randomised controlled trial of the Dutch Colorectal Cancer Group. *Lancet* **2015**, *385*, 1843–1852. [CrossRef]
8. Rochlitz, C.; Bigler, M.; von Moos, R.; Bernhard, J.; Matter-Walstra, K.; Wicki, A.; Zaman, K.; Anchisi, S.; Kung, M.; Na, K.J.; et al. SAKK 24/09: Safety and tolerability of bevacizumab plus paclitaxel vs. bevacizumab plus metronomic cyclophosphamide and capecitabine as first-line therapy in patients with HER2-negative advanced stage breast cancer—A multicenter, randomized phase III trial. *BMC Cancer* **2016**, *16*, 780. [CrossRef]
9. Robison, N.J.; Campigotto, F.; Chi, S.N.; Manley, P.E.; Turner, C.D.; Zimmerman, M.A.; Chordas, C.A.; Werger, A.M.; Allen, J.C.; Goldman, S.; et al. A phase II trial of a multi-agent oral antiangiogenic (metronomic) regimen in children with recurrent or progressive cancer. *Pediatric Blood Cancer* **2014**, *61*, 636–642. [CrossRef]
10. Kieran, M.W.; Turner, C.D.; Rubin, J.B.; Chi, S.N.; Zimmerman, M.A.; Chordas, C.; Klement, G.; Laforme, A.; Gordon, A.; Thomas, A.; et al. A feasibility trial of antiangiogenic (metronomic) chemotherapy in pediatric patients with recurrent or progressive cancer. *J. Pediatric Hematol. Oncol.* **2005**, *27*, 573–581. [CrossRef]
11. Andre, N.; Cointe, S.; Barlogis, V.; Arnaud, L.; Lacroix, R.; Pasquier, E.; Dignat-George, F.; Michel, G.; Sabatier, F. Maintenance chemotherapy in children with ALL exerts metronomic-like thrombospondin-1 associated anti-endothelial effect. *Oncotarget* **2015**, *6*, 23008–23014. [CrossRef] [PubMed]
12. Andre, N.; Abed, S.; Orbach, D.; Alla, C.A.; Padovani, L.; Pasquier, E.; Gentet, J.C.; Verschuur, A. Pilot study of a pediatric metronomic 4-drug regimen. *Oncotarget* **2011**, *2*, 960–965. [CrossRef] [PubMed]
13. Andre, N.; Rome, A.; Coze, C.; Padovani, L.; Pasquier, E.; Camoin, L.; Gentet, J.C. Metronomic etoposide/cyclophosphamide/celecoxib regimen given to children and adolescents with refractory cancer: A preliminary monocentric study. *Clin. Ther.* **2008**, *30*, 1336–1340. [CrossRef]
14. Roux, C.; Revon-Rivière, G.; Gentet, J.C.; Verschuur, A.; Scavarda, D.; Saultier, P.; Appay, R.; Padovani, L.; André, N. Metronomic Maintenance With Weekly Vinblastine After Induction With Bevacizumab-Irinotecan in Children With Low-grade Glioma Prevents Early Relapse. *J. Pediatric Hematol. Oncol.* **2021**, *43*, e630–e634. [CrossRef] [PubMed]
15. El Kababri, M.; Benmiloud, S.; Cherkaoui, S.; El Houdzi, J.; Maani, K.; Ansari, N.; Khoubila, N.; Kili, A.; El Khorassani, M.; Madani, A.; et al. Metro-SMHOP 01: Metronomics combination with cyclophosphamide-etoposide and valproic acid for refractory and relapsing pediatric malignancies. *Pediatric Blood Cancer* **2020**, *67*, e28508. [CrossRef]
16. Verschuur, A.; Heng-Maillard, M.A.; Dory-Lautrec, P.; Truillet, R.; Jouve, E.; Chastagner, P.; Leblond, P.; Aerts, I.; Honoré, S.; Entz-Werle, N.; et al. Metronomic Four-Drug Regimen Has Anti-tumor Activity in Pediatric Low-Grade Glioma; The Results of a Phase II Clinical Trial. *Front. Pharmacol.* **2018**, *9*, 00950. [CrossRef]
17. Berland, M.; Padovani, L.; Rome, A.; Pech-Gourg, G.; Figarella-Branger, D.; André, N. Sustained Complete Response to Metronomic Chemotherapy in a Child with Refractory Atypical Teratoid Rhabdoid Tumor: A Case Report. *Front. Pharmacol.* **2017**, *8*, 792. [CrossRef]
18. Sharp, J.R.; Bouffet, E.; Stempak, D.; Gammon, J.; Stephens, D.; Johnston, D.L.; Eisenstat, D.; Hukin, J.; Samson, Y.; Bartels, U.; et al. A multi-centre Canadian pilot study of metronomic temozolomide combined with radiotherapy for newly diagnosed paediatric brainstem glioma. *Eur. J. Cancer* **2010**, *46*, 3271–3279. [CrossRef]
19. Bocci, G.; Francia, G.; Man, S.; Lawler, J.; Kerbel, R.S. Thrombospondin 1, a mediator of the antiangiogenic effects of low-dose metronomic chemotherapy. *Proc. Natl. Acad. Sci. USA* **2003**, *100*, 12917–12922. [CrossRef]
20. Francia, G.; Shaked, Y.; Hashimoto, K.; Sun, J.; Yin, M.; Cesta, C.; Xu, P.; Man, S.; Hackl, C.; Stewart, J.; et al. Low-dose metronomic oral dosing of a prodrug of gemcitabine (LY2334737) causes antitumor effects in the absence of inhibition of systemic vasculogenesis. *Mol. Cancer Ther.* **2012**, *11*, 680–689. [CrossRef]
21. Ghiringhelli, F.; Menard, C.; Puig, P.E.; Ladoire, S.; Roux, S.; Martin, F.; Solary, E.; Le Cesne, A.; Zitvogel, L.; Chauffert, B. Metronomic cyclophosphamide regimen selectively depletes CD4+CD25+ regulatory T cells and restores T and NK effector functions in end stage cancer patients. *Cancer Immunol. Immunother. CII* **2007**, *56*, 641–648. [CrossRef] [PubMed]

22. Allegrini, G.; Di Desidero, T.; Barletta, M.T.; Fioravanti, A.; Orlandi, P.; Canu, B.; Chericoni, S.; Loupakis, F.; Di Paolo, A.; Masi, G.; et al. Clinical, pharmacokinetic and pharmacodynamic evaluations of metronomic UFT and cyclophosphamide plus celecoxib in patients with advanced refractory gastrointestinal cancers. *Angiogenesis* **2012**, *15*, 275–286. [CrossRef] [PubMed]
23. Bisogno, G.; De Salvo, G.L.; Bergeron, C.; Gallego Melcón, S.; Merks, J.H.; Kelsey, A.; Martelli, H.; Minard-Colin, V.; Orbach, D.; Glosli, H.; et al. Vinorelbine and continuous low-dose cyclophosphamide as maintenance chemotherapy in patients with high-risk rhabdomyosarcoma (RMS 2005): A multicentre, open-label, randomised, phase 3 trial. *Lancet. Oncol.* **2019**, *20*, 1566–1575. [CrossRef]
24. Peyrl, A.; Chocholous, M.; Kieran, M.W.; Azizi, A.A.; Prucker, C.; Czech, T.; Dieckmann, K.; Schmook, M.T.; Haberler, C.; Leiss, U.; et al. Antiangiogenic metronomic therapy for children with recurrent embryonal brain tumors. *Pediatric Blood Cancer* **2012**, *59*, 511–517. [CrossRef] [PubMed]
25. Zapletalova, D.; André, N.; Deak, L.; Kyr, M.; Bajciova, V.; Mudry, P.; Dubska, L.; Demlova, R.; Pavelka, Z.; Zitterbart, K.; et al. Metronomic chemotherapy with the COMBAT regimen in advanced pediatric malignancies: A multicenter experience. *Oncology* **2012**, *82*, 249–260. [CrossRef] [PubMed]
26. Colleoni, M.; Rocca, A.; Sandri, M.T.; Zorzino, L.; Masci, G.; Nolè, F.; Peruzzotti, G.; Robertson, C.; Orlando, L.; Cinieri, S.; et al. Low-dose oral methotrexate and cyclophosphamide in metastatic breast cancer: Antitumor activity and correlation with vascular endothelial growth factor levels. *Ann. Oncol. Off. J. Eur. Soc. Med. Oncol.* **2002**, *13*, 73–80. [CrossRef]
27. Chen, C.L.; Fuscoe, J.C.; Liu, Q.; Pui, C.H.; Mahmoud, H.H.; Relling, M.V. Relationship between cytotoxicity and site-specific DNA recombination after in vitro exposure of leukemia cells to etoposide. *J. Natl. Cancer Inst.* **1996**, *88*, 1840–1847. [CrossRef]
28. Ashley, D.M.; Meier, L.; Kerby, T.; Zalduondo, F.M.; Friedman, H.S.; Gajjar, A.; Kun, L.; Duffner, P.K.; Smith, S.; Longee, D. Response of recurrent medulloblastoma to low-dose oral etoposide. *J. Clin. Oncol. Off. J. Am. Soc. Clin. Oncol.* **1996**, *14*, 1922–1927. [CrossRef]
29. Khan, Z.; Khan, N.; Tiwari, R.P.; Sah, N.K.; Prasad, G.B.; Bisen, P.S. Biology of Cox-2: An application in cancer therapeutics. *Curr. Drug Targets* **2011**, *12*, 1082–1093. [CrossRef]
30. Gately, S.; Li, W.W. Multiple roles of COX-2 in tumor angiogenesis: A target for antiangiogenic therapy. *Semin. Oncol.* **2004**, *31*, 2–11. [CrossRef]
31. Kerbel, R.S. Improving conventional or low dose metronomic chemotherapy with targeted antiangiogenic drugs. *Cancer Res. Treat. Off. J. Korean Cancer Assoc.* **2007**, *39*, 150–159. [CrossRef] [PubMed]
32. Shu, Q.; Antalffy, B.; Su, J.M.; Adesina, A.; Ou, C.N.; Pietsch, T.; Blaney, S.M.; Lau, C.C.; Li, X.N. Valproic Acid prolongs survival time of severe combined immunodeficient mice bearing intracerebellar orthotopic medulloblastoma xenografts. *Clin. Cancer Res. Off. J. Am. Assoc. Cancer Res.* **2006**, *12*, 4687–4694. [CrossRef] [PubMed]
33. Pei, Y.; Liu, K.W.; Wang, J.; Garancher, A.; Tao, R.; Esparza, L.A.; Maier, D.L.; Udaka, Y.T.; Murad, N.; Morrissy, S.; et al. HDAC and PI3K Antagonists Cooperate to Inhibit Growth of MYC-Driven Medulloblastoma. *Cancer Cell* **2016**, *29*, 311–323. [CrossRef] [PubMed]
34. Vandenberghe, E.A.; Mecucci, C.; Delannoy, A.; Van den Berghe, H. Deletion of 5q by t(5;17) in therapy-related myelodysplastic syndrome. *Cancer Genet. Cytogenet.* **1990**, *48*, 49–52. [CrossRef]
35. Merchant, T.E.; Bendel, A.E.; Sabin, N.D.; Burger, P.C.; Shaw, D.W.; Chang, E.; Wu, S.; Zhou, T.; Eisenstat, D.D.; Foreman, N.K.; et al. Conformal Radiation Therapy for Pediatric Ependymoma, Chemotherapy for Incompletely Resected Ependymoma, and Observation for Completely Resected, Supratentorial Ependymoma. *J. Clin. Oncol. Off. J. Am. Soc. Clin. Oncol.* **2019**, *37*, 974–983. [CrossRef]
36. Esbenshade, A.J.; Kocak, M.; Hershon, L.; Rousseau, P.; Decarie, J.C.; Shaw, S.; Burger, P.; Friedman, H.S.; Gajjar, A.; Moghrabi, A. A Phase II feasibility study of oral etoposide given concurrently with radiotherapy followed by dose intensive adjuvant chemotherapy for children with newly diagnosed high-risk medulloblastoma (protocol POG 9631): A report from the Children's Oncology Group. *Pediatric Blood Cancer* **2017**, *64*, e26373. [CrossRef]
37. Michalski, J.M.; Janss, A.J.; Vezina, L.G.; Smith, K.S.; Billups, C.A.; Burger, P.C.; Embry, L.M.; Cullen, P.L.; Hardy, K.K.; Pomeroy, S.L.; et al. Children's Oncology Group Phase III Trial of Reduced-Dose and Reduced-Volume Radiotherapy With Chemotherapy for Newly Diagnosed Average-Risk Medulloblastoma. *J. Clin. Oncol. Off. J. Am. Soc. Clin. Oncol.* **2021**, *39*, 2685–2697. [CrossRef]
38. Seif, A.E.; Naranjo, A.; Baker, D.L.; Bunin, N.J.; Kletzel, M.; Kretschmar, C.S.; Maris, J.M.; McGrady, P.W.; von Allmen, D.; Cohn, S.L.; et al. A pilot study of tandem high-dose chemotherapy with stem cell rescue as consolidation for high-risk neuroblastoma: Children's Oncology Group study ANBL00P1. *Bone Marrow Transplant.* **2013**, *48*, 947–952. [CrossRef]
39. Slavc, I.; Peyrl, A.; Gojo, J.; Holm, S.; Blomgren, K.; Sehested, A.M.; Leblond, P.; Czech, T. MBCL-43. Recurrent Medulloblastoma—Long-term survival with a "MEMMAT" based antiangiogenic approach. *Neuro-Oncol.* **2020**, *22*, iii397. [CrossRef]
40. Corbacioglu, S.; Steinbach, D.; Lode, H.; Gruhn, B.; Fruehwald, M.; Broeckelmann, M. The RIST design: A molecularly targeted multimodal approach for the treatment of patients with relapsed and refractory neuroblastoma. *J. Clin. Oncol.* **2013**, *31*, 10017. [CrossRef]
41. Sun, X.; Zhen, Z.; Guo, Y.; Gao, Y.; Wang, J.; Zhang, Y.; Zhu, J.; Lu, S.; Sun, F.; Huang, J.; et al. Oral Metronomic Maintenance Therapy Can Improve Survival in High-Risk Neuroblastoma Patients Not Treated with ASCT or Anti-GD2 Antibodies. *Cancers* **2021**, *13*, 3494. [CrossRef] [PubMed]

32. Carcamo, B.; Bista, R.; Wilson, H.; Reddy, P.; Pacheco, J. Rapid Response to Lorlatinib in a Patient With TFG-ROS1 Fusion Positive Inflammatory Myofibroblastic Tumor of the Chest Wall Metastatic to the Brain and Refractory to First and Second Generation ROS1 Inhibitors. *J. Pediatric Hematol. Oncol.* **2021**, *43*, e718–e722. [CrossRef] [PubMed]
33. Hartman, L.L.R.; Oaxaca, D.M.; Carcamo, B.; Wilson, H.L.; Ross, J.A.; Robles-Escajeda, E.; Kirken, R.A. Integration of a Personalized Molecular Targeted Therapy into the Multimodal Treatment of Refractory Childhood Embryonal Tumor with Multilayered Rosettes (ETMR). *Case Rep. Oncol.* **2019**, *12*, 211–217. [CrossRef] [PubMed]
34. Doloff, J.C.; Waxman, D.J. VEGF receptor inhibitors block the ability of metronomically dosed cyclophosphamide to activate innate immunity-induced tumor regression. *Cancer Res.* **2012**, *72*, 1103–1115. [CrossRef] [PubMed]
35. Francia, G.; Emmenegger, U.; Lee, C.R.; Shaked, Y.; Folkins, C.; Mossoba, M.; Medin, J.A.; Man, S.; Zhu, Z.; Witte, L.; et al. Long-term progression and therapeutic response of visceral metastatic disease non-invasively monitored in mouse urine using beta-human choriogonadotropin secreting tumor cell lines. *Mol. Cancer Ther.* **2008**, *7*, 3452–3459. [CrossRef]
36. Tang, T.C.; Man, S.; Xu, P.; Francia, G.; Hashimoto, K.; Emmenegger, U.; Kerbel, R.S. Development of a resistance-like phenotype to sorafenib by human hepatocellular carcinoma cells is reversible and can be delayed by metronomic UFT chemotherapy. *Neoplasia* **2010**, *12*, 928–940. [CrossRef]
37. Williams, M.J.; Singleton, W.G.; Lowis, S.P.; Malik, K.; Kurian, K.M. Therapeutic Targeting of Histone Modifications in Adult and Pediatric High-Grade Glioma. *Front. Oncol.* **2017**, *7*, 45. [CrossRef]
38. Browder, T.; Butterfield, C.E.; Kraling, B.M.; Shi, B.; Marshall, B.; O'Reilly, M.S.; Folkman, J. Antiangiogenic scheduling of chemotherapy improves efficacy against experimental drug-resistant cancer. *Cancer Res.* **2000**, *60*, 1878–1886.
39. Shaked, Y.; Ciarrocchi, A.; Franco, M.; Lee, C.R.; Man, S.; Cheung, A.M.; Hicklin, D.J.; Chaplin, D.; Foster, F.S.; Benezra, R.; et al. Therapy-induced acute recruitment of circulating endothelial progenitor cells to tumors. *Science* **2006**, *313*, 1785–1787. [CrossRef]
40. Emmenegger, U.; Francia, G.; Chow, A.; Shaked, Y.; Kouri, A.; Man, S.; Kerbel, R.S. Tumors that acquire resistance to low-dose metronomic cyclophosphamide retain sensitivity to maximum tolerated dose cyclophosphamide. *Neoplasia (New York N.Y.)* **2011**, *13*, 40–48. [CrossRef]
41. Klement, G.; Baruchel, S.; Rak, J.; Man, S.; Clark, K.; Hicklin, D.J.; Bohlen, P.; Kerbel, R.S. Continuous low-dose therapy with vinblastine and VEGF receptor-2 antibody induces sustained tumor regression without overt toxicity. *J. Clin. Investig.* **2000**, *105*, R15–R24. [CrossRef] [PubMed]
42. Rochlitz, C.; von Moos, R.; Bigler, M.; Zaman, K.; Anchisi, S.; Küng, M.; Jae Na, K.; Baertschi, D.; Borner, M.M.; Rordorf, T.; et al. SAKK 24/09: Safety and tolerability of bevacizumab plus paclitaxel versus bevacizumab plus metronomic cyclophosphamide and capecitabine as first-line therapy in patients with HER2-negative advanced stage breast cancer—A multicenter, randomized phase III trial. *J. Clin. Oncol.* **2014**, *32*, 518.
43. Traore, F.; Togo, B.; Pasquier, E.; Dembele, A.; Andre, N. Preliminary evaluation of children treated with metronomic chemotherapy and valproic acid in a low-income country: Metro-Mali-02. *Indian J. Cancer* **2013**, *50*, 250–253. [CrossRef] [PubMed]
44. Pramanik, R.; Agarwala, S.; Sreenivas, V.; Dhawan, D.; Bakhshi, S. Quality of life in paediatric solid tumours: A randomised study of metronomic chemotherapy versus placebo. *BMJ Supportive Palliat. Care* **2021**. [CrossRef]
45. Qayed, M.; Cash, T.; Tighiouart, M.; MacDonald, T.J.; Goldsmith, K.C.; Tanos, R.; Kean, L.; Watkins, B.; Suessmuth, Y.; Wetmore, C.; et al. A phase I study of sirolimus in combination with metronomic therapy (CHOAnome) in children with recurrent or refractory solid and brain tumors. *Pediatric Blood Cancer* **2020**, *67*, e28134. [CrossRef]

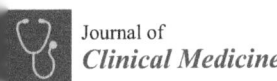

Review

Metronomic Chemotherapy for Advanced Prostate Cancer: A Literature Review

Shruti Parshad [1,2,†], Amanjot K. Sidhu [1,2,†], Nabeeha Khan [1,2,†], Andrew Naoum [1,2] and Urban Emmenegger [1,2,3,4,*]

1. Division of Medical Oncology, Odette Cancer Centre, Sunnybrook Health Sciences Centre, Toronto, ON M4N 3M5, Canada; shruti.parshad@uwaterloo.ca (S.P.); ak7sidhu@edu.uwaterloo.ca (A.K.S.); nabeeha.khan@sri.utoronto.ca (N.K.); andrew.naoum@sri.utoronto.ca (A.N.)
2. Biological Sciences Research Platform, Sunnybrook Research Institute, Sunnybrook Health Sciences Centre, Toronto, ON M4N 3M5, Canada
3. Department of Medicine, University of Toronto, Toronto, ON M5S 1A1, Canada
4. Institute of Medical Science, University of Toronto, Toronto, ON M5S 1A1, Canada
* Correspondence: urban.emmenegger@sunnybrook.ca; Tel.: +1-416-480-4928; Fax: +1-416-480-6002
† These authors contributed equally to this work.

Abstract: Metastatic castration-resistant prostate cancer (mCRPC) is the ultimately lethal form of prostate cancer. Docetaxel chemotherapy was the first life-prolonging treatment for mCRPC; however, the standard maximally tolerated dose (MTD) docetaxel regimen is often not considered for patients with mCRPC who are older and/or frail due to its toxicity. Low-dose metronomic chemotherapy (LDMC) is the frequent administration of typically oral and off-patent chemotherapeutics at low doses, which is associated with a superior safety profile and higher tolerability than MTD chemotherapy. We conducted a systematic literature review using the PUBMED, EMBASE, and MEDLINE electronic databases to identify clinical studies that examined the impact of LDMC on patients with advanced prostate cancer. The search identified 30 reports that retrospectively or prospectively investigated LDMC, 29 of which focused on mCRPC. Cyclophosphamide was the most commonly used agent integrated into 27/30 (90%) of LDMC regimens. LDMC resulted in a clinical benefit rate of 56.8 ± 24.5% across all studies. Overall, there were only a few non-hematological grade 3 or 4 adverse events reported. As such, LDMC is a well-tolerated treatment option for patients with mCRPC, including those who are older and frail. Furthermore, LDMC is considered more affordable than conventional mCRPC therapies. However, prospective phase III trials are needed to further characterize the efficacy and safety of LDMC in mCRPC before its use in practice.

Keywords: metronomic chemotherapy; metastatic castration-resistant prostate cancer; cyclophosphamide; side effects

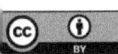

1. Introduction

Cancer is amongst the most significant contributors to disease burden worldwide, with cancer incidence expected to double by 2035 [1]. The global cancer burden is greatest in low- and middle-income countries (LMIC), in which cancer incidence is rising most rapidly, where 75% of cancer deaths occur, yet where only 5% of the global spending on cancer is directed [1]. Prostate cancer follows this general trend as the second most common malignancy in men globally [2].

Localized prostate cancer is highly curable, but metastatic prostate cancer remains a fatal condition to date [3]. While prostate cancer is diagnosed at a median age of 66, prostate cancer-related deaths occur at a median age of 80 [4].

Because prostate cancer is an androgen-driven disease, androgen deprivation therapy (ADT) is the usual first-line therapy for metastatic prostate cancer, nowadays often combined with either docetaxel chemotherapy or androgen receptor signaling inhibitors (ARSi)

such as abiraterone, apalutamide, or enzalutamide [5]. However, such patients will develop ADT-resistant prostate cancer eventually, referred to as metastatic castration-resistant prostate cancer (mCRPC), the lethal form of prostate cancer.

Docetaxel was established as the first life-prolonging and quality-of-life-improving therapy for mCRPC in 2004, providing a survival benefit of around three months [6,7]. This intravenous chemotherapeutic of the taxane family is usually administered as a three-weekly regimen at the maximum tolerated dose (MTD), which is associated with numerous acute and chronic side effects (e.g., myelosuppression, mucositis, and peripheral neuropathy). Thus, docetaxel is often not considered for older men who may have a lower tolerance than younger, healthier patients [8–11].

In recent years, abiraterone and enzalutamide have been approved as mCRPC treatment options, typically used in first line [3]. Both agents are relatively well tolerated, but acquired therapeutic resistance is the ultimate outcome of ARSi therapy in most instances [12,13]. Radium-223 and cabazitaxel chemotherapy represent treatment options for ARSi- and docetaxel-resistant mCRPC [14,15]. However, access to all these life-prolonging yet expensive prostate cancer therapies is limited, notably in LMIC [16,17]. Hence, there is a continued need for affordable mCRPC therapies, especially those suitable for the typically elderly and often patients with advanced prostate cancer who are frail. Low-dose metronomic chemotherapy (LDMC) possess many characteristics to fill this unmet need.

LDMC refers to the continuous administration of low doses of conventional chemotherapy drugs over a long period, usually via daily oral intake without scheduled treatment breaks, resulting in antiangiogenic and immunomodulatory anti-tumor effects amongst others [18]. Due to the low drug doses used, LDMC has a superior toxicity profile compared with MTD chemotherapy, including in people who are older and frail [19,20]. Furthermore, LDMC is relatively affordable owing to the use of off-patent drugs such as cyclophosphamide (CPA) and modest needs for monitoring treatment-associated side effects [21,22]. Herein, we summarize the findings of 30 studies on the role of LDMC in advanced prostate cancer.

2. Materials and Methods

2.1. Search Strategy and Study Selection

A systematic search of the PubMed, EMBASE, and MEDLINE electronic databases was conducted from inception up to 31 December 2021 to identify all relevant studies investigating the clinical impact of LDMC in patients with prostate cancer. The search strategy involved combining a methodological filter to specifically identify 'full text articles' using the search terms 'metronomic' and 'prostate cancer.' English-written literature was highly valued in the conduct of this review due to the ease of data extraction. However, non-English language was not a reason for exclusion. Additional studies were identified by screening the reference lists of review articles on LDMC. Titles and abstracts were screened for eligibility. The exclusion criteria are highlighted in Figure 1. Treatment regimens comprising at least one component administered without prespecified breaks were considered metronomic.

2.2. Data Extraction and Statistical Analysis

Two independent reviewers extracted information on study type and design, country of study, number of patients, patient demographics, treatment details, response criteria used and response rates, survival data, adverse events, and fatalities. Statistical analyses were computed using RStudio (RStudio for Macintosh, version 1.1.463). Graphs were created with Microsoft® Excel for Mac 16.45 (www.microsoft.com), Draw.io (Version 16.5.1; https://app.diagrams.net), or GraphPad Prism (Version 9.3.1; https://www.graphpad.com).

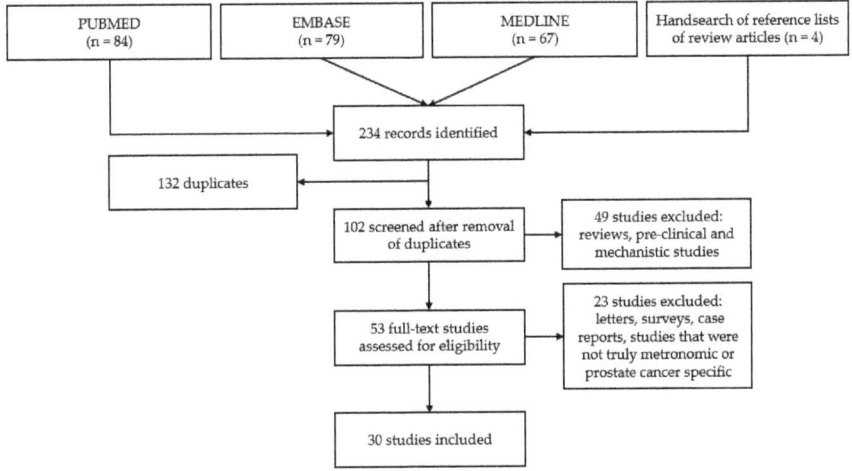

Figure 1. Flow diagram of search strategy.

3. Results

3.1. Study Selection

Among the 234 reports identified during the initial search, there were 132 duplicates, leaving 102 abstracts for screening. Following the removal of 49 studies comprising reviews, and pre-clinical and mechanistic studies, we analyzed the full text of 53 articles. A further 23 studies were excluded, including letters, surveys, case reports, and studies that were not truly metronomic or prostate cancer specific. Overall, we identified 30 studies on the clinical use of LDMC for prostate cancer, as depicted in Figure 1. Key study details are outlined in Table 1.

3.2. Study and Patient Characteristics

LDMC studies in the field of prostate cancer cover the time period from 1993 until 2019, with the majority (23/30; 77%) published from 2010 onwards (Figure 2a). More than half of the studies analyzed were conducted in Europe (17/30; 57%), notably with ten of those (33% of all studies) in Italy. Moreover, eight studies (27%) were conducted in Asia, whereas only five reports (17%) were from North America and none were from Asia or South America. Eleven studies (37%) were retrospective analyses. Among the nineteen prospective studies, two (11%) were phase I [27,36], one (5%) was phase I/II [47], and sixteen (84%) were phase II studies [22,25,26,29,30,33,34,37,38,40–43,45,48,49]. Across both prospective and retrospective phase II type studies, the majority (23/26, 88%) were single arm trials [19,21–23,25,26,28–33,35,37,38,40–42,44,48,49].

The 30 studies comprise information on 973 patients overall, with 28 (range 8 to 74) being the median number of patients per study (Figure 2b). The median patient age per trial ranged from 60 to 83 years, of which 72.8 years was the median of the reported medians (Figure 2c). Of the 30 studies included, only one reported on men with biochemically recurrent (i.e., non-metastatic and castration-sensitive) prostate cancer (Figure 3) [22]. All other studies focused on patients with mCRPC and variable treatment history. Seven (23%) studies included chemotherapy-naïve participants [25,32,33,38,45,46,48], three reported on study subjects with or without prior chemotherapy (typically docetaxel) exposure [28,31,42], and nineteen did not provide details on prior therapies other than the use of ADT [19,21,23,24,26,27,29,30,34–37,39–41,43,44,47,49].

Table 1. Study characteristics.

First Author Name	Years	Study Type	Location	N	Age, Median (Range)	Reference
Caffo et al.	2019	retrospective	Italy	8	74 (56–95)	[21]
Calcagno et al.	2016	prospective	France	14	69 (57–82)	[22]
Calvani et al.	2019	retrospective	Italy	14	75 (56–87)	[23]
Dabkara et al.	2018	retrospective	India	16	74.5 (59–83)	[24]
Derosa et al.	2014	prospective	Italy	17	72 (52–79)	[25]
Di Desidero et al.	2016	prospective	Italy	17	73 (63–86)	[26]
Di Lorenzo et al.	2007	prospective	Italy	18	67 (46–75)	[27]
Dickinson et al.	2012	retrospective	UK	21	75 (N/A)	[28]
Fontana et al.	2009	prospective	Italy	23	74.5 (54–91)	[29]
Fontana et al.	2010	retrospective	Italy	24	83 (78–92)	[19]
Gebbia et al.	2011	prospective	Italy	25	72 (56–83)	[30]
Glode et al.	2003	retrospective	USA	25	72.6 (54–88)	[31]
Hatano et al.	2011	retrospective	Japan	25	71 (49–90)	[32]
Jellvert et al.	2011	prospective	Sweden	28	60 (45–75)	[33]
Jeong & Lee	2017	prospective	Korea	28	71 (49–88)	[34]
Knipper et al.	2019	retrospective	Germany	28	78 (N/A)	[35]
Kubota et al.	2017	prospective	Japan	29	74.2 (66–88)	[36]
Ladoire et al.	2010	prospective	France	32	74 (55–88)	[37]
Lord et al.	2007	prospective	UK	35	69 (51–86)	[38]
Meng et al.	2012	retrospective	China	38	72.8 (69–78)	[39]
Nelius et al.	2010	prospective	USA	39	68 (42–85)	[40]
Nicolini et al.	2004	prospective	Italy	41	72 (62–84)	[41]
Nishimura et al.	2001	prospective	Japan	43	70 (50–82)	[42]
Noguchi et al.	2016	prospective	Japan	49	68.6 (48–80)	[43]
Orlandi et al.	2013	retrospective	USA	52	81 (52–92)	[44]
Tralongo et al.	2016	prospective	Italy	57	77 (72–82)	[45]
Vorob'ev et al.	2011	retrospective	Russia	58	72.8 * (56–85)	[46]
Wang et al.	2015	prospective	USA	58	76 (50–86)	[47]
Wozniak et al.	1993	prospective	USA	74	67 (55–78)	[48]
Yashi et al.	2014	prospective	Japan	37	75 (67.8–79.3)	[49]

* = mean; N = sample size, N/A = not available.

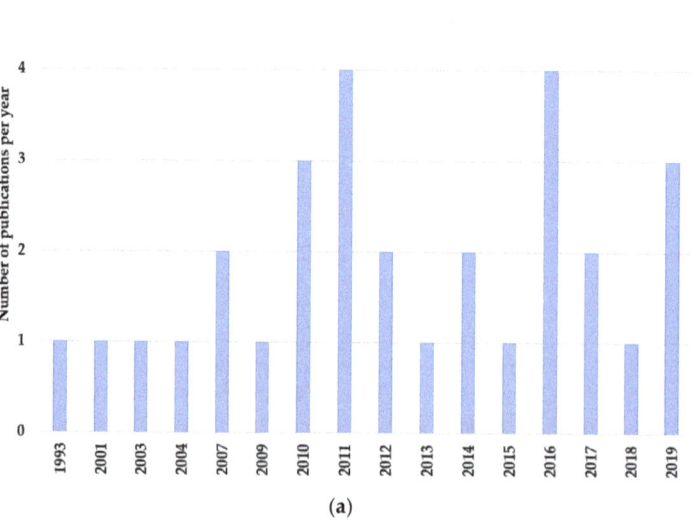

(a)

Figure 2. Cont.

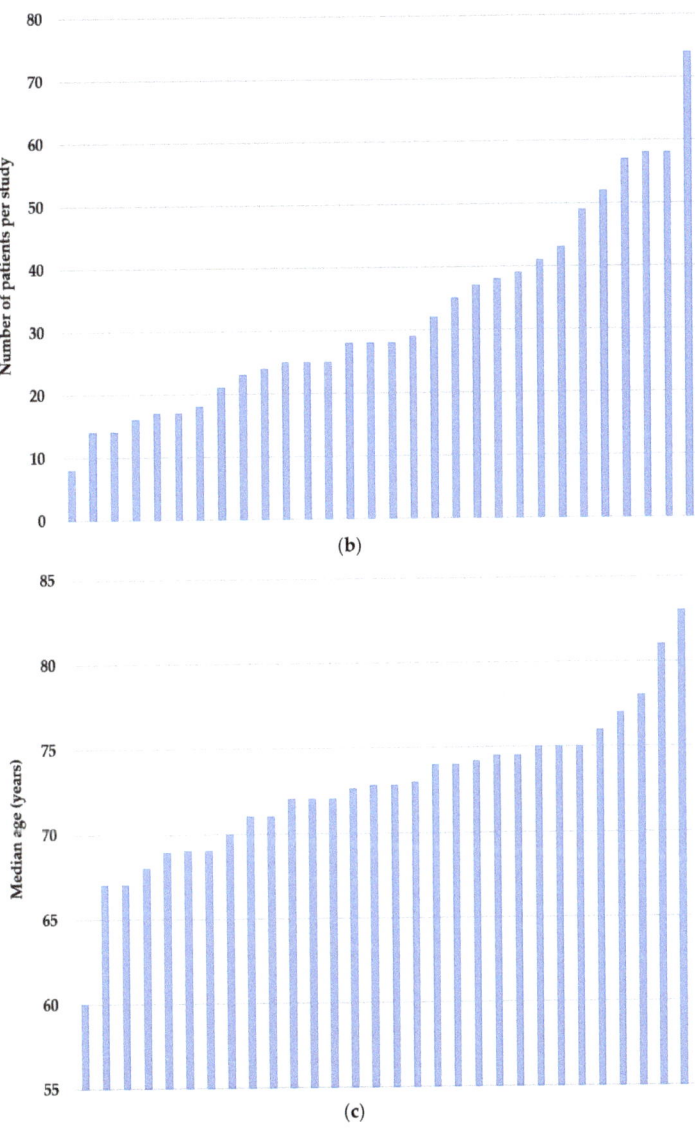

Figure 2. (**a**) Number of LDMC publications per year. (**b**) Number of patients per study. (**c**) Median patient age in years per study.

3.3. Metronomic Treatment Regimens

CPA was integrated into 27 of the 30 (90%) regimens (Figure 4) [19,21–25,27–35,37–44,46–49]. While six studies (20%) described the effects of CPA monotherapy [21,22,38,41,43,46], in the majority of reports, CPA was partnered with corticosteroids (19/30; 63.3%) [19,23–25,27,29–35,37,39,40,42,44,48,49]. Among the CPA/corticosteroid combination therapy studies, eight (27%) did not add further agents [23,24,27,31,35,37,40,49], the COX2 inhibitor celecoxib was added in three (10%) trials [19,34,44], and eight (27%) studies included other drugs (i.e., methotrexate, tegafur-uracil, etoposide, estramustine phosphate, and capecitabine) [25,29,30,32,33,39,42,48]. In two studies, CPA was combined with either thalidomide or lenalidomide (7%) [28,47].

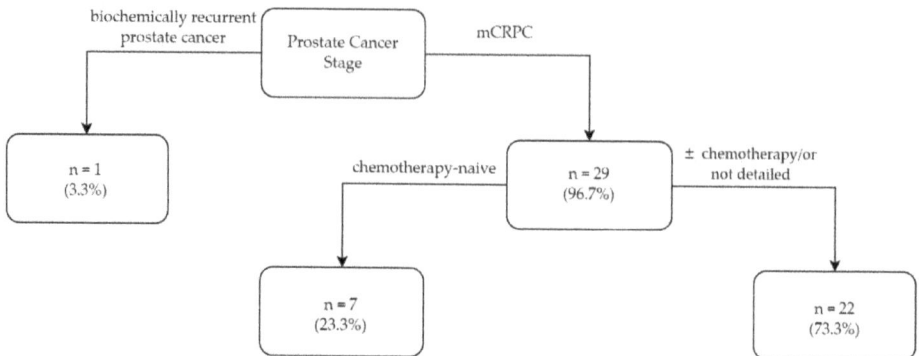

Figure 3. Prostate cancer stage of patients of LDMC studies. mCRPC: metastatic castration-resistant prostate cancer.

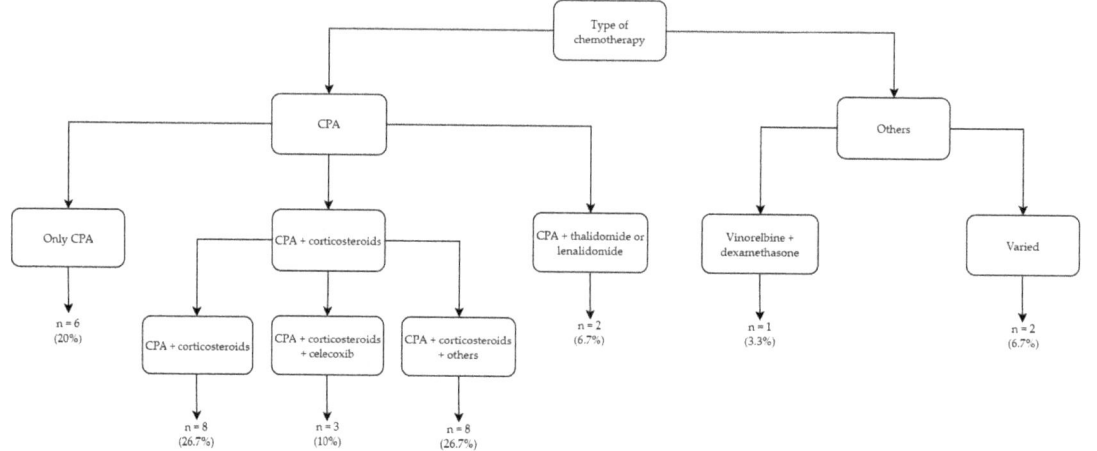

Figure 4. Details of the LDMC regimens. CPA = cyclophosphamide.

Of the studies without a CPA backbone, a variety of agents were used. Di Desidero et al. studied vinorelbine with dexamethasone [26], Kubota et al. studied cisplatin and tegafur-uracil [36], and Tralongo et al. studied docetaxel or vinorelbine [45]. Of note, 24 of 30 (80%) treatment regimens comprised oral medications only [19,21–24,26–28,31–35,37–44,46,47,49].

3.4. Outcomes

To compare the effectiveness of the various LDMC regimens used, we extracted prostate-specific antigen (PSA) response rates and clinical benefit rates. Twenty-six trials provided information regarding patients' PSA levels (Figure 5a) [19,21,22,24–34,36–42,44–47,49]. The mean ± SD PSA response rate (i.e., at least a 50% treatment-related PSA decrease compared with baseline) was 33 ± 19.1%, while another 32.2 ± 16.5% of patients achieved stable PSA readings. One third of study patients (33.5 ± 19.4%) did not experience any biochemical benefit from LDMC.

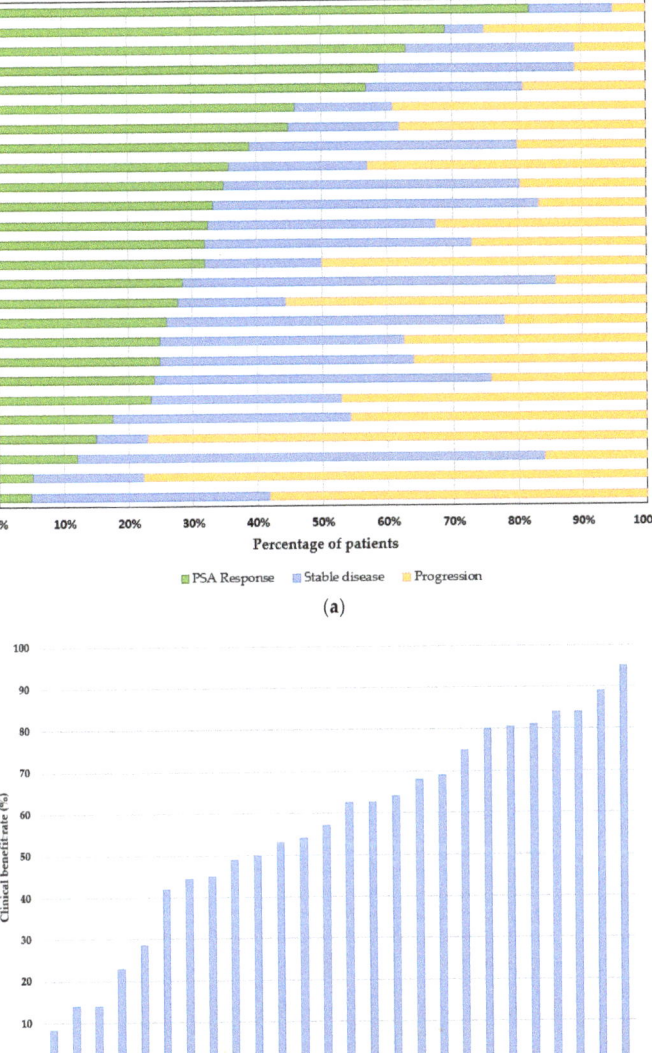

Figure 5. (a) Biochemical response assessment based on prostate specific antigen (PSA) across 26 informative studies. PSA response was defined as a ≥50% treatment-related PSA decrease compared with baseline. (b) Clinical benefit rate (%) across 26 informative studies.

The mean clinical benefit rate reported across 26 studies was 56.8 ± 24.5% (range from 8.3% to 95.0%) (Figure 5b). Of note, the publications used variable definitions of "clinical benefit", with the most common being "sustained (≥6 months) absence of biochemical, clinical, and/or radiological progression".

Twenty studies reported the median overall survival of patients on LDMC regimens [19,21,23,25,26,29–31,34–37,39–41,43,44,46,47,49]. Fontana et al. observed the shortest median survival of 3.3 (95%CI: 2.2–4.2) months [29], while Derosa et al. described the longest median survival of 33.3 (95%CI: 23–35.6) months [25]. The median of medians of reported overall survival was 16.2 months.

3.5. Toxicities and Adverse Events

Twenty of the thirty studies used varying versions of the National Cancer Institute Common Toxicity Criteria for Adverse Events (NCI-CTCAE) to grade toxicities observed among study participants undergoing LDMC [19,21–23,25–27,29,30,32,34,36–40,42–44,46]. One of the studies used criteria set by the World Health Organization (WHO) [45], while four studies reported adverse events without indicating the type of criteria used [28,47–49]. Five studies did not include information regarding toxicities and adverse events in relation to LDMC [24,31,33,35,41].

Figure 6 shows the percentage of study patients that experienced specific grade 3 or 4 (i.e. severe) toxicities reported in 15 informative clinical trials. Overall, hematological toxicities were more common than non-hematological adverse events. Instances of severe anemia were reported in nine trials, with a median of 8% of patients affected [21,27,28,34,37,38,42,43,45]. Grade 3/4 neutropenia was reported in eight studies, with a median of 5.5% of patients affected [25,27,32,37,38,43,45,47]. In the four studies listing severe lymphopenia, on average, around 20% of patients were affected. Asthenia was the most reported severe non-hematological adverse event, listed by five trials, with a median of 5.4% of patients affected [21,26,34,45,47].

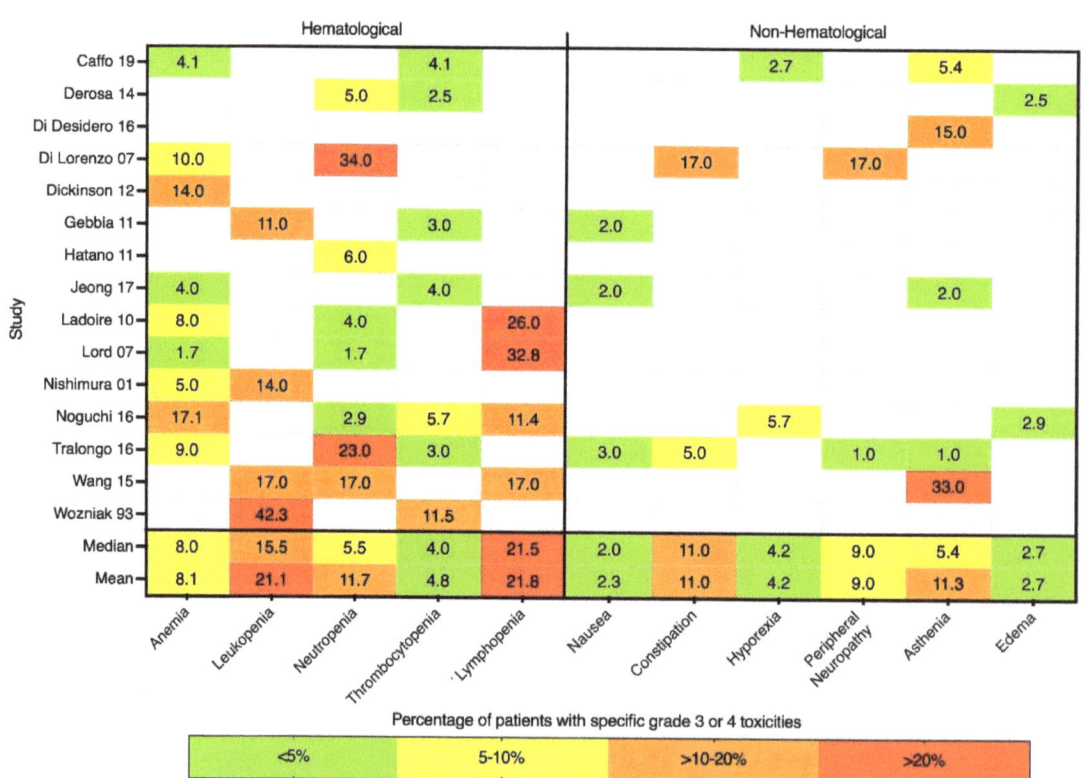

Figure 6. Heatmap of grade 3 and 4 toxicities observed in LDMC studies.

Vorob'ev et al.'s retrospective study compared the side effects of MTD docetaxel (75 mg/m^2 administered intravenously every three weeks; n = 30 patients) versus LDMC CPA (50 mg by mouth daily; n = 25 patients) [46]. There were far fewer and less severe side effects reported in the CPA cohort (using NCI-CTCAE version 3) in comparison with patients treated with docetaxel (Figure 7). While a high percentage of patients treated with docetaxel were affected by diarrhea, alopecia, grade 1–3 anemia, and grade 1–4 neutropenia, patients in the CPA cohort were primarily affected by grade 1–2 anemia and grade 1–2 neutropenia, without severe (i.e., grade 3 or 4) cytopenia. Moreover, 16.7% of the docetaxel cohort stopped treatment due to adverse events, but no patient treated with CPA discontinued treatment because of side effects. Despite the distinct toxicity profiles, the mean overall survival was similar (>15 months) for both cohorts. However, MTD docetaxel resulted in a higher PSA response rate (46.7%) than LDMC CPA (12%). MTD docetaxel treatment was also slightly favored over LDMC CPA in terms of quality of life, measured with the Functional Assessment of Cancer Therapy-Prostate (FACT-P) questionnaire, and rate of pain response, based on a visual analogue scale, although these results were not statistically significant.

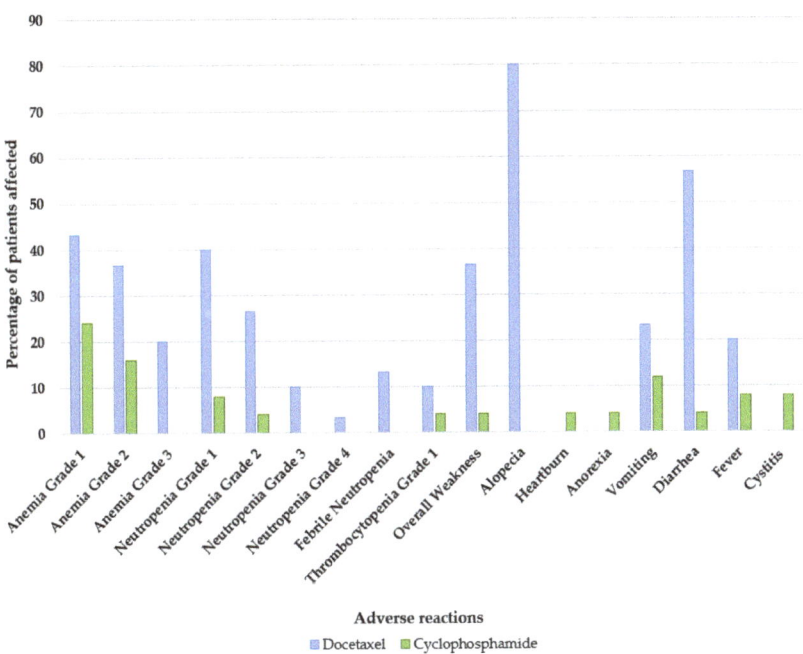

Figure 7. Depiction of the incidence of adverse events reported in patients undergoing conventional docetaxel versus metronomic cyclophosphamide therapy as reported by Vorob'ev et al., 2011 [46].

4. Discussion

The present literature review of 30 studies of LDMC for prostate cancer encompassing 973 patients illustrates several key findings. First, more than half of patients experience PSA responses or PSA stability and draw a clinical benefit from LDMC. Second, CPA is the most commonly used cytotoxic agent for metronomic purposes in prostate cancer (27/30 trials), as is the case in other cancer types [50]. The LDMC CPA studies characterize this classical alkylating agent as a convenient (oral mode of administration), well tolerated, and affordable (off-patent) treatment option that can be administered alone or in combination with other agents. Third, prostate cancer LDMC studies report low rates of severe (i.e., grade 3 or 4) adverse events. Hematological toxicity, notably lymphopenia, was more frequently observed than non-hematological adverse events. However, neither myelosuppression nor lymphopenia appear to be associated with an increased rate of infections. Furthermore, the low rate of typically mild LDMC-associated side effects compares favorably with the higher rate of adverse events seen with conventional MTD chemotherapy, including high-grade adverse events, as documented by Vorob'ev et al. [46].

Our study also reveals shortcomings and unmet needs regarding the clinical development of LDMC in prostate cancer. Foremost, there are no definite phase III clinical trials documenting the benefit of LDMC in prostate cancer, unlike in other malignancies such as breast, head and neck, and colorectal cancer [51–58]. Moreover, the majority of the LDMC prostate cancer studies were single-arm trials describing relatively small and often heterogeneous patient cohorts. Second, LDMC was almost exclusively studied in later stages of prostate cancer and often after multiple lines of prior therapies, whereas phase III trials in other tumor types suggest that LDMC might be particularly suitable for maintenance therapy in earlier tumor stages [52,55,57]. Third, there are no validated predictive markers of response to LDMC [59]. However, anecdotal evidence of responses to metronomic CPA in patients with DNA repair deficient mCRPC warrant further study [60].

In current times, with limited resources and growing expenses for the treatment of early as well as advanced prostate cancer, drug costs are becoming an increasingly important consideration when choosing treatments options [61–63]. With the incidence of cancer surging and the rising economic burden of cancer treatment worldwide, there is a need for affordable treatment options [2,64]. This is especially important for resource-limited countries, where mortality rates due to prostate cancer are rising, while decreasing in the more developed countries [65]. LDMC is an attractive treatment option in this respect. In Bocci et al.'s outcome analysis and cost comparison for conventional versus LDMC for metastatic breast cancer, LDMC was found to be more cost-effective due to several factors: LDMC (i) can be taken orally at home instead of administered during hospital visits, (ii) has lower incidences of adverse events, thereby decreasing related hospital and other healthcare visits, and (iii) is associated with lower administrative and health care provision costs due to a reduced need for medical attention [66].

Our systematic literature search did not identify studies comparing LDMC with ARSi therapy. Based on available evidence reported in the present analysis, it appears improbable that LDMC alone may provide a similar benefit to ARSi in advanced prostate cancer. Furthermore, ARSi are convenient oral albeit expensive medications that rarely result in severe side effects, even in patients who are older or frail [12,13,16,17]. However, LDMC might make ARSi therapy more affordable when integrated into intermittent ARSi regimens (e.g., LDMC maintenance therapy following ARSi induction). Aside from cost savings such LDMC use might also improve patient outcome by targeting ARSi-resistant prostate cancer cells [67,68]. Similarly, preliminary breast and ovarian cancer evidence suggests a possible role for combining LDMC using alkylating agents with poly (ADP-ribose) polymerase (PARP) inhibitors in patients with DNA-repair-deficient prostate cancer [69,70].

When extracting information from the 30 studies of LDMC for prostate cancer numerous limitations became apparent. Aside from the aforementioned lack of randomized controlled phase III trials, one third of studies were retrospective, and the majority of reports comprised relatively small single-arm studies. The definition of outcome measures such as clinical benefit rate varied across studies, rendering comparisons difficult. Not all reports contained information on adverse events. Finally, a wide variety of metronomic regimens were tested, although the use of CPA was a common denominator.

5. Conclusions

In conclusion, LDMC is a well-tolerated and cost-effective form of cancer therapy with documented anti-mCRPC effects. Because of mild toxicities and simple oral administration, LDMC can be regarded as an alternative treatment option especially for patients who are older or unfit and who are unable to tolerate conventional mCRPC therapies such as taxane chemotherapy. LDMC might also be considered in situations where ARSi are not available or affordable. Phase III trial evidence is needed to position LDMC with respect to other mCRPC therapies.

Author Contributions: Conceptualization, S.P. and U.E.; methodology, S.P. and U.E.; validation, S.P., A.K.S., N.K. and U.E; formal analysis, S.P., N.K., A.N. and U.E.; investigation, S.P., A.K.S., N.K. and U.E.; writing—original draft preparation, S.P. and A.K.S.; writing—review and editing, S.P., A.K.S., N.K., A.N. and U.E.; visualization, S.P., A.K.S. and N.K.; supervision, U.E. All authors have read and agreed to the published version of the manuscript.

Funding: The preparation of this manuscript was financially supported by the Joseph and Silvana Melara Cancer Fund, Toronto/ON, Canada.

Institutional Review Board Statement: Not applicable.

Informed Consent Statement: Not applicable.

Data Availability Statement: Not applicable.

Conflicts of Interest: The authors declare no conflict of interest.

References

1. Prager, M.G.; Braga, S.; Bystricky, B.; Qvortrup, C.; Criscitiello, C.; Esin, E.; Sonke, G.; Martínez, G.A.; Frenel, J.-S.; Karamouzis, M.; et al. Global cancer control: Responding to the growing burden, rising costs and inequalities in access. *ESMO Open* **2018**, *3*, e000285. [CrossRef] [PubMed]
2. Sung, H.; Ferlay, J.; Siegel, R.L.; Laversanne, M.; Soerjomataram, I.; Jemal, A.; Bray, F. Global Cancer Statistics 2020: GLOBOCAN Estimates of Incidence and Mortality Worldwide for 36 Cancers in 185 Countries. *CA Cancer J. Clin.* **2021**, *71*, 209–249. [CrossRef] [PubMed]
3. Sartor, O.; De Bono, J.S. Metastatic Prostate Cancer. *N. Engl. J. Med.* **2019**, *378*, 645–657. [CrossRef] [PubMed]
4. Boyle, H.; Alibhai, S.; Decoster, L.; Efstathiou, E.; Fizazi, K.; Mottet, N.; Oudard, S.; Payne, H.; Prentice, M.; Puts, M.; et al. Updated recommendations of the International Society of Geriatric Oncology on prostate cancer management in older patients. *Eur. J. Cancer* **2019**, *116*, 116–136. [CrossRef]
5. Schulte, B.; Morgans, A.K.; Shore, N.D.; Pezaro, C. Sorting Through the Maze of Treatment Options for Metastatic Castration-Sensitive Prostate Cancer. *Am. Soc. Clin. Oncol. Educ. Book* **2020**, *40*, 198–207. [CrossRef]
6. Tannock, I.F.; De Wit, R.; Berry, W.R.; Horti, J.; Pluzanska, A.; Chi, K.N.; Oudard, S.; Théodore, C.; James, N.D.; Turesson, I.; et al. Docetaxel plus Prednisone or Mitoxantrone plus Prednisone for Advanced Prostate Cancer. *N. Engl. J. Med.* **2004**, *351*, 1502–1512. [CrossRef]
7. Petrylak, D.P.; Tangen, C.M.; Hussain, M.H.; Lara, P.N.; Jones, J.A.; Taplin, M.E.; Burch, P.A.; Berry, D.; Moinpour, C.; Kohli, M.; et al. Docetaxel and Estramustine Compared with Mitoxantrone and Prednisone for Advanced Refractory Prostate Cancer. *N. Engl. J. Med.* **2004**, *351*, 1513–1520. [CrossRef]
8. Lissbrant, I.F.; Garmo, H.; Widmark, A.; Stattin, P. Population-based study on use of chemotherapy in men with castration resistant prostate cancer. *Acta Oncol.* **2013**, *52*, 1593–1601. [CrossRef]
9. Leibowitz-Amit, R.; Templeton, A.J.; Alibhai, S.M.; Knox, J.J.; Sridhar, S.S.; Tannock, I.F.; Joshua, A.M. Efficacy and toxicity of abiraterone and docetaxel in octogenarians with metastatic castration-resistant prostate cancer. *J. Geriatr. Oncol.* **2015**, *6*, 23–28. [CrossRef]
10. Horgan, A.M.; Seruga, B.; Pond, G.R.; Alibhai, S.M.; Amir, E.; De Wit, R.; Eisenberger, M.A.; Tannock, I.F. Tolerability and efficacy of docetaxel in older men with metastatic castrate-resistant prostate cancer (mCRPC) in the TAX 327 trial. *J. Geriatr. Oncol.* **2014**, *5*, 119–126. [CrossRef]
11. Khalaf, D.J.; Sunderland, K.; Eigl, B.; Kollmannsberger, C.K.; Ivanov, N.; Finch, D.L.; Oja, C.; Vergidis, J.; Zulfiqar, M.; Gleave, M.; et al. Health-related Quality of Life for Abiraterone Plus Prednisone Versus Enzalutamide in Patients with Metastatic Castration-resistant Prostate Cancer: Results from a Phase II Randomized Trial. *Eur. Urol.* **2019**, *75*, 940–947. [CrossRef] [PubMed]
12. Alibhai, S.M.H.; Breunis, H.; Hansen, A.R.; Gregg, R.; Warde, P.; Timilshina, N.; Tomlinson, G.; Joshua, A.M.; Hotte, S.; Fleshner, N.; et al. Examining the ability of the Cancer and Aging Research Group tool to predict toxicity in older men receiving chemotherapy or androgen-receptor–targeted therapy for metastatic castration-resistant prostate cancer. *Cancer* **2021**, *127*, 2587–2594. [CrossRef] [PubMed]
13. Alibhai, S.M.H.; Breunis, H.; Feng, G.; Timilshina, N.; Hansen, A.; Warde, P.; Gregg, R.; Joshua, A.; Fleshner, N.; Tomlinson, G.; et al. Association of Chemotherapy, Enzalutamide, Abiraterone, and Radium 223 With Cognitive Function in Older Men with Metastatic Castration-Resistant Prostate Cancer. *JAMA Netw. Open* **2021**, *4*, e2114694. [CrossRef] [PubMed]
14. Parker, C.; Nilsson, S.; Heinrich, D.; Helle, S.I.; O'Sullivan, J.M.; Fosså, S.D.; Chodacki, A.; Wiechno, P.; Logue, J.; Seke, M.; et al. Alpha Emitter Radium-223 and Survival in Metastatic Prostate Cancer. *N. Engl. J. Med.* **2013**, *369*, 213–223. [CrossRef] [PubMed]
15. De Bono, J.S.; Oudard, S.; Özgüroglu, M.; Hansen, S.; Machiels, J.-P.; Kocak, I.; Gravis, G.; Bodrogi, I.; Mackenzie, M.J.; Shen, L.; et al. Prednisone plus cabazitaxel or mitoxantrone for metastatic castration-resistant prostate cancer progressing after docetaxel treatment: A randomised open-label trial. *Lancet* **2010**, *376*, 1147–1154. [CrossRef]
16. Tannock, I.F. Improving Treatment for Advanced Prostate Cancer. *N. Engl. J. Med.* **2019**, *381*, 176–177. [CrossRef] [PubMed]
17. Anton, A.; Tran, B. Global Disparity in Access to Novel Therapeutics for Metastatic Prostate Cancer. *JCO Oncol. Pract.* **2022**, *18*, 57–59. [CrossRef]
18. Bocci, G.; Kerbel, R.S. Pharmacokinetics of metronomic chemotherapy: A neglected but crucial aspect. *Nat. Rev. Clin. Oncol.* **2016**, *13*, 659–673. [CrossRef]
19. Fontana, A.; Bocci, G.; Galli, L.; D'Arcangelo, M.; DeRosa, L.; Fioravanti, A.; Orlandi, P.; Barletta, M.T.; Landi, L.; Bursi, S.; et al. Metronomic cyclophosphamide in elderly patients with advanced, castration-resistant prostate cancer. *J. Am. Geriatr. Soc.* **2010**, *58*, 986–988. [CrossRef]

20. Delos Santos, K.; Sivanathan, L.; Lien, K.; Emmenegger, U. Clinical Trials of Low-Dose Metronomic Chemotherapy in Castration Resistant Prostate Cancer. In *Metronomic Chemotherapy: Pharmacology and Clinical Applications*; Springer: Berlin/Heidelberg, Germany, 2014; pp. 119–134. [CrossRef]
21. Caffo, O.; Facchini, G.; Biasco, E.; Ferraù, F.; Morelli, F.; Donini, M.; Buttigliero, C.; Calvani, N.; Guida, A.; Chiuri, V.E.; et al. Activity and safety of metronomic cyclophosphamide in the modern era of metastatic castration-resistant prostate cancer. *Futur Oncol.* **2019**, *15*, 1115–1123. [CrossRef]
22. Calcagno, F.; Mouillet, G.; Adotevi, O.; Maurina, T.; Nguyen, T.; Montcuquet, P.; Curtit, E.; Kleinclauss, F.; Pivot, X.; Borg, C.; et al. Metronomic cyclophosphamide therapy in hormone-naive patients with non-metastatic biochemical recurrent prostate cancer: A phase II trial. *Med. Oncol.* **2016**, *33*, 89. [CrossRef] [PubMed]
23. Calvani, N.; Morelli, F.; Naglieri, E.; Gnoni, A.; Chiuri, V.E.; Orlando, L.; Fedele, P.; Cinieri, S. Metronomic chemotherapy with cyclophosphamide plus low dose of corticosteroids in advanced castration-resistant prostate cancer across the era of taxanes and new hormonal drugs. *Med. Oncol.* **2019**, *36*, 80. [CrossRef] [PubMed]
24. Ganguly, S.; Dabkara, D.; Biswas, B.; Ghosh, J. Metronomic therapy in metastatic castrate-resistant prostate cancer: Experience from a tertiary cancer care center. *Indian J. Cancer* **2018**, *55*, 94. [CrossRef] [PubMed]
25. DeRosa, L.; Galli, L.; Orlandi, P.; Fioravanti, A.; Di Desidero, T.; Fontana, A.; Antonuzzo, A.; Biasco, E.; Farnesi, A.; Marconcini, R.; et al. Docetaxel plus oral metronomic cyclophosphamide: A phase II study with pharmacodynamic and pharmacogenetic analyses in castration-resistant prostate cancer patients. *Cancer* **2014**, *120*, 3923–3931. [CrossRef] [PubMed]
26. Di Desidero, T.; DeRosa, L.; Galli, L.; Orlandi, P.; Fontana, A.; Fioravanti, A.; Marconcini, R.; Giorgi, M.; Campi, B.; Saba, A.; et al. Clinical, pharmacodynamic and pharmacokinetic results of a prospective phase II study on oral metronomic vinorelbine and dexamethasone in castration-resistant prostate cancer patients. *Investig. New Drugs* **2016**, *34*, 760–770. [CrossRef] [PubMed]
27. Di Lorenzo, G.; Autorino, R.; De Laurentiis, M.; Forestieri, V.; Romano, C.; Prudente, A.; Giugliano, F.; Imbimbo, C.; Mirone, V.; De Placido, S. Thalidomide in combination with oral daily cyclophosphamide in patients with pretreated hormone refractory prostate cancer: A phase I clinical trial. *Cancer Biol. Ther.* **2007**, *6*, 313–317. [CrossRef] [PubMed]
28. Dickinson, P.D.; Peel, D.N.Y.; Sundar, S. Metronomic chemotherapy with cyclophosphamide and dexamethasone in patients with metastatic carcinoma of the prostate. *Br. J. Cancer* **2012**, *106*, 1464–1465. [CrossRef]
29. Fontana, A.; Galli, L.; Fioravanti, A.; Orlandi, P.; Galli, C.; Landi, L.; Bursi, S.; Allegrini, G.; Fontana, E.; Di Marsico, R.; et al. Clinical and Pharmacodynamic Evaluation of Metronomic Cyclophosphamide, Celecoxib, and Dexamethasone in Advanced Hormone-refractory Prostate Cancer. *Clin. Cancer Res.* **2009**, *15*, 4954–4962. [CrossRef]
30. Gebbia, V.; Serretta, V.; Borsellino, N.; Valerio, M.R. Salvage Therapy with Oral Metronomic Cyclophosphamide and Methotrexate for Castration-refractory Metastatic Adenocarcinoma of the Prostate Resistant to Docetaxel. *Urology* **2011**, *78*, 1125–1130. [CrossRef]
31. Glode, L.M.; Barqawi, A.; Crighton, F.; Crawford, E.D.; Kerbel, R. Metronomic therapy with cyclophosphamide and dexamethasone for prostate carcinoma. *Cancer* **2003**, *98*, 1643–1648. [CrossRef]
32. Hatano, K.; Nonomura, N.; Nishimura, K.; Kawashima, A.; Mukai, M.; Nagahara, A.; Nakai, Y.; Nakayama, M.; Takayama, H.; Tsujimura, A.; et al. Retrospective Analysis of an Oral Combination of Dexamethasone, Uracil plus Tegafur and Cyclophosphamide for Hormone-refractory Prostate Cancer. *Jpn. J. Clin. Oncol.* **2010**, *41*, 253–259. [CrossRef] [PubMed]
33. Jellvert, Å.; Lissbrant, I.F.; Edgren, M.; Öfverholm, E.; Braide, K.; Olvenmark, A.-M.E.; Kindblom, J.; Albertsson, P.; Lennernäs, B. Effective oral combination metronomic chemotherapy with low toxicity for the management of castration-resistant prostate cancer. *Exp. Ther. Med.* **2011**, *2*, 579–584. [CrossRef] [PubMed]
34. Jeong, Y.; Lee, J.L. Efficacy of metronomic oral cyclophosphamide with low dose dexamethasone and celecoxib in metastatic castration-resistant prostate cancer. *Asia-Pac. J. Clin. Oncol.* **2016**, *13*, 204–211. [CrossRef] [PubMed]
35. Knipper, S.; Mandel, P.; Amsberg, G.; Strölin, P.; Graefen, M.; Steuber, T. Metronomic chemotherapy with oral cyclophosphamide: An individual option for the metastatic castration-resistant prostate cancer patient? *Urol. A* **2019**, *58*, 410–417. [CrossRef]
36. Kubota, H.; Fukuta, K.; Yamada, K.; Hirose, M.; Naruyama, H.; Yanai, Y.; Yamada, Y.; Watase, H.; Kawai, N.; Tozawa, K.; et al. Feasibility of metronomic chemotherapy with tegafur-uracil, cisplatin, and dexamethasone for docetaxel-refractory prostate cancer. *J. Rural Med.* **2017**, *12*, 112–119. [CrossRef] [PubMed]
37. Ladoire, S.; Eymard, J.C.; Zanetta, S.; Mignot, G.; Martin, E.; Kermarrec, I.; Mourey, E.; Michel, F.; Cormier, L.; Ghiringhelli, F. Metronomic oral cyclophosphamide prednisolone chemotherapy is an effective treatment for metastatic hormone-refractory prostate cancer after docetaxel failure. *Anticancer Res.* **2010**, *30*, 4317–4323.
38. Lord, R.; Nair, S.; Schache, A.; Spicer, J.; Somaihah, N.; Khoo, V.; Pandha, H. Low Dose Metronomic Oral Cyclophosphamide for Hormone Resistant Prostate Cancer: A Phase II Study. *J. Urol.* **2007**, *177*, 2136–2140. [CrossRef]
39. Meng, L.-J.; Wang, J.; Fan, W.-F.; Pu, X.-L.; Liu, F.-Y.; Yang, M. Evaluation of oral chemotherapy with capecitabine and cyclophosphamide plus thalidomide and prednisone in prostate cancer patients. *J. Cancer Res. Clin. Oncol.* **2012**, *138*, 333–339. [CrossRef]
40. Nelius, T.; Klatte, T.; De Riese, W.; Haynes, A.; Filleur, S. Clinical outcome of patients with docetaxel-resistant hormone-refractory prostate cancer treated with second-line cyclophosphamide-based metronomic chemotherapy. *Med. Oncol.* **2009**, *27*, 363–367. [CrossRef]
41. Nicolini, A.; Mancini, P.; Ferrari, P.; Anselmi, L.; Tartarelli, G.; Bonazzi, V.; Carpi, A.; Giardino, R. Oral low-dose cyclophosphamide in metastatic hormone refractory prostate cancer (MHRPC). *Biomed. Pharmacother.* **2004**, *58*, 447–450. [CrossRef]

2. Nishimura, K.; Nonomura, N.; Ono, Y.; Nozawa, M.; Fukui, T.; Harada, Y.; Imazu, T.; Takaha, N.; Sugao, H.; Miki, T.; et al. Oral Combination of Cyclophosphamide, Uracil plus Tegafur and Estramustine for Hormone-Refractory Prostate Cancer. *Oncology* **2001**, *60*, 49–54. [CrossRef] [PubMed]
3. Noguchi, M.; Moriya, F.; Koga, N.; Matsueda, S.; Sasada, T.; Yamada, A.; Kakuma, T.; Itoh, K. A randomized phase II clinical trial of personalized peptide vaccination with metronomic low-dose cyclophosphamide in patients with metastatic castration-resistant prostate cancer. *Cancer Immunol. Immunother.* **2016**, *65*, 151–160. [CrossRef] [PubMed]
4. Orlandi, P.; Fontana, A.; Fioravanti, A.; Di Desidero, T.; Galli, L.; Derosa, L.; Canu, B.; Marconcini, R.; Biasco, E.; Solini, A.; et al. VEGF-A polymorphisms predict progression-free survival among advanced castration-resistant prostate cancer patients treated with metronomic cyclophosphamide. *Br. J. Cancer* **2013**, *109*, 957–964. [CrossRef] [PubMed]
5. Tralongo, P.; Bordonaro, S.; Di Mari, A.; Cappuccio, F.; Giuliano, S.R. Chemotherapy in frail elderly patients with hormone-refractory prostate cancer: A "real world" experience. *Prostate Int.* **2016**, *4*, 15–19. [CrossRef] [PubMed]
6. Vorob'Ev, N.A.; Nosov, A.K.; Vorob'Ev, A.V.; Moiseenko, B.M. Efficacy of standard docetaxel and metronomic cyclophosphamide chemotherapy in patients with hormone-resistant prostate cancer: Comparative analysis. *Probl. Oncol.* **2011**, *57*, 753–758.
7. Wang, J.; McGuire, T.R.; Britton, H.C.; Schwarz, J.K.; Loberiza, F.R.; Meza, J.L.; Talmadge, J.E. Lenalidomide and cyclophosphamide immunoregulation in patients with metastatic, castration-resistant prostate cancer. *Clin. Exp. Metastasis* **2015**, *32*, 111–124. [CrossRef] [PubMed]
8. Wozniak, A.J.; Blumenstein, B.A.; Crawford, E.D.; Boileau, M.; Rivkin, S.E.; Fletcher, W.S. Cyclophosphamide, methotrexate, and 5-fluorouracil in the treatment of metastatic prostate cancer. A southwest oncology group study. *Cancer* **1993**, *71*, 3975–3978. [CrossRef]
9. Yashi, M.; Nishihara, D.; Mizuno, T.; Yuki, H.; Masuda, A.; Kambara, T.; Betsunoh, H.; Abe, H.; Fukabori, Y.; Muraishi, O.; et al. Metronomic Oral Cyclophosphamide Chemotherapy Possibly Contributes to Stabilization of Disease in Patients with Metastatic Castration-Resistant Prostate Cancer: A Prospective Analysis of Consecutive Cases. *Clin. Genitourin. Cancer* **2014**, *12*, e197–e203. [CrossRef]
50. Lien, K.; Georgsdottir, S.; Sivanathan, L.; Chan, K.; Emmenegger, U. Low-dose metronomic chemotherapy: A systematic literature analysis. *Eur. J. Cancer* **2013**, *49*, 3387–3395. [CrossRef]
51. Crivellari, D.; Gray, K.P.; Dellapasqua, S.; Puglisi, F.; Ribi, K.; Price, K.N.; Láng, I.; Gianni, L.; Spazzapan, S.; Pinotti, G.; et al. Adjuvant pegylated liposomal doxorubicin for older women with endocrine nonresponsive breast cancer who are NOT suitable for a "standard chemotherapy regimen": The CASA randomized trial. *Breast* **2013**, *22*, 130–137. [CrossRef]
52. Colleoni, M.; Gray, K.P.; Gelber, S.; Láng, I.; Thürlimann, B.; Gianni, L.; Abdi, E.A.; Gomez, H.; Linderholm, B.K.; Puglisi, F.; et al. Low-Dose Oral Cyclophosphamide and Methotrexate Maintenance for Hormone Receptor–Negative Early Breast Cancer: International Breast Cancer Study Group Trial 22-00. *J. Clin. Oncol.* **2016**, *34*, 3400–3408. [CrossRef] [PubMed]
53. Nasr, K.E.; Osman, M.A.M.; Elkady, M.S.; Ellithy, M.A. Metronomic methotrexate and cyclophosphamide after carboplatin included adjuvant chemotherapy in triple negative breast cancer: A phase III study. *Ann. Transl. Med.* **2015**, *3*, 284. [CrossRef] [PubMed]
54. Rochlitz, C.; Bigler, M.; Von Moos, R.; Bernhard, J.; Matter-Walstra, K.; Wicki, A.; Zaman, K.; Anchisi, S.; Küng, M.; Na, K.-J.; et al. SAKK 24/09: Safety and tolerability of bevacizumab plus paclitaxel vs. bevacizumab plus metronomic cyclophosphamide and capecitabine as first-line therapy in patients with HER2-negative advanced stage breast cancer—A multicenter, randomized phase III trial. *BMC Cancer* **2016**, *16*, 780. [CrossRef] [PubMed]
55. Chen, Y.-P.; Liu, X.; Zhou, Q.; Yang, K.-Y.; Jin, F.; Zhu, X.-D.; Shi, M.; Hu, G.-Q.; Hu, W.-H.; Sun, Y.; et al. Metronomic capecitabine as adjuvant therapy in locoregionally advanced nasopharyngeal carcinoma: A multicentre, open-label, parallel-group, randomised, controlled, phase 3 trial. *Lancet* **2021**, *398*, 303–313. [CrossRef]
56. Patil, V.; Noronha, V.; Dhumal, S.B.; Joshi, A.; Menon, N.; Bhattacharjee, A.; Kulkarni, S.; Ankathi, S.K.; Mahajan, A.; Sable, N.; et al. Low-cost oral metronomic chemotherapy versus intravenous cisplatin in patients with recurrent, metastatic, inoperable head and neck carcinoma: An open-label, parallel-group, non-inferiority, randomised, phase 3 trial. *Lancet Glob. Health* **2020**, *8*, e1213–e1222. [CrossRef]
57. Simkens, L.H.J.; van Tinteren, H.; May, A.; Tije, A.J.T.; Creemers, G.-J.M.; Loosveld, O.J.L.; de Jongh, F.E.; Erdkamp, F.L.G.; Erjavec, Z.; van der Torren, A.M.E.; et al. Maintenance treatment with capecitabine and bevacizumab in metastatic colorectal cancer (CAIRO3): A phase 3 randomised controlled trial of the Dutch Colorectal Cancer Group. *Lancet* **2015**, *385*, 1843–1852. [CrossRef]
58. Hagman, H.; Frödin, J.-E.; Berglund, Å.; Sundberg, J.; Vestermark, L.W.; Albertsson, M.; Fernebro, E.; Johnsson, A. A randomized study of KRAS-guided maintenance therapy with bevacizumab, erlotinib or metronomic capecitabine after first-line induction treatment of metastatic colorectal cancer: The Nordic ACT2 trial. *Ann. Oncol.* **2016**, *27*, 140–147. [CrossRef]
59. Cramarossa, G.; Lee, E.K.; Sivanathan, L.; Georgsdottir, S.; Lien, K.; Santos, K.D.; Chan, K.; Emmenegger, U. A systematic literature analysis of correlative studies in low-dose metronomic chemotherapy trials. *Biomarkers Med.* **2014**, *8*, 893–911. [CrossRef]
60. Ling, H.H.; Lin, Y.-C. Metronomic Oral Cyclophosphamide in 2 Heavily Pretreated Patients with Metastatic Castration-resistant Prostate Cancer With Homologous Recombination Deficiency (HRD): A Case Report. *Clin. Genitourin. Cancer* **2018**, *17*, 157–160. [CrossRef]
61. Mittmann, N.; Liu, N.; Cheng, S.Y.; Seung, S.J.; Saxena, F.E.; Hong, N.J.L.; Earle, C.C.; Cheung, M.C.; Leighl, N.B.; Coburn, N.G.; et al. Health system costs for cancer medications and radiation treatment in Ontario for the 4 most common cancers: A retrospective cohort study. *CMAJ Open* **2020**, *8*, E191–E198. [CrossRef]

62. Trogdon, J.G.; Falchook, A.D.; Basak, R.; Carpenter, W.R.; Chen, R.C. Total Medicare Costs Associated with Diagnosis and Treatment of Prostate Cancer in Elderly Men. *JAMA Oncol.* **2019**, *5*, 60–66. [CrossRef] [PubMed]
63. Parmar, A.; Timilshina, N.; Emmenegger, U.; Smoragiewicz, M.; Sander, B.; Alibhai, S.; Chan, K.K. A cost-utility analysis of apalutamide for metastatic castration-sensitive prostate cancer. *Can. Urol. Assoc. J.* **2021**, *16*, E126–E131. [CrossRef] [PubMed]
64. Simsek, C.; Esin, E.; Yalcin, S. Metronomic Chemotherapy: A Systematic Review of the Literature and Clinical Experience. *J. Oncol.* **2019**, *2019*, 5483791. [CrossRef] [PubMed]
65. Center, M.M.; Jemal, A.; Lortet-Tieulent, J.; Ward, E.; Ferlay, J.; Brawley, O.; Bray, F. International Variation in Prostate Cancer Incidence and Mortality Rates. *Eur. Urol.* **2012**, *61*, 1079–1092. [CrossRef]
66. Bocci, G.; Tuccori, M.; Emmenegger, U.; Liguori, V.; Falcone, A.; Kerbel, R.S.; Del Tacca, M. Cyclophosphamide-methotrexate 'metronomic' chemotherapy for the palliative treatment of metastatic breast cancer. A comparative pharmacoeconomic evaluation. *Ann. Oncol.* **2005**, *16*, 1243–1252. [CrossRef]
67. Mason, N.T.; Burkett, J.M.; Nelson, R.S.; Pow-Sang, J.M.; Gatenby, R.A.; Kubal, T.; Peabody, J.W.; Letson, G.D.; McLeod, H.L.; Zhang, J. Budget Impact of Adaptive Abiraterone Therapy for Castration-Resistant Prostate Cancer. *Am. Health Drug Benefits* **2021**, *14*, 15–20.
68. West, J.B.; Dinh, M.N.; Brown, J.S.; Zhang, J.; Anderson, A.R.; Gatenby, R.A. Multidrug Cancer Therapy in Metastatic Castrate-Resistant Prostate Cancer: An Evolution-Based Strategy. *Clin. Cancer Res.* **2019**, *25*, 4413–4421. [CrossRef]
69. Kummar, S.; Wade, J.L.; Oza, A.; O'Sullivan, C.G.; Chen, A.P.; Gandara, D.R.; Ji, J.; Kinders, R.J.; Wang, L.; Allen, D.; et al. Randomized phase II trial of cyclophosphamide and the oral poly (ADP-ribose) polymerase inhibitor veliparib in patients with recurrent, advanced triple-negative breast cancer. *Investig. New Drugs* **2016**, *34*, 355–363. [CrossRef]
70. Rivkin, S.E.; Moon, J.; Iriarte, D.S.; Bailey, E.; Sloan, H.L.; Goodman, G.E.; Bondurant, A.E.; Velijovich, D.; Wahl, T.; Jiang, P.; et al. Phase Ib with expansion study of olaparib plus weekly (Metronomic) carboplatin and paclitaxel in relapsed ovarian cancer patients. *Int. J. Gynecol. Cancer* **2019**, *29*, 325–333. [CrossRef]

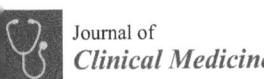

Review

Metronomic Therapy in Oral Squamous Cell Carcinoma

Nai-Wen Su [1,2] and Yu-Jen Chen [2,3,4,*]

1. Department of Internal Medicine, Division of Hematology and Medical Oncology, MacKay Memorial Hospital, No. 92, Sec. 2, Zhongshan N. Rd., Taipei City 10449, Taiwan; medicine_su@hotmail.com
2. Department of Nursing, MacKay Junior College of Medicine, Nursing and Management, Taipei City 112021, Taiwan
3. Department of Radiation Oncology, Mackay Memorial Hospital, No. 45, Minsheng Rd., Tamsui District, New Taipei City 25160, Taiwan
4. Department of Medical Research, China Medical University Hospital, Taichung 40402, Taiwan
* Correspondence: chenmdphd@gmail.com; Tel.: +886-2-2809-4661

Abstract: Metronomic therapy is characterized by drug administration in a low-dose, repeated, and regular manner without prolonged drug-free interval. The two main anticancer mechanisms of metronomic therapy are antiangiogenesis and immunomodulation, which have been demonstrated in several delicate in vitro and in vivo experiments. In contrast to the traditional maximum tolerated dose (MTD) dosing of chemotherapy, metronomic therapy possesses comparative efficacy but greatly-decreases the incidence and severity of treatment side-effects. Clinical trials of metronomic anticancer treatment have revealed promising results in a variety cancer types and specific patient populations such as the elderly and pediatric malignancies. Oral cavity squamous cell carcinoma (OCSCC) is an important health issue in many areas around the world. Long-term survival is about 50% in locally advanced disease despite having high-intensity treatment combined surgery, radiotherapy, and chemotherapy. In this article, we review and summarize the essence of metronomic therapy and focus on its applications in OCSCC treatment.

Keywords: metronomic; oral cancer; oral squamous cell carcinoma

1. Introduction

Head and neck squamous cell carcinoma (HNSCC), the sixth most common cancer worldwide, comprises heterogenous groups of tumors arising from the oral cavity, oropharynx, hypopharynx, and larynx [1]. In Taiwan, South–Central Asia, and parts of Europe, oral cavity squamous cell carcinoma (OCSCC) has a higher incidence (9–22 per 100,000) than tumors arising from other sites [2]. Smoking, alcohol consumption, and betel nut use are the major contributors in OCSCC carcinogenesis [3]. More importantly, OCSCC patients exposed to these traditional carcinogens tend to have poorer treatment outcomes than human papillomavirus (HPV)-related HNSCC patients [4]. In addition, the long-term (5 year) survival rate is unsatisfactory (approximately 50%). According to the GLOBOCAN 2018 report, 117,384 of the 354,846 newly diagnosed OCSCC patients died from the disease [5]. Therefore, OCSCC poses a considerable burden to the healthcare systems in different regions [6–11]. The majority of OCSCC patients present with a locally advanced disease, and the main therapeutic strategy is tumor wide excision plus radical neck dissection, followed by adjuvant radiotherapy with or without chemotherapy [12,13]. This high-intensity treatment program results in significant acute or chronic adverse events [14]. Locoregional relapse and secondary primary HNSCC [15,16] are the most common recurrent patterns and curable if amenable to local treatment. However, the prognosis is grave once the disease is metastatic or attains platinum-refractory status. Although the therapeutic armamentarium is expanding, for example, anti-epidermal growth factor receptor (EGFR) monoclonal antibody and immune checkpoint inhibitors have been developed, the median overall survival is approximately 10–14 months [17–21].

The most important chemotherapeutic agent in OCSCC treatment is platinum. In platinum-based concurrent chemoradiotherapy or palliative chemotherapy, administration of the maximum tolerated dose (MTD) of cisplatin(100 mg/m^2 every 3 weeks) is generally considered a gold standard regimen [12,13,17]. The development of platinum-resistant OCSCC is an important factor that leads to treatment failure. Existence of cancer stem cells [22,23], increased angiogenesis [24,25], and unfavorable immune profile in the microenvironment [26,27] are the proposed mechanisms that contribute to platinum-resistant OCSCC and predict poor prognosis. Moreover, the MTD of cisplatin (100 mg/m^2) is deemed as a highly toxic regimen because it has significant side-effects such as nephrotoxicity, ototoxicity, and neurotoxicity [28,29]. Therefore, novel therapeutic strategies are necessary to improve OCSCC treatment outcomes a step further [30]. Metronomic chemotherapy, one of the potentially promising treatments, is being studied and utilized in clinical practice for a variety of cancer types, including OCSCC [31–37]. The unique dosing schedule stems from preclinical studies, which have revealed the advantages of overcoming drug resistance and antiangiogenesis effects [38,39]. Clinically, metronomic chemotherapy induces drug sensitivity and, most importantly, it is accompanied by minimal adverse effects [40]. In this article, we briefly review the mechanism of action and clinical development of metronomic therapies in OCSCC.

2. History of Metronomic Therapy

Since the appearance of cytotoxic chemotherapeutic agents in the early 1960s, they have been playing a critical role in cancer treatment. The use of MTD to obtain the highest possible cancer cell killing is the mainstream method to calculate the chemotherapy dose [41]. The MTD chemotherapy originated from the great success of a pediatric leukemia treatment model [42]. However, MTD chemotherapy imposes great damage to the rapidly proliferating normal tissues such as hematopoietic or gastrointestinal epithelial cells. To limit the toxic effects and permit patient recovery, MTD chemotherapy should be administered with 3–4 weeks of drug-free interval only. Regrowth of the residual cancer cells is inevitable [43]. Moreover, complete eradication of cancer cells is rarely achieved with MTD chemotherapy owing to the development of drug resistance [44]. Decades of cancer research has revealed that cancer cells possess multiple genetic alterations and could have genomic evolution that contributes to resistance [45,46]. The cancer treatment is far more complex because components of the tumor microenvironment, such as immune cells, endothelial cells, and fibroblasts, communicate and relay pro-survival signals to malignant cells [47–49]. This adds more obstacles to our goal of cure or long-term disease control with MTD chemotherapy.

To evaluate the biological effects of administered chemotherapy, other than MTD, one unique dosing schedule—metronomic chemotherapy—was studied in preclinical cell and animal models. Metronomic dosing was defined as administration of low doses (1/3–1/10 of MTD) cytotoxic agents at more frequent intervals (no prolonged drug-free breaks) [50]. Initially, the metronomic chemotherapy was reported to inhibit cancer-associated angiogenesis and consequently promote tumor regression [51,52]. Simultaneously, Broder et al. demonstrated that this low-dose and frequent administration aids in overcoming drug resistance [53]. This regimen is more attractive because it has a lower toxicity profile than MTD [54]. In the following decade, more studies focused on the biological effects of metronomic chemotherapy.

3. Metronomic Therapy: Mechanisms of Action

3.1. Antiangiogenic Effects

Neoangiogenesis takes a central role during the growing phase of the primary tumor and supports the establishment of distant metastatic deposits. It has long been proposed as a potential target in cancer treatment [55,56]. Chemotherapeutic agents were found to have antiangiogenesis effects in a preclinical study, although the dosing schedule matters in this phenomenon [57]. Tumor-associated vascular endothelial cells are genetically more stable than cancer cells. This is one of the possible explanations why metronomic chemotherapy more specifically causes endothelial cell apoptosis and less resistance development. Other proposed molecular mechanisms are the suppression of endothelial progenitor cell mobilization from the bone marrow [58] and an increase in the expression of thrombospondin-1 (TSP-1), which is an endogenous antiangiogenic factor [59]. Recently, metronomic chemotherapy was found to normalize the defective tumor vasculature [60]. Cyclophosphamide is the prototype of a chemotherapeutic agent possessing antiangiogenic property when administered in the metronomic schedule [61]. The same biological activity was proven for other agents such as taxanes, camptothecin, and vinca alkaloids in a variety of cancer types [62,63]. On the contrary, some studies have suggested that chemotherapeutic agents might induce acute mobilization of the bone marrow-derived circulating endothelial progenitor cells (EPCs), homing viable tumors and promoting their growth. Studies have provided evidence that coadministration of antiangiogenic agents might work in a synergistic fashion with chemotherapy for the suppression of tumor and emergence of resistance [64–67].

3.2. Immunomodulatory Effects

During the process of carcinogenesis and tumor progression, cancer cells may evade the immunosurveillance through the release of cytokines (such as transforming growth factor, vascular endothelial growth factor (VEGF), and interleukin-6) and recruitment of precancerous immune cells (such as regulatory T cell (Treg), myeloid derived suppressor cells (MDSC), and tumor associated macrophage-2) [68]. Studies have shown that the MTD of some traditional chemotherapeutic agents have immunomodulatory effects such as the induction of immunogenic cell death [69]. Through low-dose metronomic chemotherapy, studies found that different agents can deplete Treg and suppress MDSC [70–73]. In addition, it can promote dendritic cell maturation, an important step to educate the naïve cytotoxic T cells [74]. Some metronomic agents cause cell death and favorably promote the release of "eat me" signals (such as damage-associated molecular patterns, calreticulin, and high-mobility group box 1) [75]. All of these phenomena can possibly activate our immune cells to attack the tumor. However, our immune system is dynamic and, therefore, some study results might be controversial and require further clinical validation [76,77].

3.3. Inhibition of Cancer Stem Cells

Cancer cells, like their normal counterparts, contain a minority portion of cells that possess the ability of self-renewal and differentiation. These specific cancer cells are called cancer stem cells (CSCs), which are detected mainly with the expression of specific cell surface markers ($CD24^+$, $CD44^+$, or $CD133^+$; alone or combined expression) [78]. CSCs have been strongly linked to chemoresistance or radio resistance and, consequently, anticancer treatment failure [79,80]. A few studies have revealed that metronomic chemotherapy can decrease the CSC population [81–83]. Vives et al. demonstrated that MTD chemotherapy followed by metronomic maintenance therapy with gemcitabine and cyclophosphamide successfully eliminated the CSCs in pancreatic cancer and ovarian cancer orthotopic models, respectively [84]. Incorporation of metronomic chemotherapy into or combined with current cancer treatment may aid in a further reduction in CSC-related resistance.

4. Metronomic Therapy in OCSCC
4.1. Preclinical Evidence

Although metronomic therapy has been applied in clinical trials or daily oncological practice, only one chemotherapeutic agent, S-1, has been tested completely in both in vitro and in vivo models. S-1 is composed of three compounds. One compound is a 5-fluorouracil (5-FU) prodrug, tegafur. The other two are gimeracil (inhibits the 5-FU degradation) and oteracil (lowers the gastrointestinal toxicity of 5-FU) [85]. In an in vitro study, Ferdous et al. first demonstrated that more frequent 5-FU dosing (16h treatment, 8h rest vs. 96h treatment, 48h rest or 48h treatment, 24h rest) did not result in more cytotoxic cell death according to 3-(4, 5-dimethyl-2-thiazolyl)-2, 5-diphenyl-2H tetrazolium bromide assay. However, functional evaluations revealed that oral cancer treatment with more frequent 5-FU dosing (16h treatment, 8h rest) showed the highest expression of TSP-1 (antiangiogenesis molecule) and lowest expression of VEGF and CD44 (CSC marker). In the in vivo xenograft model, the usual S-1 schedules were 4weeks on followed by 2 weeks off and 2weeks on followed by 1weekoff, which were the same as the standard regimens in human. The metronomic dosing was 1dayon followed by 1dayoff. The results revealed that all three regimens resulted in similar tumor volume reductions. The nude mice in the two standard regimen groups had a lower weight than those in the metronomic treatment group. The xenograft tumors in the metronomic treatment group showed increased TSP-1 and decreased VEGF expression, which was consistent with the findings of the in vitro study. In addition, a reduction in CD44 expression was observed. The number of endothelial cells (based on CD31 expression) and the micro vessel density (MVD) both decreased in the metronomic treatment group tumors. The results of S-1 treatment in an oral tongue cancer model revealed that metronomic dosing resulted in comparable tumor inhibition. Considering the proof-of-concept viewpoint, metronomic dosing of S-1 demonstrated antiangiogenesis and cancer stem cell elimination effects. According to our knowledge, a variety of compounds extracted from traditional Chinese medicine possess anticancer effects [86]. Some of the studies have tested compounds in xenograft models with daily administration, which mimicked the metronomic dosing schedule. Most studies had a long treatment duration ranging from 3–8 weeks and no significant side-effects [87–93]. In our previous studies, we treated the oral cancer-bearing mice with cordycepin, a major biological compound from *Cordyceps sinensis*, alone or in combination with radiotherapy for 8 weeks. No weight loss was observed, and the hematological, renal, and hepatic functions were preserved [92,93].

4.2. Clinical Evidence

In the past two decades, the concept of metronomic therapy was translated into real practice, and clinical trials have finally proven its effectiveness and better tolerability in a variety of cancers [94–97] and specific populations [98,99]. Oral chemotherapeutic agents are the central pillars in most studies with different combinations, including targeted therapy [100], vascular disrupting agent [101], and even noncytotoxic agent [102]. We found two main clinical settings for the use of metronomic therapy in OCSCC; one was adjuvant/maintenance therapy after curative intent surgery or chemoradiotherapy, and the other was a palliative therapy in recurrent/metastatic status.

Three studies used metronomic fluorouracil drugs in adjuvant/maintenance therapy. Lin et al. conducted a prospective cohort study and reported that 80 OCSCC patients with stage III–IVa (T3–T4a and/or N0–N1) diseases received curative intent surgery. Forty patients received metronoic UFUR (each capsule contains tegafur 100 mg and uracil 224 mg) with a fixed dose of tegafur 150 mg/m^2/day for 1 year, and another 40 patients were observational controls. The 4year disease-free survival (DFS) of the metronomic group versus the control group was 85.6% and 75.9% (p = 0.02). Simultaneously, they performed laboratory correlation by detecting the change in CEP (circulating endothelial precursor) cells, a marker of angiogenesis activity. The results revealed that patients treated with metronomic UFUR had a significant reduction in the detectable viable CEP cells, which might implicate an antiangiogenesis mechanism behind the survival benefits. The toxicities were mild and manageable, with skin rash (5%) being the most common side-effect, followed by hematological side-effects (2.5%) and nausea/vomiting (2.5%) [103]. Hsieh et al. [104] conducted a retrospective study of 356 stage III and IV OCSCC patients. All the patients received curative surgery followed by chemoradiotherapy, which suggested a more advanced disease condition. A total of 114 patients received tegafur/uracil (tegafur: 100–400 mg/day) as adjuvant therapy for 1–2 years if tolerable. The survival endpoints revealed that 5-year overall survival (OS) and DFS were 65% versus 48% (HR = 0.54, p = 0.0008) and 57% versus 41% (HR = 0.62, p = 0.0034) in the metronomic and control groups, respectively. In addition, longer UFUR treatment duration (≥12 months) and higher dose (300–400 mg/day) contributed to better survival benefits. The metronomic UFUR treatment seemed to decrease the occurrence of distant metastasis (OR = 4.3, p = 0.0015) compared with no UFUR treatment. Moreover, the toxicities were mild and well-tolerated, with skin rash (3.5%) being the most common side-effect. Another study used low-dose S-1 as adjuvant chemotherapy in locally advanced HNSCC patients [105]. The study retrospectively reviewed 52 stage III/IVa/IVb HNSCC patients who completed curative treatment and confirmed no residual tumor. Sixteen out of 52 patients had oral cancer. The S-1 dose was half of the usual standard dose (40 mg/day for body surface area (BSA) < 1.25 m^2; 50 mg/day for 1.25 m^2 ≤ BSA < 1.5 m^2; 60 mg/day for BSA ≥ 1.5 m^2) and was administered for 2 years. Forty-three (82.7%) patients received S-1 continuously for 2 years without dose reduction. Hematological toxicity was found in 98.1% of the patients; however, only two (3.8%) patients were grade 3. Nonhematological toxicity was found in 15 (28.8%) patients, and all cases were grade 1. The 3year DFS and OS rates were 82.6% and 94%, respectively.

Three studies examined the effectiveness and toxicity profiles using metronomic therapy in recurrent/metastatic OCSCC patients. Patil et al. conducted a prospective randomized phase II clinical trial, comparing metronomic chemotherapy with single agent (three-weekly cisplatin (75 mg/m^2)) in recurrent/metastatic HNSCC patients. The metronomic chemotherapy consisted of weekly oral methotrexate (MTX; 15 mg/m^2) and daily celecoxib (200 mg twice daily) [106]. MTX is one of the commonly used chemotherapeutic agents in HNSCC [107]. Celecoxib, a nonsteroidal anti-inflammatory agent, was found to have an antiangiogenesis effect in preclinical experiments [108,109]. A total of 110 patients were enrolled in the study, with 57 randomized to the metronomic arm and 53 to the cisplatin arm. The primary oral cancer patients accounted for 75–77% of the cohort in both the groups. The metronomic arm had a significantly longer progression-free survival (PFS; median PFS: 101 vs. 66 days, p = 0.014) and OS (median OS: 249 vs. 152 days, p = 0.02) compared with the cisplatin arm. Moreover, the response rate (RR) and clinical beneficial rate were better in the metronomic arm compared with the cisplatin arm: 12.3% versus 1.9% and 54.4% versus 32.1%, respectively. Fewer grade 3–4 adverse events were noted in the metronomic arm compared with the cisplatin arm (18.9% vs. 31.4%, p = 0.14), without statistical significance [110]. Due to the promising results of the phase II study, the same group did an open-label, parallel-group, noninferiority, randomized phase 3 trial. The treatments of the experimental arm and control arm were still MTX plus celecoxib versus three-weekly cisplatin (75 mg/m^2). Overall, 418 patients (211 in the oral metronomic chemotherapy group and 207 in the intravenous cisplatin group) were included in the per-protocol analysis. At a median follow-up of 15.73 months, the primary endpoint, median overall survival, was 7.5 months in the oral metronomic chemotherapy group compared with 6.1 months in the intravenous cisplatin group (HR ratio for death 0.775; 95% confidence interval 0.616–0.974, p =0.029). Grade 3 or higher adverse events were observed in 37(19%) of 196 patients in the oral metronomic chemotherapy group versus 61(30%) of 202 patients in the cisplatin group [111]. This was the first phase III study to demonstrate that metronomic chemotherapy resulted in better survival and a preferable toxicity profile in recurrent/metastatic head and neck cancer. Actually, the oral cavity cancers consisted of about 80% of the overall population. The study design and its results undoubtedly added a more solid evidence to the application of metronomic treatment in OCSCC. In another study, a single arm phase I/II trial, Patil et al. determined the dose and evaluated the efficacy of triple metronomic chemotherapy in platinum-refractory oral cancer patients [110]. The regimen included fixed dose erlotinib (an anti-EGFR tyrosine kinase inhibitor; 150 mg/day) and celecoxib (200 mg twice daily). In phase I, they first determined the optimal biological dose (OBD) of MTX by de-escalating from weekly 15 mg/m^2 and found 9 mg/m^2 to be the OBD. Overall, 91 patients were enrolled in the study. The median PFS and OS were 4.6 and 7.17 months, respectively. The overall best RR was 42.9%, which was superior to the second line treatment (RR = 2.2–13.6%) in platinum-refractory HN-

SCC [18,19,107]. The most common grade 3–4 toxicity was hyponatremia (14.8%), followed by elevation of aspartate transaminase (AST) and alanine transaminase (ALT) levels (4.5% and 5.7%, respectively).

5. Advantages and Limitations of Metronomic Therapy in OCSCC

Our data review revealed that metronomic therapy does achieve comparable disease control rate in OCSCC and has a favorable toxicity profile compared with standard systemic chemotherapy, such as platinum. However, more solid and high-level evidence (e.g., randomized phase III trials) is required to consolidate the role of metronomic therapy. In addition, we found that the optimal metronomic dosage for OCSCC is not well defined. Pharmacodynamic and pharmacokinetic analysis of the metronomic dosing might provide valuable information for determining the optimal dose [112–114]. Considering the viewpoint of healthcare economics, metronomic therapy truly curtails the cost [115]. The reasons for cost reduction are as follows: (1) metronomic agents are not newly developed, (2) enteral administration is performed, and (3) less high-grade toxicities occur that might avoid additional supportive agents or admission. These advantages of metronomic therapy might relieve the soaring healthcare cost and facilitate patients in areas with insufficient medical resources [116]. Although the enteral route for metronomic agents brings convenience and at-home treatment, it should be noted that some OCSCC patients have difficulty in swallowing. This issue matters and affects patient compliance if metronomic chemotherapy is used as adjuvant/maintenance therapy in OCSCC, which might last for 1–2 years [103,104].

6. Future Perspectives of Metronomic Therapy in OCSCC

Antiangiogenesis and immunomodulation are the two main mechanisms of action of metronomic therapy [117]. As far as we understand, these two mechanisms might have synergistic effects with contemporary immunotherapy [118,119]. Some preliminary experiments using combined metronomic chemotherapy and vaccine or oncolytic virus in advanced cancers have been reported [120,121]. Although not in OCSCC, some ongoing clinical trials are studying the use of current immune checkpoint inhibitor and metronomic chemotherapy combination in lung cancer (NCT03801304), breast cancer (NCT03007992), pediatric tumors (NCT03585465), and sarcomas (NCT02406781). The results are eagerly awaited, and this strategy can hopefully be tested in OCSCC patients.

7. Conclusions

Oral squamous cell carcinoma is a heterogenous disease with a high unmet medical requirement. The cure rate and accompanied complications have not improved despite high-intensity treatment. Metronomic therapy provides an alternative treatment choice in contrast to traditional chemotherapy. Its mechanism of action is as follows: angiogenesis inhibition, immunomodulation, and overcoming drug resistance. A comparative disease control rate and superior toxicity profile are its advantages. It is widely applicable in clinical patient care. However, randomized phase III trials comparing it with the standard care are required to demonstrate its effectiveness. We can anticipate that more studies focusing on metronomic therapy with novel agent combination, such as immunotherapy, will be conducted in the future and translated into clinical treatment benefits.

Author Contributions: Conceptualization, N.-W.S. and Y.-J.C.; writing—original draft preparation, N.-W.S.; writing—review and editing, Y.-J.C. All authors have read and agreed to the published version of the manuscript.

Funding: This work was supported by the Ministry of Science and Technology (grant number: MOST 109-2314-B-195-003-MY3) and MacKay Memorial Hospital (grant numbers: MMH-E-109-13, MMH-E-110-13, TTMMH-109-05, and TTMMH-110-01), Taiwan.

Conflicts of Interest: The authors declare no conflict of interest.

References

1. Chow, L.Q.M. Head and neck cancer. *N. Engl. J. Med.* **2020**, *382*, 60–72. [CrossRef] [PubMed]
2. Ferlay, J.; Soerjomataram, I.; Dikshit, R.; Eser, S.; Mathers, C.; Rebelo, M.; Parkin, D.M.; Forman, D.; Bray, F. Cancer incidence and mortality worldwide: Sources, methods and major patterns in GLOBOCAN 2012. *Int. J. Cancer* **2015**, *5*, e359–e386. [CrossRef] [PubMed]
3. Hashim, D.; Genden, E.; Posner, M.; Hashibe, M.; Boffetta, P. Head and neck cancer prevention: From primary prevention to impact of clinicians on reducing burden. *Ann. Oncol.* **2019**, *30*, 744–756. [CrossRef] [PubMed]
4. Taberna, M.; Mena, M.; Pavon, M.A.; Alemany, L.; Gillison, M.L.; Mesia, R. Human papillomavirus-related oropharyngeal cancer. *Ann. Oncol.* **2017**, *28*, 2386–2398. [CrossRef] [PubMed]
5. Bray, F.; Ferlay, J.; Soerjomataram, I.; Siegel, R.L.; Torre, L.A.; Jemel, A. Global cancer statistics 2018: GLOBOCAN estimates of incidence and mortality worldwide for 36 cancers in 185 countries. *CA: Cancer J. Clin.* **2018**, *68*, 394–424. [CrossRef] [PubMed]
6. Schwam, Z.G.; Judson, B.L. Improved prognosis for patients with oral cavity squamous cell carcinoma: Analysis of the National Cancer Database 1998–2006. *Oral Oncol.* **2016**, *52*, 45–51. [CrossRef]
7. Capote-Moreno, A.; Brabyn, P.; Munoz-Guerra, M.F.; Sastre-Perez, J.; Escorial-Hernandez, V.; Rodriquez-Campo, F.J.; Garcia, T.; Naval-Gias, L. Oral squamous cell carcinoma: Epidemiology study and risk factor assessment based on a 39-year series. *Int. J. Oral. Maxillofac. Surg.* **2020**, *29*, S0901–5027(20)30100–4. [CrossRef] [PubMed]
8. Zanoni, D.K.; Montero, P.H.; Migliacci, J.C.; Shah, J.P.; Wong, R.J.; Ganly, I.; Patel, S.G. Survival outcomes after treatment of cancer of the oral cavity (1985–2015). *Oral Oncol.* **2019**, *9*, 115–121. [CrossRef]
9. Van Dijk, B.A.C.; Brands, M.T.; Geurts, S.M.E.; Merkx, M.A.W.; Roodenburg, J.L.N. Trends in oral cavity cancer incidence, mortality, survival and treatment in the Netherlands. *Int. J. Cancer* **2016**, *139*, 574–583. [CrossRef] [PubMed]
10. Mummudi, N.; Agarwal, J.P.; Chatterjee, S.; Mallick, I.; Ghosh-Laskar, S. Oral cavity cancer in the Indian subcontinent–challenges and opportunities. *Clin. Oncol.* **2019**, *30*, 520–528. [CrossRef]
11. Cheng, Y.J.; Tsai, M.H.; Chiang, C.J.; Tsai, S.T.; Liu, T.W.; Lou, P.J.; Liao, C.T.; Lin, J.C.; Chang, J.T.C.; Tsai, M.H.; et al. Adjuvant radiotherapy after curative surgery for oral cavity squamous cell carcinoma and treatment effect of timing and duration on outcome -a Taiwan Cancer Registry national database analysis. *Cancer Med.* **2018**, *7*, 3073–3083. [CrossRef]
12. Bernier, J.; Domenge, C.; Ozsahin, M.; Matuszewska, K.; Lefebvre, J.L.; Griener, R.H.; Giralt, J.; Maingon, P.; Rolland, F.; Bolla, M.; et al. Postoperative irradiation with or without concomitant chemotherapy for locally advanced head and neck cancer. *N. Engl. J. Med.* **2004**, *350*, 1945–1952. [CrossRef] [PubMed]
13. Cooper, J.S.; Pajak, T.F.; Forastiere, A.A.; Jacobs, J.; Campbell, B.H.; Saxman, S.B.; Kish, J.A.; Kim, H.E.; Cmelak, A.J.; Rotman, M.; et al. Postoperative concurrent radiotherapy and chemotherapy for high-risk squamous-cell carcinoma of the head and neck. *N. Engl. J. Med.* **2004**, *350*, 1937–1944. [CrossRef] [PubMed]
14. Machtay, M.; Moughan, J.; Trotti, A.; Garden, A.S.; Weber, R.S.; Cooper, J.S.; Forastiere, A.; Ang, K.K. Factors associated with severe late toxicity after concurrent chemoradiation for locally advanced head and neck cancer: An RTOG analysis. *J. Clin. Oncol.* **2008**, *26*, 2582–3589. [CrossRef] [PubMed]
15. Liao, C.T.; Wallace, C.G.; Lee, L.Y.; Hsueh, C.; Lin, C.Y.; Fan, K.H.; Wang, H.M.; Ng, S.H.; Lin, C.H.; Tsao, C.K.; et al. Clinical evidence of field cancerization in patients with oral cavity cancer in betel quid chewing area. *Oral Oncol.* **2014**, *50*, 721–731. [CrossRef]
16. Min, S.K.; Choi, S.W.; Lim, J.; Park, J.Y.; Jung, K.W.; Won, Y.J. Second primary cancers in patients with oral cavity cancer included in the Korea Central Cancer Registry. *Oral Oncol.* **2019**, *95*, 16–28. [CrossRef] [PubMed]
17. Vermorken, J.B.; Mesia, R.; Rivera, F.; Remenar, E.; Kawecki, A.; Rotty, S.; Erfan, J.; Zabolotnyy, D.; Kienzer, H.R.; Cupissol, D.; et al. Platinum-based chemotherapy plus cetuximab in head and neck cancer. *N. Engl. J. Med.* **2008**, *359*, 1116–1127. [CrossRef]
18. Ferris, R.L.; Blumenschein, G.; Fayette, J.; Guigay, J.; Licitra, C.L.; Harrington, K.; Kasper, S.; Vokes, E.E.; Even, C.; Worden, F.; et al. Nivolumab for recurrent squamous-cell carcinoma of the head and neck. *N. Engl. J. Med.* **2016**, *375*, 1856–1867. [CrossRef]
19. Cohen, E.E.W.; Soulieres, D.; Le Tourneau, C.; Dinis, J.; Licitra, L.; Ahn, M.J.; Soria, A.; Machiels, J.P.; Mach, N.; Mehra, R.; et al. Pembrolizumab versus methotrexate, docetaxel, or cetuximab for recurrent or metastatic head-and-neck squamous cell carcinoma (KEYNOTE-040): A randomized, open-label, phase 3 study. *Lancet* **2019**, *393*, 156–167. [CrossRef]
20. Burtness, B.; Harrington, K.J.; Greil, R.; Soulieres, D.; Tahara, M.; deCastro, G.; Psyrri, A.; Baste, N.; Neupane, P.; Bratland, A.; et al. Pembrolizumab alone or with chemotherapy versus cetuximab with chemotherapy for recurrent or metastatic squamous cell carcinoma of the head and neck (KEYNOTE-048): A randomized, open-label, phase 3 study. *Lancet* **2019**, *394*, 1915–1928. [CrossRef]
21. Szturz, P.; Vermorken, J.B. Management of recurrent and metastatic oral cavity cancer: Raising the bar a step higher. *Oral Oncol.* **2020**, *101*, 104492. [CrossRef] [PubMed]
22. Hu, J.; Mirshahidi, S.; Simental, A.; Lee, S.C.; De Andrade Filho, P.A.; Peterson, N.R.; Duerksen-Hughes, P.; Yuan, X. Cancer stem cell self-renewal as a therapeutic target in human oral cancer. *Oncogene* **2019**, *38*, 5440–5456. [CrossRef] [PubMed]
23. Naik, P.P.; Das, D.N.; Panda, P.K.; Mukhopadhyay, S.; Sinha, N.; Praharaj, P.P.; Agarwal, R.; Bhutia, S.K. Implications of cancer stem cells in developing therapeutic resistance in oral cancer. *Oral Oncol.* **2016**, *62*, 122–135. [CrossRef]
24. Sakata, J.; Hirosue, A.; Yoshida, R.; Kawahara, K.; Matsuoka, Y.; Yamamoto, T.; Nakamoto, M.; Hirayama, M.; Takahashi, N.; Nakamura, T.; et al. HMGA2 contributes to distant metastasis and poor prognosis by promoting angiogenesis in oral squamous cell carcinoma. *Int. J. Mol. Sci.* **2019**, *20*, 2473. [CrossRef]

25. Li, C.; Fan, J.; Song, X.; Zhang, B.; Chen, Y.; Li, C.; Mi, K.; Ma, H.; Song, Y.; Tao, X.; et al. Expression of angiopoietin-2 and vascular endothelial growth factor receptor-3 correlates with lymphangiogenesis and angiogenesis and affects survival of oral squamous cell carcinoma. *PLoS ONE* **2013**, *8*, e75388. [CrossRef]
26. Boxberg, M.; Leising, L.; Steiger, K.; Jesinghaus, M.; Alkhamas, A.; Mielke, M.; Pfarr, N.; Gotz, C.; Wolff, K.D.; Weichert, W.; et al Tumor microenvironment in oral squamous cell carcinoma. *J. Immunol.* **2019**, *202*, 278–291. [CrossRef] [PubMed]
27. Gasparoto, T.H.; de Souza Malaspina, T.S.; Benevides, L.; de Melo, E.J.F., Jr.; Costa, M.R.S.N.; Damante, J.H.; Ikoma, M.R.V.; Garlet, G.P.; Cavassani, K.A.; da Silva, J.S.; et al. Patients with oral squamous cell carcinoma are characterized by increased frequency of suppressive regulatory T cell in the blood and tumor microenvironment. *Cancer Immunol. Immunother.* **2010**, *59*, 819–828. [CrossRef]
28. Walsh, L.; Gillham, C.; Dunne, M.; Fraser, I.; Hollywood, D.; Armstrong, J.; Thirion, P. Toxicity of cetuximab versus cisplatin concurrent with radiotherapy in locally advanced head and neck squamous cell cancer (LAHNSCC). *Radiother. Oncol.* **2011**, *98*, 38–41. [CrossRef]
29. Mackiewicz, J.; Rybarczyk-Kasiuchnicz, A.; Lasinska, I.; Mazur-Roszak, M.; Swiniuch, D.; Michalak, M.; Kazmierska, J.; Studniarek, A.; Krokowicz, L.; Bajon, T. The comparison of acute toxicity in 2 treatment courses: Three-weekly and weekly cisplatin treatment administered with radiotherapy in patients with head and neck squamous cell carcinoma. *Medicine* **2017**, *96*, e9151. [CrossRef]
30. Sinha, N.; Mukhopadhyay, S.; Das, D.N.; Panda, P.K.; Bhutia, S.K. Relevance of cancer initiating/stem cells in carcinogenesis and therapy resistance in oral cancer. *Oral Oncol.* **2013**, *49*, 854–862. [CrossRef] [PubMed]
31. Filippi, R.; Lombardi, P.; Depetris, I.; Fenocchio, E.; Quara, V.; Chila, G.; Aglietta, M.; Leone, F. Rationale for the use of metronomic chemotherapy in gastrointestinal cancer. *Expert Opin. Pharmacother.* **2018**, *19*, 1451–1463. [CrossRef] [PubMed]
32. Cazzaniga, M.E.; Cortesi, L.; Ferzi, A.; Scaltriti, L.; Cicchiello, M.; Torre, S.D.; Villa, F.; Giordano, M.; Verusio, C.; Gambaro, A.R.; et al. Metronomic chemotherapy in triple-negative breast cancer: The future is now? *Int. J. Breast Cancer* **2017**, *2017*, 1683060. [CrossRef] [PubMed]
33. Lambrescu, I.; Fica, S.; Martins, D.; Spada, F.; Cella, C.; Bertani, E.; Rubino, M.; Gibelli, B.; Bonomo, G.; Funicelli, L.; et al. Metronomic and metronomic-like therapies in neuroendocrine tumors—Rationale and clinical perspectives. *Cancer Treat Rev.* **2017**, *55*, 46–56. [CrossRef] [PubMed]
34. Woo, I.S.; Jung, Y.H. Metronomic chemotherapy in metastatic colorectal cancer. *Cancer Lett.* **2017**, *400*, 319–324. [CrossRef]
35. Romiti, A.; Falcone, R.; Roberto, M.; Marchetti, P. Tackling pancreatic cancer with metronomic chemotherapy. *Cancer Lett.* **2017**, *394*, 88–95. [CrossRef]
36. Romiti, A.; Falcone, R.; Roberto, M.; Marchetti, P. Current achievements and future perspectives of metronomic chemotherapy. *Investig. New Drugs* **2017**, *35*, 359–374. [CrossRef]
37. Gourd, E. Metronomic chemotherapy option for advanced oral cancer. *Lancet Oncol.* **2019**, *20*, e614. [CrossRef]
38. Kerbel, R.S. A decade of experience in developing preclinical models of advanced- or early-stage spontaneous metastasis to study antiangiogenic drugs, metronomic chemotherapy, and the tumor microenvironment. *Cancer J.* **2015**, *21*, 274–283. [CrossRef]
39. Natale, G.; Bocci, G. Does metronomic chemotherapy induce tumor angiogenic dormancy? A review of available preclinical and clinical data. *Cancer Lett.* **2018**, *432*, 28–37. [CrossRef]
40. Wichmann, V.; Eigeliene, N.; Saarenheimo, J.; Jekunen, A. Recent clinical evidence on metronomic dosing in controlled clinical trials: A systemic literature review. *Acta. Oncol.* **2020**, *59*, 775–785. [CrossRef] [PubMed]
41. Frei, E.; Canellos, G.P. Dose: A critical factor in cancer chemotherapy. *Am. J. Med.* **1980**, *69*, 585–594. [CrossRef]
42. Skipper, H.E.; Schabel, F.M.; Mellett, L.B.; Montgomery, J.A.; Wilkoff, L.J.; Lloyd, H.H.; Brockman, R.W. Implications of biochemical, cytokinetic, pharmacologic, and toxicologic relationships in the design of optimal therapeutic scheduled. *Cancer Chemother. Rep.* **1970**, *54*, 431–450.
43. Kareva, I.; Waxman, D.J.; Klement, G.L. Metronomic chemotherapy: An attractive alternative to maximum tolerated dose therapy that can activate anti-tumor immunity and minimize therapeutic resistance. *Cancer Lett.* **2015**, *358*, 100–106. [CrossRef] [PubMed]
44. Bukowski, K.; Kciuk, M.; Kontek, R. Mechanisms of multidrug resistance in cancer chemotherapy. *Int. J. Mol. Sci.* **2020**, *21*, 3233. [CrossRef]
45. Hanahan, D.; Weinberg, R.A. Hallmarks of cancer: The next generation. *Cell* **2011**, *144*, 646–674. [CrossRef] [PubMed]
46. Dagogo-Jack, I.; Shaw, A.T. Tumor heterogeneity and resistance to cancer therapies. *Nat. Rev. Clin. Oncol.* **2018**, *15*, 81–94. [CrossRef] [PubMed]
47. Chen, S.H.; Chang, J.Y. New insights into mechanisms of cisplatin resistance: From tumor cells to microenvironment. *Int. J. Mol. Sci.* **2019**, *20*, 4136. [CrossRef] [PubMed]
48. Qu, Y.; Dou, B.; Tan, H.; Feng, Y.; Wang, N.; Wang, D. Tumor microenvironment-driven non-cell-autonomous resistance to antineoplastic treatment. *Mol. Cancer* **2019**, *18*, 69. [CrossRef] [PubMed]
49. Tan, Q.; Saggar, J.K.; Yu, M.; Wang, M.; Tannock, I.F. Mechanisms of drug resistance related to the microenvironment of solid tumors and possible strategies to inhibit them. *Cancer J.* **2015**, *21*, 254–262. [CrossRef]
50. Gasparini, G. Metronomic scheduling: The future of chemotherapy? *Lancet Oncol.* **2001**, *2*, 733–740. [CrossRef]
51. Bocci, G.; Nicolaou, K.C.; Kervel, R.S. Protracted low-dose effects on human endothelial cell proliferation and survival in vitro reveal a selective antiangiogenic window for various chemotherapeutic drugs. *Cancer Res.* **2002**, *62*, 6938–6943.
52. Gately, S.; Kerbel, R.S. Antiangiogenic scheduling of lower dose cancer chemotherapy. *Cancer J.* **2001**, *7*, 427–436.

3. Browder, T.; Butterfield, C.E.; Kraling, B.M.; Shi, B.; Marshall, B.; O'Reilly, M.S.; Folkman, J. Antiangiogenic scheduling of chemotherapy improves efficacy against experimental drug-resistant cancer. *Cancer Res.* **2000**, *60*, 1878–1886. [PubMed]
4. Emmenegger, U.; Man, S.; Shaked, Y.; Francia, G.; Wong, J.W.; Hicklin, D.J.; Kerbel, R.S. A comparative analysis of low-dose metronomic cyclophosphamide reveals absent or low-grade toxicity on tissues highly sensitive to the toxic effects of maximum tolerated dose regimens. *Cancer Res.* **2004**, *64*, 3994–4000. [CrossRef] [PubMed]
5. Folkman, J. Tumor angiogenesis: Therapeutic implications. *N. Engl. J. Med.* **1971**, *285*, 1182–1186. [CrossRef] [PubMed]
6. Ramjiawana, R.R.; Griffioen, A.W.; Duda, D.G. Anti-angiogenesis for cancer revisited: Is there a role for combinations with immunotherapy? *Angiogenesis* **2017**, *20*, 185–204. [CrossRef] [PubMed]
7. Hanahan, D.; Bergers, G.; Bergsland, E. Less is more, regularly: Metronomic dosing of cytotoxic drugs can target tumor angiogenesis in mice. *J. Clin. Investig.* **2000**, *105*, 1045–1047. [CrossRef] [PubMed]
8. Bertolini, F.; Paul, S.; Mancuso, P.; Monestiroli, S.; Gobbi, A.; Shaked, Y.; Kerbel, R.S. Maximum tolerable dose and low-dose metronomic chemotherapy have opposite effects on the mobilization and viability of circulating endothelial progenitor cells. *Cancer Res.* **2003**, *63*, 4342–4346. [PubMed]
9. Bocci, G.; Francia, G.; Man, S.; Lawler, J.; Kerbel, R.S. Thrombospondin 1, a mediator of the antiangiogenic effects of low-dose metronomic chemotherapy. *PNAS* **2003**, *100*, 12917–12922. [CrossRef]
10. Mpekris, F.; Baish, J.W.; Stylianopoulos, T.; Jain, R.K. Role of vascular normalization in benefit from metronomic chemotherapy. *Proc. Natl. Acad. Sci. USA* **2017**, *114*, 1994–1999. [CrossRef]
11. Penel, N.; Adenis, A.; Bocci, G. Cyclophosphamide-based metronomic chemotherapy: After 10 years of experience, where do we stand and where are we going? *Crit. Rev. Oncol. Hematol.* **2012**, *82*, 40–50. [CrossRef]
12. Vacca, A.; Iurlaro, M.; Ribatti, D.; Minischetti, M.; Nico, B.; Ria, R.; Pellegrino, A.; Dammacco, F. Antiangiogenesis is produced by nontoxic doses of vinblastine. *Blood* **1999**, *94*, 4143–4155. [CrossRef]
13. Wang, J.; Lou, P.; Lesniewski, R.; Henkin, J. Paclitaxel at ultra low concentrations inhibits angiogenesis without affecting cellular microtubule assembly. *Anticancer Drugs* **2003**, *14*, 13–19. [CrossRef]
14. Klement, G.; Huang, P.; Mayer, B.; Green, S.K.; Man, S.; Bohlen, P. Differences in therapeutic indexes of combination metronomic chemotherapy and anti-VEGFR-2 antibody in multidrug-resistant human breast cancer xenografts. *Clin. Cancer Res.* **2002**, *8*, 221–232.
15. Shaked, Y.; Bertolini, F.; Man, S.; Rogers, M.S.; Cervi, D.; Foutz, T.; Rawn, K.; Voskas, D.; Dumont, D.J.; Ben-David, y.; et al. Genetic heterogeneity of the vasculogenic phenotype parallels angiogenesis; Im plications for cellular surrogate marker analysis of antiangiogenesis. *Cancer Cell* **2005**, *7*, 101–111. [CrossRef]
16. Shaked, Y.; Ciarrocchi, A.; Franco, M.; Lee, C.R.; Man, S.; Cheung, A.M.; Hicklin, D.J.; Chaplin, D.; Foster, F.S.; Benezra, R.; et al. Therapy-induced acute recruitment of circulating endothelial progenitor cells to tumors. *Science* **2006**, *313*, 1785–1787. [CrossRef]
17. Shaked, Y.; Henke, E.; Roodhart, J.M.L.; Mancuso, P.; Langenberg, M.H.G.; Colleoni, M.; Daenen, L.G.; Man, S.; Xu, P.; Emmenegger, U.; et al. Rapid chemotherapy-induced acute endothelial progenitor cell mobilization: Implications for antiangiogenic drugs as chemosensitizing agents. *Cancer Cell* **2008**, *14*, 263–273. [CrossRef] [PubMed]
18. Biziota, E.; Mavroeidis, L.; Hatzimichael, E.; Pappas, P. Metronomic chemotherapy: A potent macerator of cancer by inducing angiogenesis suppression and antitumor immune activation. *Cancer Lett.* **2017**, *100*, 243–251. [CrossRef]
19. Chen, Y.L.; Change, M.C.; Cheng, W.F. Metronomic chemotherapy and immunotherapy in cancer treatment. *Cancer Lett.* **2017**, *400*, 282–292. [CrossRef] [PubMed]
20. Ghiringhelli, F.; Menard, C.; Puig, P.E.; Ladoire, S.; Roux, S.; Martin, F.; Solary, E.; Cesne, A.L.; Zitvogel, L.; Chauffert, B. Metronomic cyclophosphamide regimen selectively depletes CD4+CD25+ regulatory T cells and restores T and NK effector functions in end stage cancer patients. *Cancer Immunol. Immunother.* **2007**, *56*, 41–48. [CrossRef] [PubMed]
21. Banissi, C.; Ghiringhelli, F.; Chen, L.; Carpentier, A.F. Treg depletion with a low-dose metronomic temozolomide regimen in a rat glioma model. *Cancer Immunol. Immunother.* **2009**, *58*, 1627–1634. [CrossRef] [PubMed]
22. Kodumudi, K.N.; Woan, K.; Gilvary, D.L.; Sahakian, E.; Wei, S.; Djeu, J.Y. A novel chemoimmunomodulating property of docetaxel: Suppression of myeloid-derived suppressor cells in tumor bearers. *Clin. Cancer Res.* **2010**, *16*, 4583–4594. [CrossRef]
23. Peereboom, D.M.; Alban, T.J.; Grabowski, M.M.; Alvarado, A.G.; Otvos, B.; Bayik, D.; Roversi, G.; McGraw, M.; Huang, P.; Mohammadi, A.M.; et al. Metronomic capecitabine as an immune modulator in glioblastoma patients reduces myeloid-derived suppressor cells. *JCI Insight* **2019**, *4*, e130748. [CrossRef] [PubMed]
24. Tanaka, H.; Matsushima, H.; Mizomoto, N.; Takashima, A. Classification of chemotherapeutic agents based on their differential in vitro effects on dendritic cells. *Cancer Res.* **2009**, *69*, 6978–6986. [CrossRef]
25. Aymeric, L.; Apetoh, L.; Ghiringhelli, F.; Tesniere, A.; Martins, I.; Kroemer, G.; Smyth, M.J.; Zitvogel, L. Tumor cell death and ATP release prime dendritic cells and efficient anticancer immunity. *Cancer Res.* **2010**, *70*, 855–858. [CrossRef]
26. Michaud, M.; Martins, I.; Sukkurwala, A.Q.; Adjemian, S.; Ma, Y.; Pellegatti, P.; Shen, S.; Kepp, O.; Scoazec, M.; Mignot, G.; et al. Autophagy-dependent anticancer immune responses induced by chemotherapeutic agents in mice. *Science* **2011**, *3345*, 1573–1577. [CrossRef]
27. Ge, Y.; Domschke, C.; Stoiber, N.; Schott, S.; Heil, J.; Rom, J.; Blumenstein, M.; Thum, J.; Sohn, C. Metronomic cyclophosphamide treatment in metastasized breast cancer patients: Immunological effects and clinical outcome. *Cancer Immunol. Immunother.* **2012**, *61*, 353–362. [CrossRef] [PubMed]

78. Nguyen, L.V.; Vanncer, R.; Dirks, P.; Eaves, C.J. Cancer stem cells: An evolving concept. *Nat. Rev. Cancer* **2012**, *12*, 133–143. [CrossRef] [PubMed]
79. Arnold, C.R.; Mangesius, J.; Skvortsova, I.I.; Ganswindt, U. The role of cancer stem cells in radiation resistance. *Front. Oncol.* **2020**, *10*, 164. [CrossRef]
80. Nunes, T.; Hamdan, D.; Leboeuf, C.; El Bouchtaoui, M.; Gaoihan, G.; Nguyen, T.T.; Meles, S.; Angeli, E.; Rtajczak, P.; Lu, H.; et al. Targeting cancer stem cells to overcome chemoresistance. *Int. J. Mol. Sci.* **2018**, *19*, 4036. [CrossRef]
81. Chen, T.S.; Hsu, C.C.; Pai, V.C.; Liao, W.Y.; Huang, S.S.; Tan, K.T.; Yen, C.J.; Hsu, S.C.; Chen, W.Y.; Shan, Y.S.; et al. Metronomic chemotherapy prevents therapy-induced stromal activation and induction of tumor-initiating cells. *J. Exp. Med.* **2016**, *213*, 2967–2988. [CrossRef]
82. Folkins, C.; Man, S.; Xu, P.; Shaked, Y.; Hicklin, D.J.; Kerbel, R.S. Anticancer therapies combining antiangiogenic and tumor cell cytotoxic effects reduce the tumor stem-like cell fraction in glioma xenograft tumors. *Cancer Res.* **2007**, *67*, 3560–3564. [CrossRef]
83. Kerbel, R.S.; Shaked, Y. The potential clinical promise of 'multimodality' metronomic chemotherapy revealed by preclinical studies of metastatic disease. *Cancer Lett.* **2017**, *400*, 293–304. [CrossRef]
84. Vives, M.; Ginesta, M.M.; Gracova, K.; Graupera, M.; Casanovas, O.; Capella, G.; Serrano, T.; Laquente, B.; Vinals, F. Metronomic chemotherapy following the maximum tolerated dose is an effective anti-tumour therapy affecting angiogenesis, tumour dissemination and cancer stem cells. *Int. J. Cancer* **2013**, *133*, 2464–2472. [CrossRef] [PubMed]
85. Ferdous, T.; Harada, K.; Kin, T.; Harada, T.; Ueyama, Y. Efficacy of schedule-dependent metronomic S-1 chemotherapy in human oral squamous cell carcinoma cells. *Int. J. Oncol.* **2013**, *43*, 271–279. [CrossRef]
86. Xiang, Y.; Guo, Z.; Zhu, P.; Chen, J.; Huang, Y. Traditional Chinese medicine as a cancer treatment: Modern perspectives of ancient but advanced science. *Cancer Med.* **2019**, *8*, 1958–1975. [CrossRef] [PubMed]
87. Chen, Y.W.; Lin, G.J.; Chia, W.T.; Lin, C.K.; Chuang, Y.P.; Sytwu, H.K. Triptolide exerts anti-tumor effect on oral cancer and KB cells in vitro and in vivo. *Oral Oncol.* **2009**, *45*, 562–568. [CrossRef] [PubMed]
88. Chang, K.W.; Hung, P.S.; Lin, I.Y.; Hou, C.P.; Chen, L.K.; Tsai, Y.M.; Lin, S.C. Curcumin upregulates insulin-like growth factor binding protein-5 (IGFBP-5) and C/EBPα during oral cancer suppression. *Int. J. Cancer.* **2010**, *127*, 9–20. [CrossRef]
89. Yang, J.; Ren, X.; Zhang, L.; Li, Y.; Cheng, B.; Xia, J. Oridonin inhibits oral cancer growth and PI3K/Akt signaling pathway. *Biomed. Pharmacother.* **2018**, *100*, 226–232. [CrossRef]
90. Yang, C.Y.; Lin, C.K.; Hsieh, C.C.; Tsao, C.H.; Lin, C.S.; Peng, B.; Chen, Y.T.; Ting, C.C.; Chang, W.C.; Lin, G.J.; et al. Anti-oral cancer effects of triptolide by downregulation of DcR3 in vitro, in vivo, and in preclinical patient-derived tumor xenograft model. *Head Neck* **2019**, *41*, 1260–1269. [CrossRef]
91. Yang, C.Y.; Tsao, C.H.; Hsieh, C.C.; Lin, C.K.; Lin, C.S.; Li, Y.H.; Chang, W.C.; Chen, J.C.; Lin, G.J.; Sytwu, H.K.; et al. Downregulation of Jumonji-C domain-containing protein 5 inhibits proliferation by silibinin in the oral cancer PDTX model. *PLoS ONE* **2020**, *15*, e0236101. [CrossRef]
92. Su, N.W.; Wu, S.H.; Chi, C.W.; Liu, C.J.; Tsai, T.H.; Chen, Y.J. Metronomic cordycepin therapy prolongs survival of oral cancer-bearing mice and inhibits epithelial-mesenchymal transition. *Molecules* **2017**, *22*, 629. [CrossRef]
93. Su, N.W.; Wu, S.H.; Chi, C.W.; Chen, Y.J. Cordycepin, isolated from medicinal fungus Cordyceps sinensis, enhances radiosensitivity of oral cancer associated with modulation of DNA damage repair. *Food Chem. Toxicol.* **2019**, *124*, 400–410. [CrossRef]
94. Montagna, E.; Palazzo, A.; Maisonneuve, P.; Cancello, G.; Iorfida, M.; Sciandivasci, A.; Esopsito, A.; Cardillo, A.; Mazza, M.; Munzone, E.; et al. Safety and efficacy study of metronomic vinorelbine, cyclophosphamide plus capecitabine in metastatic breast cancer: A phase II trial. *Cancer Lett.* **2017**, *400*, 276–281. [CrossRef] [PubMed]
95. Clarke, J.L.; Iwamoto, F.M.; Sul, J.; Panageas, K.; Lassman, A.B.; DeAngelis, L.M.; Hormigo, A.; Nolan, C.P.; Gavrilovic, I.; Karimi, S.; et al. Randomized phase II trial of chemoradiotherapy followed by either dose-dense or metronomic temozolomide for newly diagnosed glioblastoma. *J. Clin. Oncol.* **2009**, *27*, 3861–3867. [CrossRef] [PubMed]
96. Papanikolaou, X.; Szymonifka, J.; Rosenthal, A.; Heuck, C.J.; Mitchell, A.; Johann Jr., D.; Keller, J.; Waheed, S.; Usmani, S.Z.; Rhee, F.V.; et al. Metronomic therapy is an effective salvage treatment for heavily pretreated relapsed/refractory multiple myeloma. *Heamatologica.* **2013**, *98*, 1147–1153. [CrossRef] [PubMed]
97. Mir, O.; Domont, J.; Cioffi, A.; Bonvalot, S.; Boulet, B.; Le Pechoux, C.; Terrier, P.; Spielmann, M.; Le Cesne, A. Feasibility of metronomic oral cyclophosphamide plus prednisolone in elderly patients with inoperable or metastatic soft tissue sarcoma. *Eur. J. Cancer* **2011**, *47*, 515–519. [CrossRef] [PubMed]
98. Camerini, A.; Puccetti, C.; Donati, S.; Valsuani, C.; Petrella, M.C.; Tartarelli, G.; Puccinelli, P.; Amoroso, D. Metronomic oral vinorelbine as first-line treatment in elderly patients with advanced non-small cell lung cancer: Results of a phase II trial (MOVE trial). *BMC Cancer* **2015**, *15*, 359. [CrossRef] [PubMed]
99. Pramanik, R.; Agarwala, S.; Gupta, Y.K.; Thulkar, S.; Vishnubhatla, S.; Batra, A.; Dhawan, D.; Bakhshi, S. Metronomic chemotherapy vs. best supportive care in progressive pediatric solid malignant tumors: A randomized clinical trial. *JAMA Oncol.* **2017**, *3*, 1222–1227. [CrossRef]
100. Hsu, C.H.; Shen, Y.C.; Lin, Z.Z.; Chen, P.J.; Shao, Y.Y.; Ding, Y.H.; Hsu, C.; Cheng, A.L. Phase II study of combining sorafenib with metronomic tegafur/uracil for advanced hepatocellular carcinoma. *J. Hepatol.* **2010**, *53*, 126–131. [CrossRef]
101. Barber, E.L.; Zsiros, E.; Lurain, J.R.; Rademaker, A.; Schink, J.C.; Neubauer, N.L. The combination of intravenous bevacizumab and metronomic oral cyclophosphamide is an effective regimen for platinum-resistant recurrent ovarian cancer. *J. Gynecol. Oncol.* **2013**, *24*, 258–264. [CrossRef] [PubMed]

102. Perroud, H.A.; Alasino, C.M.; Rico, M.J.; Mainetti, L.E.; Pezzotto, S.M.; Rozados, V.R.; Scharovsky, O.G. Metastatic breast cancer patients treated with low-dose metronomic chemotherapy with cyclophosphamide and celecoxib: Clinical outcomes and biomarkers of response. *Cancer Chemother. Pharmacol.* **2016**, *77*, 365–374. [CrossRef]
103. Lin, J.S.; Cheng, C.Y.; Liu, C.J. Oral uracil and tegafur as postoperative adjuvant metronomic chemotherapy in patients with advanced oral squamous cell carcinoma. *J. Dent. Sci.* **2015**, *10*, 408–413. [CrossRef]
104. Hsieh, M.Y.; Chen, G.; Chang, D.C.; Chien, S.Y.; Chen, M.K. The impact of metronomic adjuvant chemotherapy in patients with advanced oral cancer. *Ann. Surg. Oncol.* **2018**, *25*, 2091–2097. [CrossRef]
105. Furusaka, T.; Tanaka, A.; Mstsuda, H.; Ikeda, M. Consecutive daily low-dose S-1 adjuvant chemotherapy after radial treatment for squamous cell carcinoma in head and neck cancer. *Acta. Otolaryngol.* **2011**, *131*, 1099–1103. [CrossRef]
106. Patil, V.M.; Moronha, V.; Jashi, A.; Muddu, V.K.; Dhumal, S.; Bhosale, B.; Arya, S.; Juvekar, S.; Banavali, S.; D'Cruz, A.; et al. A prospective randomized phase II comparing metronomic chemotherapy with chemotherapy (single agent cisplatin), in patients with metastatic, relapsed or inoperable squamous cell carcinoma of head and neck. *Oral Oncol.* **2015**, *51*, 279–286. [CrossRef] [PubMed]
107. Machiels, J.P.H.; Haddad, R.I.; Fayette, J.; Licitra, L.F.; Tahara, M.; Vermorken, J.B.; Clement, P.M.; Gauler, T.; Cupissol, D.; Grau, J.J.; et al. Afatinib versus methotrexate as second-line treatment in patients with recurrent or metastatic squamous-cell carcinoma of the head and neck progressing on or after platinum-based therapy (LUX-Head & Neck 1): An open-label, randomized phase 3 trial. *Lancet Oncol.* **2015**, *16*, 583–594. [CrossRef]
108. Khan, Z.; Khan, N.; Tiwari, R.P.; Sah, N.K.; Prasad, G.B.; Bisen, P.S. Biology of Cox-2: An application in cancer therapeutics. *Curr. Drug Targets* **2011**, *12*, 1082–1093. [CrossRef]
109. Jones, M.K.; Wang, H.; Peskar, B.M.; Levin, E.; Itani, R.M.; Sarfeh, I.J.; Tarnawski, A.S. Inhibition of angiogenesis by nonsteroidal anti-inflammatory drugs: Insight into mechanisms and implications for cancer growth and ulcer healing. *Nat. Med.* **1999**, *12*, 1418–1423. [CrossRef]
110. Patil, V.M.; Noronha, V.; Joshi, A.; Dhumal, S.; Mahimkar, M.; Bhattacharjee, A.; Gota, V.; Pandey, M.; Menon, N.; Mahajan, A.; et al. Phase I/II study of palliative triple metronomic chemotherapy in platinum-refractory/early-failure oral cancer. *J. Clin. Oncol.* **2019**, *37*, 3032–3041. [CrossRef]
111. Patil, V.; Noronha, V.; Dhumal, S.B.; Joshi, A.; Menon, N.; Bhattacharjee, A.; Kulkarni, S.; Ankathi, S.K.; Mahajan, A.; Sable, N.; et al. Low-cost oral metronomic chemotherapy versus intravenous cisplatin in patients with recurrent, metastatic, inoperable head and neck carcinoma: An open-label, parallel-group, non-inferiority, randomized, phase 3 trial. *Lancet Glob Health* **2020**, *8*, e1213–e1222. [CrossRef]
112. Allegrini, G.; Falcone, A.; Fioravanti, A.; Barletta, M.T.; Orlandi, P.; Loupakis, F.; Cerri, E.; Masi, G.; Di Paolo, A.; Kerbel, R.S.; et al. A pharmacokinetic and pharmacodynamic study on metronomic irinotecan in metastatic colorectal cancer patients. *Br. J. Cancer* **2008**, *98*, 1312–1319. [CrossRef] [PubMed]
113. Allegrini, G.; Di Desidero, T.; Barletta, M.T.; Fioravanti, A.; Oralandi, P.; Canu, B.; Chericoni, S.; Loupakis, F.; Di Paolo, A.; Masi, G.; et al. Clinical, pharmacokinetic and pharmacodynamic evaluations of metronomic UFT and cyclophosphamide plus celecoxib in patients with advanced refractory gastrointestinal cancers. *Angiogenesis* **2012**, *15*, 257–286. [CrossRef] [PubMed]
114. Di Desidero, T.; Oralandi, P.; Fioravanti, A.; Cremolini, C.; Loupakis, F.; Marmorino, F.; Antoniotti, C.; Masi, G.; Lonardi, S.; Bergamo, F.; et al. Pharmacokinetic analysis of metronomic capecitabine in refractory metastatic colorectal cancer patient. *Investig. New Drugs* **2018**, *36*, 709–714. [CrossRef]
115. Andre, N.; Banavali, S.; Snihur, Y.; Pasquier, E. Has the time come for metronomics in low-income and middle-income countries? *Lancet Oncol.* **2013**, *14*, e239–e248. [CrossRef]
116. Del Tacca, M. Cyclophosphamide-methotrexate 'metronomic' chemotherapy for the palliative treatment of metastatic breast cancer. A comparative pharmacoeconomic evaluation. *Ann. Oncol.* **2005**, *16*, 1243–1452. [CrossRef]
117. Benzekry, S.; Pasquier, E.; Barbolosi, D.; Lacarelle, B.; Barlesi, F.; Andre, N.; Ciccolini, J. Metronomic reloaded: Theoretical models bringing chemotherapy into the era of precision medicine. *Semin. Cancer Biol.* **2015**, *35*, 53–61. [CrossRef]
118. Guo, F.; Cui, J. Anti-angiogenesis: Opening a new window for immunotherapy. *Life Sci.* **2020**, *258*, 118163. [CrossRef]
119. Kareva, I. A combination of immune checkpoint inhibition with metronomic chemotherapy as a way of targeting therapy-resistant cancer cells. *Int. J. Mol. Sci.* **2017**, *18*, 2134. [CrossRef]
120. Liikanen, I.; Ahtiainen, L.; Hirvinen, M.L.; Bramante, S.; Cerullo, V.; Nokisalmi, P.; Hemminki, O.; Diaconu, I.; Pesonen, S.; Koski, A.; et al. Oncolytic adenovirus with temozolomide induces autophagy and antitumor immune responses in cancer patients. *Mol. Ther.* **2013**, *21*, 1212–1223. [CrossRef] [PubMed]
121. Ellbaek, E.; Engell-Noerregaard, L.; Iversen, T.Z.; Froesig, T.M.; Munir, S.; Hadrup, S.R.; Andersen, M.H.; Svane, I.M. Metastatic melanoma patients treated with dendritic cell vaccination, interleukin-2 and metronomic cyclophosphamide: Results from a phase II trial. *Cancer Immunol. Immunother.* **2012**, *61*, 1791–1804. [CrossRef] [PubMed]

MDPI
St. Alban-Anlage 66
4052 Basel
Switzerland
www.mdpi.com

Journal of Clinical Medicine Editorial Office
E-mail: jcm@mdpi.com
www.mdpi.com/journal/jcm

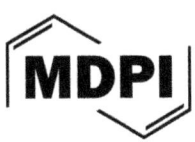

Disclaimer/Publisher's Note: The statements, opinions and data contained in all publications are solely those of the individual author(s) and contributor(s) and not of MDPI and/or the editor(s). MDPI and/or the editor(s) disclaim responsibility for any injury to people or property resulting from any ideas, methods, instructions or products referred to in the content.